Disease
and Class

**HEALTH
AND MEDICINE
IN AMERICAN
SOCIETY**
series editors
Judith Walzer Leavitt
Morris Vogel

Disease and Class

TUBERCULOSIS AND THE SHAPING OF MODERN NORTH AMERICAN SOCIETY

Georgina D. Feldberg

 RUTGERS UNIVERSITY PRESS
NEW BRUNSWICK, NEW JERSEY

Feldberg, Georgina, D., 1956–
    Disease and class : tuberculosis and the shaping of modern North
American society / Georgina D. Feldberg.
        p.   cm. — (Health and medicine in American society)
    Includes bibliographical references and index.
    ISBN 0–8135–2217–X (cloth : alk. paper). — ISBN 0–8135–2218–8
(pbk. : alk. paper)
    1. Tuberculosis—Government policy—United States—History.
2. Tuberculosis—Government policy—Canada—History. I. Title.
II. Series.
    [DNLM: 1. Tuberculosis—history—North America. 2. Tuberculosis—
prevention & control—North America. 3. BCG Vaccine—history—
North America.   WF 11 DA2 F3d 1995]
RC310.5.F45   1995
614.5'42'0973—dc20
DNLM/DLC
for Library of Congress   95–15169
                                                                            CIP

British Cataloging-in-Publication information available

For my parents, with love, respect, and thanks

Contents

Illustrations

Acknowledgments

During the long period of this book's gestation, I have often looked forward to the moment when I might thank all those who have helped to make it possible. Now, the task of adequately cataloguing and capturing many and varied contributions is not easy, for words alone cannot possibly discharge my numerous personal and professional debts. My first debt is to my teachers, Barbara Rosenkrantz and Allan Brandt, who supervised the thesis from which this book evolved. Professor Rosenkrantz's course on the history of the Great White Plague sparked my interest in this subject, and the experience of being her student and her teaching and research assistant informed my historical approach. This book continues to bear the imprint of the lessons she and Professor Brandt taught.

Judy Leavitt and Morris Vogel patiently facilitated the transition from dissertation to book. Their supportive and thoughtful criticisms were invaluable and provided an important benchmark against which to judge the comments and suggestions of other readers. Marlie Wasserman and Karen Reeds guided the production of the manuscript with fortitude and humor. Pamela Fischer, who copyedited the manuscript, was also a pleasure to work with. She caught and contained errors—mechanical, human, and electronic—that continually escaped the author's tired gaze, and her comments and queries helped me clarify my interpretations.

Librarians and archivists from across North America diligently hunted for lost and hidden records. Staff in the general, reference, archival, and rare-book collections at Harvard, the University of Pennsylvania, York University, the University of Toronto, Dalhousie, McGill, Queen's, the University of Western Ontario, the National Library of Medicine, the

Academy of Medicine of Toronto, the Free Library at Saranac Lake, the Center for Disease Control, the Provincial Archives of Ontario, the City of Toronto Archives, and the Provincial Archives of Manitoba made the task of research easier. So did staff in other public and private institutions. I would particularly like to thank Tom Horrocks and his staff at the Library of the College of Physicians of Philadelphia; Beth Horrocks at the American Philosophical Society; Elora South and Linda Querec, custodians of the Public Health Service records at the National Archives; Diane Schiasson at the Canadian National Archives, Ottawa; Florence Berg and Ken Gibilesco of Merck, Sharp and Dohme; Joan Rudin and Doris Schally at Smith-Kline and French; Audrey Ashby and Evelyn Armstrong at Wyeth. My colleague Tom Cohen generously shared his family's collection of papers pertaining to the Eagleville Sanatorium and tuberculosis-control efforts in Pennsylvania.

I have presented segments of this work at the Academy of Medicine of Toronto, Brown University, Clemson University, the University of Toronto, the Memorial University of Newfoundland, the American Society for the History of Medicine, the Canadian Society for the History of Medicine, the Canadian Science and Technology Historical Association, the History of Science Society, and the International Society for the History of Medicine. The questions these audiences raised helped cast my work in a different light. I wish particularly to thank Ruth Schwartz Cowan and Judy Walzer Leavitt for comments they made at the 1991 meeting of the History of Science Society on my analysis of the gendered nature of tuberculosis and its treatments. Colleagues both at home and abroad—Susan Lawrence, Naomi Rogers, Harriet Rosenberg, Jim and Jennifer Connor, Jacalyn Duffin, Paul Axelrod, Shelly Romalis, Robert Macbeth, Paula Caplan, Rusty Shteir, Jay Cassel, Susan Solomon, Ted Madger—helped me formulate and refine ideas, interpretations, and drafts. They variously sustained my writing with personal and scholarly advice, solace, laughter, and especially chocolate. I owe a special debt to Kathryn McPherson, who has been a loyal, diligent, and supportive critic, colleague, and friend.

Financial support from Harvard University and Radcliffe College, the College of Physicians of Philadelphia, York University, and the Hannah Institute defrayed research costs. So did the generosity of friends who opened their homes: Cynthia Heath Sunderland; Nancy Netzer and Bob Silberman; Janet Golden and Eric Schneider; Arthur and Phyllis Ezra; William and Susan Lasser; Renée Matalon and Stephen Marcus; Mary Vipond and Bill Butler; Reid and Dorothy Vipond.

George Comstock, Stuart Houston, and Shirley Ferebee Woolpert made the task of negotiating medical and public records less daunting by sharing their knowledge, experience, and reflections and bringing to life a long cast of characters.

John Dawson and the Department of Instructional Technologies at York University assisted with the reproduction of illustrations.

I could not have completed this work without my office staff and graduate research assistants: Randee Holmes, Rosanna Moretti, Yasmin Rahman, and Tracy Shannon. In particular, Tracy organized the final manuscript with her expert research and superb secretarial skills. She undertook such tedious tasks as cross-checking references and abbreviations with no greater complaint than "Do I really have to list this on my c.v. and let others know I can do this work?"

And then there is Rob, who has truly and unfailingly been my partner, my guide, and my friend. He has helped in more ways than I can possibly acknowledge, serving variously and so generously as proofreader, housekeeper, research assistant, chauffeur, cook, errand boy, critic, and editor. Even more than for his actions I thank him for the wry humor that has kept my work in perspective.

Last though not least, I thank my families, especially my grandmother Mutti, my brother Ralph, and above all my parents, who value books, helped steer me along this path, and prodded me forward.

Abbreviations

ACTR	Associate Committee on Tuberculosis Research of the NRCC
AMA	American Medical Association
APHA	American Public Health Association
ATS	American Trudeau Society
BCG	bacillus Calmette Guérin
BIA	Bureau of Indian Affairs (United States)
CMA	Canadian Medical Association
CPP	College of Physicians of Philadelphia
CTA	Canadian Tuberculosis Association
MRC	Medical Research Committee of the NTA
NASPT	National Association for the Study and Prevention of Tuberculosis
NIH	National Institutes of Health
NRCC	National Research Council of Canada
NTA	National Tuberculosis Association
PHS	Public Health Service (United States)
USBC	United States Bureau of the Census
USDA	United States Department of Agriculture
USDHEW	United States Department of Health, Education and Welfare

Disease
and Class

Tuberculosis as a Different Kind of Disease

When I began this study of tuberculosis in 1982, few of those with whom I spoke understood my interest in the disease. TB, after all, had long been eradicated, and AIDS and cancer had replaced it as threats. Now, this is no longer the case. As the front-page headlines of North American newspapers report that "TB Is Back with Strains That Are Deadlier," Americans openly puzzle over its resurgence.[1] The eradication of tuberculosis had seemed one of the great triumphs of modern medicine. Known commonly as "the First Cause of Nineteenth-Century Deaths," "the Great White Plague," "the Captain of All Men of Death," TB had all but disappeared from public view by the 1960s. Confident that this disease was "dead," the public and private American hospitals and agencies responsible for tuberculosis control closed, disbanded, and consigned their records to remote storage depots. However, reports of tuberculosis associated with immigration, new drug resistant strains, and AIDS have challenged the image of TB as a historical relic. Epidemics in New York, Boston, and other major American cities belie the myth that TB is dead; observations that the epidemiology of AIDS seems to replicate that of TB and that AIDS patients frequently develop tuberculosis fuel both professional and popular concern about the disease; and the recognition that TB, like AIDS, serves as a metaphor for other social ills has inspired varied historical analyses.

This book explores the historical context of contemporary American experiences with tuberculosis. To many, the resurgence of TB, like the advent of AIDS, represents a failure of biomedicine—a failure to adapt to changing bacterial strains or new population bases. But contemporary experience also reflects a series of social reactions to disease and the health-care policy decisions that accommodated those reactions to scientific and epidemiological change. Specifically, the problematical reemergence of drug-resistant strains of TB must also be explored in the context of decisions that the United States Public Health Service (PHS) made, in the 1930s, 1940s, and 1950s, to mount a crusade based on hygienic measures and chemoprophylaxis rather than vaccination. Discussion of bacillus Calmette Guérin (BCG), a vaccine developed during the 1920s and used throughout the world, has been conspicuously absent from the contemporary American debate over tuberculosis control. As the popular press ponders the causes of the new wave of TB and weighs alternatives for control, it makes little mention of BCG, even in its reports of efforts to develop a vaccine against tuberculosis. Historians have also ignored the vaccine. The relative merits of BCG and whether vaccination would have produced a different result are not the questions here. Clio—the muse of history—has no prophetic powers. Instead, Clio can help us to understand the constellation of epidemiological, scientific, and sociopolitical events that shaped a particular series of decisions, and, in this sense, she can help us move beyond the obvious question of what went wrong to an analysis of the intersections of disease, biomedicine, history, and society. Those intersections form the substance of this book.

Our surprise at the resurgence of TB is based in the false premise that tuberculosis essentially disappeared with Queen Victoria. TB ranked well into the twentieth century as "the costliest of communicable diseases,"[2] and, in real terms and against the backdrop of other infections, it posed a significant American public health problem. Both in epidemiological and economic terms tuberculosis easily earned the appellation "costliest" of diseases. In 1949, as polio cases rose to the "epidemic" rate of 30/100,000, the tuberculous case rate exceeded 90/100,000; in 1951 alone, there were over 119,000 new cases of tuberculosis. Tuberculous mortality also exceeded that for polio almost threefold; while 9.7/100,000 Americans died of polio in 1949, tuberculosis claimed 28/100,000.[3] And well into this century TB sapped the strength of the nation by disrupting families and industries and creating dependency that cost millions of dollars in lost revenues and welfare payments. In 1950, public spending on tuberculosis ranked second only to that spent on venereal disease.[4]

Yet, unlike polio, tuberculosis did not etch its fearful imprint on the public imagination. The millions of Americans whom tuberculosis affected included none other than Eleanor Roosevelt, who in 1962 died from the reactivation of a tuberculous lesion she acquired in 1919, scarcely a year before her husband contracted polio.[5] Whereas polio immediately brings to mind the image of FDR in a wheelchair, Eleanor Roosevelt never championed or embodied the American campaign against TB. Tuberculosis remained so hidden a part of Eleanor Roosevelt's life that references to it appear only fleetingly in her biographies and autobiographies.

And while Americans eagerly sought an antipolio vaccine, they did not rush to vaccinate against tuberculosis.[6] In 1949 Americans anxiously watched the polio case rate climb, and journalists, voluntary agencies, and public health officials, haunted by the specter of the disabled FDR, exhorted the scientific community to produce a preventive vaccine. In contrast, from 1924 on representatives of the PHS and of the American Trudeau Society (ATS) actively resisted vaccination against tuberculosis with BCG—an attenuated bovine tubercle bacillus that Albert Calmette and Camille Guérin developed at the Pasteur Institute in Lille, France. In 1948, the ATS dismissed the need for a vaccination program against TB with the declaration that "the most effective methods of controlling tuberculosis in the general population are (a) further improvement of living conditions and the general health."[7] Again, in 1960, the PHS reiterated this position.[8]

American opposition to BCG vaccine stood curiously at odds with both domestic and international policy. Between 1924 and 1960, extensive epidemiological and clinical testing demonstrated BCG to be 80 percent effective. The World Health Organization approved its use; twenty-four nations enforced compulsory programs of BCG vaccination; and an additional seventy-eight—including the closest neighbor of the United States, Canada—implemented voluntary vaccination programs. By 1960 a majority of American physicians and laymen also thought vaccines to be among the greatest triumphs of modern medicine. The fights against vaccination waged during the eighteenth, nineteenth, and early twentieth centuries had been laid aside during the 1940s and 1950s as knowledge of the bacterial agents of disease provided the theoretical and practical bases needed to produce vaccines safely, efficiently, and effectively.[9] "Immunization is the most ideal and usually cheapest medical tool to which we can look for the control of a disease," Surgeon General Jesse Steinfeld advised at a 1971 conference on immunization against tuberculosis. But he issued a caveat: not in the case of TB.[10]

In these ways and others, American social and medical responses to tuberculosis differed markedly from responses to polio and other major infections; those differences, which demarcate American tuberculosis policy, guide this book, for they help to explain both the peculiar contours of the American campaign and the historical lessons to be learned.

That tuberculosis was "different" should come as little surprise. Some historians and epidemiologists have long recognized and discussed its unique status. They have argued that the eradication of tuberculosis, a disease born and bred of poverty, owed far less to magic bullets or vaccines than to extramedical factors such as public health activities and changing social conditions. Richard Harrison Shryock, Marion Torchia, René Dubos, and many others have skillfully argued that the successful conquest of tuberculosis owed much to social interventions.

However, this view of tuberculosis as different stands in marked contrast to the other standard historical portrait. In his essay on the etiology of tuberculosis, Robert Koch not only identified the microbial agents of disease but also proclaimed that "one has been accustomed until now to regard tuberculosis as the outcome of social misery, and to hope by relief of distress to diminish the disease. But in the future struggle against this dreadful plague of the human race one will no longer have to contend with an indefinite something, but with an actual parasite whose life conditions are for the most part known or can easily be still further investigated."[11] Historians, such as George Rosen, often mark Koch's identification of the tubercle bacillus as the starting point of the new "bacteriologic, immunologic and chemotherapeutic period." If, as Rosen suggests, Koch's elucidation of the etiological role of the tubercle bacilli empowered physicians to combat TB through rational attacks on specific microbes, American physicians did not always welcome the opportunity to control infectious disease "unswervingly without being sidetracked by considerations of social policy."[12] Clear and compelling as the laboratory evidence might seem, the medical response to that evidence was often ambivalent.

Well into the twentieth century, American physicians held fast to an etiology that included microbes but also found room for malnutrition, unemployment, crowding, the living conditions in slums, and other social ills. Like Allen Krause, professor of pathology at Johns Hopkins University and the director of its Kenneth Dows Tuberculosis Laboratories, they continued to link their preventative and therapeutic strategies to the relief of distress with the argument that "[t]he solution of the tuberculosis problem is partly dependent on the removal of other evils and inequalities which constitute, no doubt, a more fundamental social problem than does tuberculosis itself."[13] Drawing on a metaphor of seed and soil, a majority of the physicians and public health workers who led the American campaign against tuberculosis continued to recognize that poverty and social misery contributed to the development of that disease. And they argued, again and again, that tubercle bacilli could not alone cause tuberculosis. Thus, Steinfeld formed part of a venerable tradition whose interest in the sociological dimensions of tuberculosis cannot be dismissed so easily as a last resort, a diversion from biomedical priorities, the empty lament of those who had no alternative—or as so much rhetorical window dressing hung to conceal the shortcomings of science.

This book explores the implicit differences between tuberculosis and other infectious diseases, such as polio, by charting the paths that American physicians and public health officials took to control TB in the years bounded by Jean-Antoine Villemin's work on the inoculability of tuberculosis in 1861 and the ultimate rejection of BCG in 1960. My purpose is twofold. Since the 1970s, tuberculosis has attracted much attention from historians, sociologists, physicians, and epidemiologists who have appreciated the value of an "externalist," or social-historical, approach. Their analyses, which serve as the basis for the observation that tuberculosis was different, have tended, however, either to ignore or to deemphasize the roles of physicians. Arguing that tuberculosis was a disease of poverty, they have shifted attention to nurses and other alternative practitioners, to patients, and to improvements in public health and the standard of living. Or they have assessed the ways in which institutional, sociopolitical, and other extrascientific influences constrained or facilitated medical progress.[14] Implicit in these analyses is the assumption that medicine and social reform are dichotomous, for these critics of modern medicine, like its champions, accept that bacteriology fundamentally altered modern Western medical practice. They argue that American physicians, ravished by science, moved swiftly and systematically away from policies that encouraged moral reform or the modification of individual behavior toward the public application of procedures that directly attacked microorganisms. They condemn the shortcomings of modern medicine's narrow appeal to specific etiologies and quick technological fixes, which disassociate the social from the biological dimensions of disease.[15] Or, alternatively, they condemn the social considerations, biases, or prejudices that corrupted biomedicine.

Lost in these ventures are the voices of physicians who chose to follow a path other than the traditional one—who turned to the laboratory but continued to acknowledge the importance of social circumstances, and who let those circumstances shape their clinical/therapeutic and experimental judgment. The first purpose of this book, then, is to demonstrate, through the history of tuberculosis, that many such physicians existed and to restore their voices to the historical score. I argue that the definition of tuberculosis as a social problem did not necessarily cast it as an extramedical problem. I argue as well that the failure of state policy and institutions to support materially the rhetoric of social reform, rather than a socially conscious medicine, limited the success of American TB control efforts. If these are historiographic points, they are also political ones, for current efforts to reform medical education and practice can benefit much from the resuscitation and reevaluation of traditions of socially informed medicine.

The second purpose of this book is to understand why, in the case of tuberculosis, American physicians chose "the road less traveled" and did not rush to embrace the quick technological fix—why, instead of grasping for vaccines, they continually insisted that "tuberculosis is part a sociological as well as a biological problem."[16] This choice distinguishes the American campaign against TB and also provides a point of comparison for other diseases like AIDS. To understand why Americans took the path that they did, one needs to explore the links between medical campaigns against TB and middle-class programs of social reform not as they worked side by side but as they intersected and intertwined at both symbolic and substantive levels.

The generations of physicians who attempted to control TB in the years bounded by 1860 and 1960 confronted a series of social, political-economic, and scientific challenges that consolidated the middle-class state. During this century, a rural country became increasingly urbanized, and an agrarian economy gave way to an industrial one. Slavery was abolished. Blacks and women entered the waged workforce in ever increasing numbers. Science became the paramount form of explanation, and technology the preferred vehicle of change. Organized medicine and the pharmaceutical manufacturers with whom it allied itself gained professional and economic power. The state acquired new responsibilities for the control of poverty, disease, and disorder.

Efforts to control tuberculosis formed a fundamental part of these processes, and the explanation for why American physicians treated tuberculosis "differently" is consequently tied to the varied social and scientific challenges that gave rise to the American middle classes. Exactly who and what the American middle classes comprise remain the subject of considerable scholarly debate, but while sociologists, anthropologists, and historians disagree on the precise definition of this class, its bounds, and its points of formation, they have generally agreed that it must be understood in the context of its relations to the material forces of production. Because the middle class neither worked with its hands nor garnered capital, those relations are to the dissemination of symbolic or intellectual property— in other words, knowledge and social institutions, particularly medicine and the state.[17] In this sense, the formation of the middle class can be understood as ideological: it comprised a series of material, symbolic, and institutional reactions to profound and disconcerting changes, and it represented an effort to make sense of those changes.[18]

Experiences with disease were one of the sites around which the middle classes formed, and tuberculosis played a particularly critical role in shaping the middle-class order. A wasting disease, characterized by the development of growths in the lungs, joints, and other tissues, the disease posed specific material and economic threats. TB sapped the strength of its victims and exacted a physical toll that frequently curtailed their ability to work at home or outside. The limited participation of tuberculous men and women in the domestic and waged economies formed a consistent concern for each of the generations that attempted to eradicate tuberculosis.

Like plague before it and AIDS after it, tuberculosis also summoned up images and myths that gave shape to human experience. The explanations offered for patterns of susceptibility to tuberculosis defined social roles, framed social differences, and betrayed assumptions about deviance. As mid-nineteenth century American physicians puzzled over the changing epidemiology of TB, they did so while watching the demise of an agrarian order and the emergence of an urban working class. Defining health as the habits of the male pioneer—indeed, equating health with those habits—they invoked tuberculosis to render intelligible the experiences of blacks, urban industrial workers, and all others who did not participate in the rugged, outdoor life. In the years that bounded the turn of the century, physicians also confronted the direct economic and social threats that female and immigrant workers posed, and their examinations of differential susceptibility to TB probed the changing status of women. In the interwar years tuberculosis symbolized the needs of a postwar economy in which patterns of industrial production had shifted. After World War II, children, the elderly, and the indigent replaced women as the most serious social challenge, and explanations for TB reflected this change.

Tuberculosis also intersected with the institutional structures that gave the middle classes shape, most particularly medicine, science, and the state. The formation of the middle-class order was, as Robert Wiebe suggested in 1967, a "search for order" in which scientific knowledge and institutions came increasingly to dominate American culture.[19] The scientific transformations that occurred in the century bounded by 1860 and 1960 had particular significance for American campaigns against TB. In 1861, when Villemin first demonstrated the inoculability of consumption, few Americans found his arguments compelling. By 1960, the bacterial hypothesis of tuberculosis that Koch had articulated in 1882 seemed so prescient and clear that opposition to it appeared backward and unthinkable.

Over the course of a hundred years, scientific knowledge had changed, but so had its authority. American efforts to control tuberculosis occurred in the context of these changes. The disease created a market for bacteriological and pharmacological knowledge. It fostered scientific research programs within public health and pharmaceutical laboratories, sanatoria, and voluntary agencies. In this sense, tuberculosis helped to build the institutions of modern middle class life, and while it prevented millions of Americans from seeking gainful employment, it generated numerous opportunities for biomedical work that allowed North American women and men to change or secure their economic and social status. Hence, TB is a prism that refracts the beam of middle class formation into its constituent bands, and the specific colors of those bands illuminate the goals of the American campaign against TB. Medical responses to TB were themselves ideological; they intersected with and indeed formed part of the broader effort to consolidate the status of the American middle classes.[20]

The question of whether tuberculosis was different is clearly central to this work but so is the ancillary question of how different Americans were. To probe the nature and extent of American distinctiveness, I compare American and Canadian campaigns against tuberculosis. The American response to BCG, curiously at odds with policy adopted throughout the world, seems particularly puzzling when contrasted with that of Canada. While substantive and significant differences in national identity exist, the United States and Canada resemble one another politically, geographically, culturally, and demographically, and they shared experiences with tuberculosis. Both nations are young, industrialized, developed democracies. Both operate under a federal system in which, during the period under investigation, responsibility for public health was informal, diffuse, and divided between national and local levels of government. Their populations are a mix of European, African, Asian, and Native American stocks. In both countries, tuberculous mortality declined during the first half of this century, but remained significant for immigrants and Native Americans. Yet in 1925, almost two decades before the American government began to determine policy for the use of BCG, the National Research Council of Canada (NRCC) began to test and develop the vaccine. The NRCC approved BCG for use soon thereafter. Quebec began an extensive vaccination program in 1930; after 1946, every province implemented BCG vaccination.

A full comparison of American and Canadian experiences and policies is well beyond the scope of this book, but examination of key differences and their historical roots prevents one from lapsing into simple affirmations of American exceptionalism. The comparative perspective clarifies the meanings American physicians attached to experiences with TB and reveals the ways in which the control of tuberculosis formed part of a larger material, institutional, and ideological effort to shape the middle-class state.

The chapters that follow pursue these various themes in an effort to explain the "different" American response to TB, which was exemplified in the decision not to vaccinate with BCG. Each chapter explores the interplay of intellectual, institutional, professional, and ideological concerns in American and Canadian reactions to pivotal episodes in the history of tuberculosis control. In this sense, the history of tuberculosis developed here is different, in both emphasis and scope, from that presented in other recent studies of tuberculosis—such as Barbara Bates's *Bargaining for Life* or Sheila Rothman's *Living in the Shadow of Death*.[21] Comparative, and focused on the years between 1920 and 1960, this book differs further in that it is more a history of disease, physicians, and society than of patients or institutions; and it emphasizes the social and policy bases, rather than the purely scientific bases for medical practices.

Chapter One provides the historical backdrop through a discussion of patterns of disease and medical responses to those patterns in the era that followed Villemin's early suggestion that tuberculosis was an infectious disease and that immediately preceded Koch's identification of the tubercle bacillus. This chapter examines the ways in which the classification of tuberculosis as a "diathetic" disease—one with both physiological and environmental causes—allowed regular physicians to consolidate their professional status and marshall their defenses against sectarian and empiricist rivals but at the same time to issue prescriptive statements that rendered intelligible the social and economic changes of the Civil War era.

Chapter Two articulates the American reactions to the first significant scientific challenges to nineteenth-century understandings of tuberculosis: Koch's bacterial hypothesis and his tuberculin cure. From the vantage of the "bacteriologic, immunologic and chemotherapeutic period," Koch's postulates seemed so compelling that opposition to them was unthinkable; yet contemporary American physicians reacted with considerable skepticism. Similarly, long after Koch's tuberculin had lost favor in Europe and Canada, American physicians remained loyal to it and continued to use it. Chapter Two evaluates those reactions and explores the roots of American opposition to BCG in the efforts to consolidate the scientific and professional status of medicine, to build the institutions essential to medicine's economic security, and to reconcile practical and conceptual difficulties in a metaphor of "seed and soil." This metaphor, which a range of American physicians adopted, accommodated the new evidence of Koch's bacillus to patterns of disease and gave rise to a therapeutic strategy designed to build resistance. Chapter Three provides an analysis of the varied initiatives to build resistance developed in sanatoria, voluntary agencies, and governmental institutions during the years bounding the first World War. Through analysis of the special measures taken to combat the intersecting problems of spit and degeneracy, it also explores the intersections among medicine, gender, and the agenda of social reform.

Chapters Four, Five, and Six bring us to BCG—to an analysis of the epidemiological trials that affirmed the association of tuberculosis with poverty and to the efforts governmental agencies made to grapple with an agenda that called for attacking simultaneously the biological and the social causes of disease. These chapters place in epidemiological and institutional context the persistent cry that vaccination was "not enough." As these chapters show, peculiarly American definitions of disease and unique reactions to Koch's bacillus, to medical professionalism and institutions, and to the state, economic development, and poverty all shaped the American experience with tuberculosis. But so did the illusion that we had conquered this disease. The Conclusion consequently assesses the "disappearance" of tuberculosis from public view, from both policy and history.

CHAPTER 1

Disease and the Agrarian Order: Tuberculosis before Koch

Jean-Antoine Villemin's experimental demonstration of the inoculability of tuberculosis, published in 1861, attracted little attention from Americans.[1] Villemin's work promised to shed new light on the causes of consumption—otherwise known as phthisis, pulmonary tuberculosis, or TB; yet, on the eve of the Civil War, contagion seemed an implausible explanation for the distribution of the leading cause of European and North American deaths. Few diseases shaped the contours of American life more dramatically than tuberculosis, which claimed between a seventh and a quarter of all who died during the first half of the nineteenth century.[2] But though it affected all North Americans, tuberculosis did so differently than did other major infections. Consumption differed from typhoid, cholera, and smallpox in its presentation, course, and, most important, distribution. This was not a gruesome, disfiguring malady. Characterized as a wasting condition, in an era when frailty and pallor symbolized beauty, consumption seemed actually to render its victims more interesting and attractive. Beware phthisis, classic medical texts warned, "the intellect frequently remains bright and active; . . . the feelings are usually cheerful and buoyant."[3] Consumption differed further from cholera, smallpox, or typhoid in that it was not epidemic. Chronic in its course, it existed in all places at all times.

Most important, however, as those who collected statistics soon noted, TB was unlike other infections in that it affected some populations and individuals preferentially. Concern about differential susceptibility dominated American discussions of tuberculosis from the mid-nineteenth century onward, and as each generation attempted to make sense of this preferential, or differential, susceptibility, the explanations they offered reflected and reinforced their uncertainties about a changing scientific and social order. In the decades that bounded the Civil War, medical writings exposed apprehensions about professional status, regional rivalries, and the growth of industrial cities, and they foreshadowed persistent American concerns with the social dimensions of disease.

American interest in consumption took shape with the new republic. As part of a broad effort to map national riches, estimate strengths, and anticipate weaknesses, the founders of the United States collected numbers. Statistics about disease formed part of their efforts to construct a national identity, for healthfulness seemed as fundamental a characteristic of the country as liberty.[4] Claims for the salubrity of the American climate, designed to promote the national interest and attract new settlers, needed substantiation; conversely, the many diseases that threatened American well-being demanded systematic attention. Through local studies like Benjamin Rush's of Philadelphia or regional surveys like Daniel Drake's of the Mississippi Valley, physicians simultaneously reaffirmed the healthfulness of the United States and warned against those conditions and diseases that threatened their country's well-being.

Phthisis, or consumption, figured prominently among the threats. During the early years of the republic, missionaries, cataloguers, and physicians commented frequently on consumption, and their accounts revealed two distinct but interrelated concerns. First, the absolute number of consumptive cases and deaths troubled surveyors like C. F. Volney, who found the disease so pervasive that it seemed the "direct offspring of the American soil and climate."[5] Second, the recognition that consumption affected some populations preferentially was also troubling. In an article entitled "Dr. Rush's Thoughts upon the Cause and Cure of Pulmonary Consumption," the *Boston Medical and Surgical Journal* remarked that this disease "is unknown among the Indians of North America. It is scarcely known by those citizens of the United States who live in the *first* stage of civilized life, and who have lately obtained the title of the *first settlers*. . . . It is less common in country places than in cities, and increases in both with intemperance and sedentary modes of life. . . . Women, who sit more than men, and whose work is connected with less exertion, are most subject to the consumption."[6] As they developed inventories of American experiences with disease, Samuel Forry, Drake, and other eminent physicians likewise observed that consumption was "more common in the South," among women, and among slaves.[7]

These twin concerns about prevalence and differential susceptibility dominated early-nineteenth-century discussions of consumption, but by the start of the Civil War the balance between them shifted. Through the first half of the century, increases in mortality and morbidity preoccupied both medical and lay writers. Anecdotal accounts from frontier and city alike, and more systematic reviews of bills of mortality, drew attention to "the great prevalence of tuberculous diseases."[8] Convinced that their health was deteriorating, Americans fixed their attention on consumption, which weekly reports of deaths, like those included in the *Boston Medical and Surgical Journal*, indicated was on the rise. Refined mortality data, included after 1830 in the federal census, fueled these fears. While consumption regularly claimed one-tenth of the deaths that occurred in Boston in the 1830s, by 1842 it accounted for close to one-seventh.[9] Lemuel Shattuck's *Report of the Sanitary Commission of Massachusetts, 1850*, one of the first systematic reviews of American vital statistics, lent further numerical credence to these fears. Designed both to improve record-keeping and to ensure that these data were applied to pragmatic, political ends, Shattuck investigated "the circumstances under which consumption operates."[10] Through this effort, Shattuck demonstrated that consumption took its toll everywhere, ranked as the first cause of American deaths, and claimed between fourteen and twenty-five deaths per hundred. Numerous studies published in the decade that followed Shattuck's report confirmed that in Philadelphia, New York, and Baltimore, New Orleans and Atlanta, in California, Missouri, and Florida, consumption caused 15 to 30 percent of all deaths.[11]

The apprehensions about the prevalence of consumption that dominated early-nineteenth-century medical writings persisted through the second half of the century as tuberculosis continued to head the bills of mortality. However, though consumption retained its rank as the first cause of American deaths, after 1850 the tuberculous death rate began to fall. Whether as a result of changing definitions of disease, new methods of record-keeping, or actual changes in mortality, the number of recorded deaths dropped by almost one-third between 1850 and 1890.

The Americans who applauded this decline also noted how inconsistent and nonuniform it was, and as they did so, their attention shifted to marked geographical and social variations in experience. Statistics collected during the middle years of the nineteenth century affirmed and drew new attention to the ways in which the incidence of tuberculosis varied with geographical location, occupation, race, and gender. Shattuck's *Report* highlighted the extent to which the causes of consumption "press[ed] most heavily upon cities and populous villages."[12] Echoing his teacher, Rush, the Virginia-born and Mississippi-bred Samuel Cartwright claimed the disease to be almost unknown "among the early pioneers of our western and southern wilderness" and blamed its increase on city life.[13] Medical statistics of the U.S. Army, compiled by a Dr. Coolidge, showed consumption to be far more prevalent in the South Atlantic region than anywhere else on the continent. In contrast, data from the seventh census suggested that consumptive mortality was far lower in Alabama, Louisiana, Georgia, and South Carolina than in Massachusetts or Maine.[14]

DIFFERENTIAL SUSCEPTIBILITY AND PROFESSIONAL POLITICS

Heated debates about the sources of differential susceptibility dominated both popular and medical literature from the mid-nineteenth century onward. In the decades that bounded the Civil War, these debates reflected, in the first instance, deep-seated medical conflicts over etiology and therapy. Through the first half of the nineteenth century, regular American physicians generally ascribed disease to constitutional imbalance. Consumption, they agreed, represented a cluster of diseases in which the tissues formed small tumors known as tubercles. However, as American physicians began their move away from doctrines of therapeutic specificity toward rationalism, empiricism, and universalism, sharp conflicts ensued over the causes of tubercularization. Through the first half of the nineteenth century, most prominent American physicians ascribed consumption to environment, to unhealthy living in damp, dark surroundings. Both statistical information and shifting medical knowledge, however, also lent credence to the etiological roles of heredity and contagion. "The reality of hereditary influence on the production of phthisis is so universally admitted, that it would seem a sort of scientific heresy to doubt it," a reviewer for the *Boston Medical and Surgical Journal* noted in 1844.[15] A desire to systematize the knowledge that underlay their profession and to ground practice on empirical and experimental data also led physicians to reflect on the contagiousness of consumption. Contingent contagionism, which allowed for the interplay of environment and germs, offered to some a plausible explanation for patterns of tubercular disease, and by the 1840s medical journals began regularly to report the results of "inoculation" experiments.[16]

Debates over the causes of consumption rooted in a contested professional terrain also cultivated therapeutic rivalries. The skepticism that led many American physicians of this period to question heroic depletion and to advocate, instead, the healing powers of nature and sectarian remedies, left its mark on consumption. Despite protestations to the contrary, most nineteenth century physicians believed consumption to be incurable. "Like philosopher's stone," a reviewer for the *Boston Medical and Surgical Journal* lamented in 1843, "a cure for consumption will continue, we apprehend, to be a desideratum for ages yet to come. . . . Medicine has never yet accomplished it, neither has any system of regimen, nor change of climate had any other than a temporary modifying influence, and death has ultimately asserted his power over human agencies."[17] This sense of ultimate impotence tempered the optimism of allopathic and homeopathic practitioners alike. Amidst the omnipresent debates over bloodletting, blistering, and purging, even the most ardent advocates of medical intervention doubted its usefulness to consumptives. "Dr. Rush," the *Boston Medical and Surgical Journal* suggested, questioned whether "bloodletting, emetics, blisters, setons or issues" were of any use to consumptives. "Not one of them all," he maintained, "has ever, I believe, cured a single consumptive."[18]

This widespread pessimism about the physician's ability to treat consumption cut right to the core of medical identity during a period of professional reorganization and consolidation. Buffeted by competition from sectarian practitioners and from those within their own ranks who subscribed to alternative philosophies of practice, regular mid-nineteenth century American physicians began to alter their prescriptive advice. Samuel George Morton, who in 1834 had advocated bleeding from the arm as "indispensable" and likely to "save the patient from the most hopeless consequences," and who advised his colleagues also to apply spirits of turpentine, sugars of lead, and carefully managed blistering, insisted just three years later that "bleeding, mercury and confinement to house are utterly inadmissible."[19]

Morton did not entirely abandon the use of medicines. He continued to prescribe digitalis, prussic acid, narcotics, and other preparations of their ilk, but the weight of his text and of his prescriptions shifted toward exercise, diet, clothing, and a change of climate. By the 1850s, this had become a common shift. The best course of treatment for consumption, advised Leonidas Lawson's classic text, billed as the first major American study of phthisis pulmonalis to follow Morton's, was "due regulation of exercise, diet, clothing, change of climate; and, in certain cases, a general tonic course of medication."[20] Two years later, when he addressed the New York Academy of Medicine, Austin Flint similarly extolled the values of "change of habits with respect to exercise and outdoor life."[21]

Appeals to diet, hygiene, and a change of climate served regular physicians in three distinct ways. First, the hypothesis that where and how one lived had an influence on health bolstered the beleaguered systemic tradition, for it allowed physicians to tailor their therapies to individual circumstance and need. Second, in the form that it took during the middle decades of the nineteenth century, the climatic theory of consumption also allowed for a more empiricist approach to therapeutics. Third, as Americans compiled statistics about geographical variations in the incidence of consumption, they came to recognize that some regions of the country—particularly the Southwest—appeared healthier than others, and this observation allowed for a standardization of treatment. If mid-nineteenth-century American physicians could agree on nothing else, they agreed that consumptives could improve their condition through travel, exercise, and other changes of habit. Celebrations of the advantages that travel to the Southwest, a sea voyage, or strenuous outdoor exercise exerted dominated the regular medical literature and captured diverse practitioners.

The appeal to climate also broke down barriers among regular physicians who employed medicines, those who extolled the healing powers of nature, and sectarians, most particularly homeopaths. No physician could, in good faith, simply allow consumption to take its course and hope that time and circumstance alone would cure. However, if advocates of the healing power of nature could not invoke its authority in precisely this sense, both they and their opponents in the regular ranks maintained that nature, as embodied by the natural environment, could and did alter the course of consumptive disease. The best treatment for acutely ill slaves, Cartwright suggested in 1854, was to return them "to an imitation of barbarism in the woods or fields"; for whites, he similarly advocated a return to the healthy habits of the early settlers.[22] This reification of nature provided a compelling and uniting therapeutic stratagem. It appealed to a wide range of regular physicians, but it also brought regular and sectarian practitioners together.

Just as the orthodoxy of the regular ranks faced the challenge of empiricists and "trusters" in nature, so all regular physicians recognized the professional challenge of sectarian practitioners, whose gentler medicines seemed a welcome alternative to heroic depletion. Rather than prescribing blisters and leeches, homeopaths preferred highly attenuated doses of sulphur and arsenicum, or albuminous matter, which allowed for intervention but lacked the intensity of regular cures.[23] However, though nonorthodox therapies were less harsh, they were not obviously more effective. Homeopaths might boast that Dr. Samuel Gregg had joined their ranks when he discovered that regular medicine could not cure his daughter of consumption. But much as they rejoiced in Gregg's conversion, and that of others like him, they had to confess that despite the best homeopathic effort the girl died.[24] Similarly, Dr. Charles Cullis of Boston had to explain why fully half of the patients admitted to his homeopathic consumptives home had died during the first five years of its existence.[25] Rhetoric aside, homeopathic remedies proved little more successful than allopathic ones, and they held relatively limited appeal. The casebooks of homeopathic practitioners, as reported in national homeopathic journals, rarely included accounts of consumptive patients.[26] Moreover, few patients actually entered Cullis's home, which based its appeal as much on its promise to treat the indigent as to treat them homeopathically. Thus, where the threat of cholera led North Americans to turn in droves to irregulars, the threat of tuberculosis seemed not to, and homeopaths well understood this hesitancy.

Sectarians recognized their limited ability to cure consumption. Just as the *Boston Medical and Surgical Journal*'s reviewer doubted the efficacy of standard medicinal treatments, so William Hawley confessed to the Homoeopathic Society of the State of New York: "I suppose every man who has undertaken to practice the art of healing, feels at times a want of satisfaction in the use of remedies, and a sense of uncertainty as to the curative action of drugs, such as to lead him sometimes, if not often, into a condition of skepticism in regard to medicine which makes his daily labor a weariness to the flesh."[27] But homeopaths confronted their limitations differently than allopaths did. When faced with the limited efficacy of their armamentarium, allopaths began to critique the principles on which they based their cures and to shift their practices. Homeopaths, in contrast, found new strength in failure. Rather than dismissing traditional homeopathic procedures, Hawley clung to the principles of attenuation, and he extolled "the wisdom of allowing remedies to exhaust their action before repetition in such chronic cases, as well as to demonstrate the efficacy of high attenuations, even when the lower have failed."[28] Similarly, though homeopathy failed to cure Gregg's daughter, he nonetheless professed himself "more devoted to his profession and the truths of homeopathy."[29]

Homeopaths did not simply become more ardent practitioners of attenuation however. They too recognized the need to attract consumptive patients, and like allopaths they attempted to capture their market by borrowing some of what the competition had to offer. Diatribes against the "aping of allopathic measures in treating disease" and the "insane use of poultices . . . and other expedients that may be reconcilable with allopathic medication, but in the hands of an intelligent homeopath are simply useless and ridiculous" became increasingly common as homeopaths struggled against the formal and informal restrictions state medical societies imposed on their practice.[30] But if homeopaths aped the allopathic effort to apply poultices and "parboil" their patients with excessive doses, they also borrowed the allopaths' advice to travel. Longtime advocates of "regulation" of the bodily functions, mid-nineteenth-century American homeopaths came increasingly to emphasize the influence of climate on bodily integrity. Whereas homeopaths of the 1840s and 1850s emphasized the need to dose their patients so as to redress imbalances in albumen and other bodily fluids, those of the 1860s advised patients to avoid sickness by seeking healthy lives in healthy locales.[31]

Thus, in the years that immediately preceded the Civil War, medical discussions of consumption formed part of larger disputes over etiology, therapy, and professional authority. Regular physicians' attempts to use licensing and organization "to protect the public against the specious encroachments of empiricism, and place the medical profession as far as practicable upon an elevated and honorable platform" fell short in the face of their inability to prevent or to cure consumptive disease.[32] In reality, neither regulars nor sectarians could offer consumptives much, yet, in their efforts to capture new medical markets and establish professional autonomy, each group decried the impotence of its rival. And in their efforts to attract consumptive patients, accommodate intellectual changes within their own ranks, and respond to the practical challenge of competition, regulars and sectarians alike modified their therapeutic practices.

Caught between clinical, statistical, and experimental evidence that supported various hereditary and environmental causes of phthisis, American physicians reconciled their differences by categorizing consumption as a diathetic disease.[33] This classification marked consumption as a general systemic condition shaped by both the physical and moral attributes of individuals. The diathesis—a "constitutional predisposition to a particular form of disease" located in the anatomical structure of the tissues— might be congenital, or it might be acquired by living wrongly or in the wrong place. The label *diathetic* thus provided regular physicians with a compromise position that allowed them to acknowledge a multiplicity of causes, among them germs. It allowed as well for therapeutic efforts that reconciled conflicting medical doctrines. Rather than lamenting their lack of definite knowledge about the causes of consumption or their inability to employ specific preventives and cures, regular physicians could direct their prescriptions toward the diathesis, and that focus allowed them to capitalize on the interplay of physiological and environmental factors that their competition had identified as so critical.

NORTH AND SOUTH: RACE, REGION, AND SUSCEPTIBILITY

Debates over the causes of differential susceptibility reflected tensions between competing medical interests, but as they focused attention on the diathesis, American physicians also betrayed their unease about a changing American order. Expositions of differences in the health of their regions had long served to distinguish North from South. Though Northerners and Southerners agreed that a hot, humid climate—and the habits of life it inspired—fostered agues, malaria, yellow fever, and a host of other peculiar diseases, Northerners used this evidence to bolster their claims to superiority, while Southerners traditionally employed it in the cause of distinctiveness.[34] On the eve of the Civil War, mortality data from the seventh census challenged the status quo and shifted the terms of debate. Compiled under the direction of Superintendent J.D.B. DeBow, it upset the image of the healthy North and allowed Southerners to strengthen the case for their climate, their way of life, and their "peculiar institutions." Consumption played no small part in this process.

Southern culture had no greater champion than the Louisianian DeBow, whose *Review* promoted and publicized the special Southern causes of slavery and cotton. A professor of commerce, political economics, and statistics, DeBow had also served as director of Louisiana's State Bureau of Statistics. He was consequently adept in the use of the tools of political arithmetic, and, when appointed to the census in 1852, DeBow employed these tools in the interests of his region. He expressly shifted the analytical framework of the census to investigate race, geography, and gender.[35] In contrast to contemporaries, who had regularly accepted the evidence that their states were poor, diseased, and debauched but who manipulated the evidence to advance the cause of Southern distinctiveness, DeBow denied the validity of Northern claims to superiority. He laid open the essential premise from which Northerners had begun—that a temperate climate was superior—with evidence that the prevalence of epidemic diseases and the poverty that bred them were far less in the South than had previously been thought. His analysis of the 1850 data, published in 1854 as *A Statistical View of the United States*, suggested that the South had been much maligned, for in DeBow's estimate the most recent census clearly demonstrated that most Southern diseases were nowhere near as prevalent or fatal as supposed, and many other diseases, consumption among them, occurred more often in the North.

If contemporary data vindicated the South, so also, it seemed, did history. In addition to reviewing the findings of the seventh census, DeBow compared the most recent data with every census after 1790. Subsequent publication of the collected mortality statistics refuted old prejudices, grounded in earlier military surveys and the works of Forry and Drake, which condemned the unhealthfulness of the South. Clearly, the errors of the earlier statistics affected a wide range of diseases, but they seemed particularly egregious in the case of consumption. Whereas Drake, Forry, and the military surveyors had suggested that consumption was more common in the South, the 1850 census indicated that it occurred only a quarter as often. This disease claimed one-sixth of all American deaths and one-quarter of those in New England, but it took one in nineteen in Louisiana and only one in thirty-six in Georgia. If the seventh census could be believed, consumption was undeniably a disease of the North, and it levied a far greater toll than malaria, yellow fever, or any other distinctively Southern disease.

Northerners did not passively accept DeBow's reformulation of either the past or the present. Denial and dismissal served as the first lines of defense; and as Northern critics worked and reworked the mortality data of the seventh census, they repeatedly cited methodological flaws in the collection of data, in the analysis, and in the interpretation. Put simply, Northerners were convinced that DeBow had erred, that consumption still proved more fatal in the South. Their counterclaims, launched in medical and lay journals of the Civil War era, began from the received wisdom that Southern climates were generally unhealthy—how else could one explain the great prevalence of malaria and yellow fever?—and hot, humid weather was especially fatal to those in the last stages of consumptive disease. To support these assertions, they cited local mortality figures, which testified to the great number of consumptive deaths in New Orleans, Charleston, Atlanta, and other Southern cities.

Such criticisms invited pat rejoinders, which Southerners readily marshaled. Some kept the debate at a statistical and methodological level. Others defended the healthfulness of their climate by pointing to the regularity with which Northern physicians advised consumptive patients to travel South or to the frequency with which Northern consumptives sought the North Carolina hills or the South Carolina coast. In a particularly compelling refutation of Northern efforts to dismiss DeBow, the Louisianian physician Bennet Dowler made both arguments. Northern physicians and popular opinion, he wrote in 1857, "favor the South as a residence for consumptives, . . . while the South rarely, if ever sends a consumptive North for the benefits of its climate." Yet more than this anecdotal evidence, Dowler found compelling the numerical finding that consumption always favored the South and decreased in fatality as one crossed the northern lateral.[36]

Dowler also appreciated that differential susceptibility to consumption had political cachet. DeBow's *Statistical View* cut to the core of American identity. Framed in the literature of transcendentalist New England, the image of American health propounded during the first half of the nine-

teenth century was an image of Northern health, predicated on the merits of Northern climate, society, and politics. By the mid-1850s, in the face
of statistical assessments like Shattuck's, which quantified increases in
mortality, and European commentaries, which with increasing frequency
exposed the "supposed degeneration of the physical condition" of Americans, this image was hard to sustain.[37] The implication of the seventh census, that New England could compete with neither the European
homeland nor its Southern rival, seemed to add insult to injury. Perturbed
Northern politicians, statisticians, and physicians consequently struggled
to defend their states against charges of degeneracy by disputing the data
of the census and challenging DeBow's interpretation. Southerners, like
Dowler, seized the opportunity to manipulate DeBow's data to their own
political ends. As Dowler noted, regional differences in consumption bespoke the need for a complete reassessment of the national order. "If
Maine, for instance, loses nine times more than Georgia in proportion to
the whole mortality," he wrote in 1857, "life insurance, life itself, and the
material interests of property and of the population, as well as the prophylactic and curative influences of climate become topics of permanent
importance, and the well being of society demands that these things should
be known as a guide to conduct."[38] In the years that followed, Dowler,
along with fellow Southern physicians, statisticians, politicians, and po-
lemicists, ensured that DeBow's data were probed and applied as guides
to conduct. The evidence that their region was relatively immune to consumption, they recognized, could affirm the virtues of the Southern climate and way of life, and also justify an agrarian, slave-holding order.

Dowler coupled his 1857 defense of DeBow with a response to a commentary on consumption in the South that had been issued on behalf of
a Northern "insurance company," and the juxtaposition of these two pieces
betrays the ways in which discussions of differential susceptibilities articulated regional rivalries. Both Dowler's essay and the Northern promotional
literature to which it responded carried a political edge. The promotional
literature had two purposes. First, it aimed to establish how ridden with
consumption, yellow fever, and other "plagues" the South really was. Second, it attempted to make this point by relying heavily on the testimony
of Southerners themselves, in this case, one Dr. Barton of Louisiana—
presumably E. H. Barton of the New Orleans Sanitary Commission.
Dowler's response contained the standard, substantive refutations: that
Barton had little evidence, that the evidence he could marshal was flawed
and outdated, that European data and the seventh census clearly demonstrated that if one took the slave-holding states as the limit to the South,
"the ratio of deaths to the number of people is generally lower in the South

than the North."[39] But mortality statistics, he alleged, made "the case worse for the South, as to consumption, than the reality warrants; because the popular opinion in favor of the South as a residence for consumptives sends a vast number of such patients to the Southern States, swelling the bills of mortality."[40] If discrepancies in the number of consumptive deaths that occurred in rural and urban areas within the South itself could be attributed to migration, Dowler asked how much more so could regional differences have the same cause? Surveyors, he claimed, observed an excessive number of consumptive deaths in his region only because Northern physicians constantly exported their patients to the South.

Migration unfairly inflated estimates of mortality, but, from the Southern perspective, it also obscured the real cause of ill health—Northern exploitation—for which the Southern climate and way of life had become scapegoats. The migration of Northern consumptives thus represented yet another of the many situations in which Northern injustice forced the South to bear an unfair burden. Southern physicians charged again and again that mortality from phthisis "is vastly increased by strangers who come here to die of this terrible disease. The wards of our Charity Hospital show an annual influx of phthisis patients from all parts of the country, who come here only to die."[41] Through this analysis, the North, rather than any factor intrinsic to the South, emerged as the true cause of poor Southern health.

As the debate evolved, Southerners not only shifted critical attention from South to North but also used the epidemiology of consumption to make their case for Southern ways. Dowler became a particularly ardent participant in this effort, and he exemplified the Southern effort to recast alleged weaknesses as strengths. He turned attention first to malaria and yellow fever, the emblems of the fragile Southern constitution and of the behaviors and conditions that left the South prey to disease. Drawing ammunition from the seventh census, Dowler disputed earlier estimates of the prevalence of these diseases but once again moved quickly away from discussion of actual rates to the significance of those rates. "It may be thought," he wrote, "that what the South gains in consumption it loses to yellow fever and other diseases," but new mortality data demonstrated this claim to be patently untrue. More significant, however, when compared to consumption, "cholera and yellow fever sink into insignificance, seeing that consumption sweeps into the tomb from $1/4$ to $1/5$ of all the population in some districts, its victims generally in the prime of life." Here, Dowler identified consumption, rather than the distinctively Southern diseases, as the real threat to the United States, and he also began to reframe the earlier debate over these diseases. Whereas yellow fever had traditionally been employed against the cause of the South, Dowler now implied that it might actually work to the South's advantage, for yellow fever seemed to protect against consumption. At the height of a yellow fever epidemic, he suggested, both the number of consumptive deaths and the total number of deaths that occurred in New Orleans were far fewer than in Boston.[42] Two other Southern physicians, William Hutson Ford and E. M. Pendleton, of Sparta, Georgia, elaborated on and refined these analyses of the relationship between consumption and the distinctively Southern diseases. In the years that followed, each proposed that an antagonism between malaria, yellow fever, and consumption allowed Southerners to better withstand the great white plague.[43]

If malaria and yellow fever protected against consumption—the true threat to American health—so Southerners argued did their other unique institutions, most particularly slavery. By the early 1860s, physicians had amassed a varied and rich literature on the "special needs" of slaves. Some of this literature attempted to make sense of the differential susceptibility and mortality, some to assess the medical care that slaves would need, and much to justify the institution of slavery itself. Few Northerners or Southerners doubted that blacks experienced disease differently than did whites, but though blacks clearly suffered from a specific range of ailments that never afflicted whites, and suffered more acutely, they were often portrayed as healthier. The African's superior resistance to malaria and heat underpinned these claims; so did a romanticized rendering of slave life. As an editorialist for the *Boston Medical and Surgical Journal* noted early in the century, slaves "are probably more temperate in the use of spirituous liquors and more abstemious in their mode of living than whites of the same class. Hence they are for the most part healthy, and when sick ordinarily require less active evacuations than the white."[44] This language captured pervasive and enduring sentiments that Southerners clung to long after most Northerners had abandoned them. Before, during, and after the Civil War, Southern judges, politicians, and, most important, physicians repeatedly asserted that "coloreds" were healthier, worked harder, and lived longer in the South.[45]

The distribution of consumption, as revealed once again in DeBow's seventh census, made the best case for the benefits of life under slavery. Southerners commonly believed that blacks suffered from a distinctive form of consumption, known as "negro consumption"; indeed, this peculiar form of the disease served often to justify a distinctive system of medical education that looked beyond the "causes, prevention and cure of the maladies of the white race in cold climates" or a specialized slave medicine.[46] Southerners also accepted that slaves commonly suffered from pulmonary affections, but DeBow's census indicated that they were far less susceptible than whites to ordinary, pulmonary consumption. Having tabulated phthisical deaths by region, DeBow demonstrated that throughout the South phthisis claimed far fewer blacks than whites. In Virginia, for example, consumption accounted for roughly one in ten white deaths but only one in sixteen slave deaths. In Alabama, the white to slave ratio of consumptive deaths was one in eighteen to one in thirty-eight. Here, the distinction between "negro" and slave deaths became key, for though DeBow's data suggested that slaves rarely succumbed to consumption, it further indicated that Northern whites and free blacks had no such immunity. Among these populations, mortality rates were virtually identical.[47]

The variations in mortality of free blacks and slaves became particularly useful to Southern medical writers, led by Cartwright and Josiah Nott, who invoked their medical knowledge and authority to justify slavery. In the years that immediately preceded the Civil War, both Cartwright and Nott wrote prolifically on the subject of medicine and slavery; between 1851 and 1862, Cartwright alone published fourteen articles on the subject in DeBow's celebrated *Review*. In these, Cartwright attempted to advocate for secession, a cause to which he had only recently converted. Virginia-born, Cartwright had trained in Philadelphia with Rush before returning to practice in both Alabama and Mississippi. Winner of Harvard's Boylston Prize and a true democrat, he stood between North and South, and his essays on yellow fever and cholera were widely acclaimed throughout the country. But Cartwright was also committed to doctrines of the separate and inferior creation of "negro races" and of state rights—opinions that many Northerners found less convincing—and these scientific and political opinions ultimately led him to support secession. Similarly, Nott, a native of Columbia, South Carolina, had studied in Philadelphia. Celebrated for his articles on the instincts of races, he gained particular renown for his work on the separate creation of black and white races, and these doctrines underpinned his discussions of slavery.

The premise of separate origins informed both Cartwright's and Nott's analyses of the "peculiar negro diseases," and both invoked the obvious racial differences between blacks and whites as the first and simplest explanation for their distinctive reactions to disease. This was the stock in trade of antebellum physicians, who viewed distinctive black responses to yellow fever, malaria, and other diseases as yet another ostensibly unique racial feature; who measured their skill by their ability to minister to the special needs of slaves; and who believed that the physician could make no greater error than to treat "negroes" as though they were "white men in black skins."[48]

Yet Cartwright in particular did not restrict his analysis to physiological or physical differences; he also ascribed the good health of the South's slaves to the conditions under which they lived. His appeal to environment was consistent with a mid-nineteenth-century understanding of heredity, in which nature and nurture easily interplayed, but it also served to affirm the virtues of the Southern order. Cartwright's narrative betrayed his extreme paternalism and his desire to vindicate "the peculiar institution." Only plantation owners, he argued, appreciated the true nature of slaves, and only they would ensure that blacks received the care of properly trained medical practitioners who fully understood the therapeutic and diagnostic significance of racial variations. Plantation life, Cartwright further proposed, ensured that Africans accommodated their diet and habits to the American habitat, for in his experience they were inherently unable to care for themselves. But Cartwright also understood plantation life to be good for slaves because of the discipline and habits it imposed. Under slavery, he wrote, blacks were "made to labor and exercise, which makes the lungs perform the duty of vitalizing the blood more perfectly than is done when they are left free to indulge in idleness. It is the red, vital blood, sent to the brain, that liberates their mind when under white man's control; and it is the want of a sufficiency of red,vital blood that chains their mind to ignorance and barbarism when in freedom."[49] From Cartwright's perspective, plantation life provided a particularly potent deterrent to consumption, for by the mid-nineteenth century American physicians almost unanimously agreed that the etiology of this disease included those conditions that impeded digestion, respiration, and circulation.

Cartwright's celebration of the plantation glorified not only slavery but also the agrarian order. If he believed the outdoor life good for slaves, he found it similarly good for whites. In language borrowed almost verbatim from his teacher Rush, who suggested that consumption occurred rarely among the Indians and "first settlers" of North America, Cartwright wrote "that among the early pioneers of our western and southern wilderness, pulmonary consumption was almost unknown."[50] Cartwright's analysis of the reasons for the pioneers' apparent immunity to consumption served as a starting point for the condemnations of the urbanized, industrial North that resounded in antebellum writings. It was not the "sturdy stock" of the pioneers that accounted for their healthfulness, he maintained, for they fared ill in cities. Rather, it was their adherence to a rugged, industrious, outdoor life, a life lived in harmony with nature.[51]

This rejection of the industrial order seemed, to Cartwright, to account for increased consumptive mortality among all Americans who chose city life, and these included, especially, free blacks.

Patterns of differential mortality, critical to the antebellum defense of slavery, became in the years that followed the Civil War, increasingly important in Southern attempts to expose the fallacies of emancipation. The mortality of blacks, the *Southern Journal of Medical Science* reported in 1866, had more than doubled in Charleston and other Southern cities, to the point that it exceeded threefold the mortality of whites.[52] Nowhere, subsequent accounts proclaimed, was the deterioration of black health so apparent as in mortality from tubercular diseases. In Richmond, Virginia, Thomas Atkinson noted in 1873, "the most marked difference between the diseases of the two races is in *the far greater prevalence and mortality of tubercular diseases amongst the blacks.*"[53] Summarizing data culled from numerous sources, Atkinson presented evidence that the free blacks who inhabited the major Southern cities, and Northern cities like New York as well, had grown increasingly susceptible to tuberculosis. Not only did they suffer from this disease more often than previously, but they suffered to a greater extent than whites.

Physicians attributed this "excessive death-rate among negroes"[54] to varied causes. The hereditarian/environmental debate persisted as Northern commentators regularly attributed excessive mortality to "the general insalubrity of the sections of the city inhabited by [blacks], the crowded condition of their dwellings, insufficient nourishment, and the other influences of poverty,"[55] while Southerners more typically cited the "habitual improvidence" of the black races.[56] However, Reconstructionism and Reconstructionist practice became increasingly frequent targets for both Northern and Southern critics. Emancipation had not gone far enough, a commentator for the *Medical Times and Gazette* charged, for Northerners behaved hypocritically and inconsistently. Their emancipatory rhetoric did not match their actions. "The despised race—who only become 'our colored brethren' for platform purposes," he suggested, suffered materially "at the hands of Yankee soldiers" who, when confronted with scarcity, met their own needs first. This commentator used mortality among freedmen as an opportunity to implore American statesmen to "find a far nobler sphere of operations in ameliorating the miserable condition of slaves, to whom they have given freedom, than in political cabals."[57]

Southerners took a still harder line. Nott and Atkinson did not simply implore Reconstructionists to demonstrate their superior virtue by taking better care of freed slaves; rather, they seized the evidence for deteriorating health to advance racist creeds and advocate resurrection of the economic practices of the Old South. The condition of freedmen, Nott argued in his 1866 essay on the instincts of races, attested to the failure of emancipation. The slave population, he argued, had been "the best cared for, most comfortable, contented, and increasing labor population in the world"; it had also been "more intelligent, more moral, more christianized, more useful in the progress of civilization than this race had ever been in its native or in foreign lands in freedom." Free blacks, in contrast, were "dying from the effects of indolence" and falling into degradation, improvidence, licentiousness, and "physical and moral rot." The general decline in black health seemed to Nott to confirm the race's inferior status, for he could find no "excuse" other than "origins" for the blacks' historical failure to thrive or inability to advance with freedom.[58]

Atkinson, like Nott, invoked the racial determinants of health, but he provided a less essentialist explanation for the deteriorating health of free blacks. Rather than ascribing increases in consumption to inherent racial characteristics, Atkinson blamed Northern physicians who committed "great errors in the treatment of the diseases of the negro."[59] This case for Southern medical distinctiveness quickly evolved into a plea for the resurrection of the Old Southern order. With language strongly reminiscent of that used by his antebellum colleagues, Atkinson accused his Northern colleagues of viewing the South through the "mists of prejudice," as exemplified in the *Boston Medical and Surgical Journal*'s out-of-hand dismissal of his logic. Northerners might depict Southern institutions as the enemy, he argued, but they were really the transported African's true friend. Southern medicine served as a prime example, for it alone preserved the health of slaves. So too had the conditions of life on the plantation. "During slavery, when a negro was seldom content with less than six pounds of fat pork per week, and was otherwise well fed, and well clothed," Atkinson wrote, "consumption was comparatively seldom seen among them, but since their emancipation I have seen more of them than the whites fall victims to it."[60]

Atkinson found little merit in the Northern effort to link the incidence of consumption to the conditions under which free blacks lived and worked; however, other Southerners were less resistant than he. They too accepted the free blacks' greater susceptibility to consumption as evidence in favor of distinctive Southern medical practice and of the paternalism of the plantation, but they also employed this evidence to make a more general case for the agrarian order. Whereas slaves had worked at healthful, outdoor activities, the standard apology read, Reconstruction reduced blacks to employment in cities and towns as "boot blacks, scavengers, waiters in hotels and steamboats, and other positions subordinate to the whites."[61] Physicians predicted two consequences of this change in work patterns. The first was a "gradual extinction" of the black race, through poverty, unhealthy habits, and the "widening field of white labor."[62] The second was the more general demise of the Southern economy—of cotton and agricultural production. These foundations of the Southern order, Nott maintained in a stunningly contorted piece of logic, could not survive without slaves even though Nott believed blacks to have an "instinctual" aversion to agriculture. Thus, he argued, in order to preserve the Southern economy, one needed to preserve slavery.

The plea for preservation of the agrarian order also became an indictment of Northern employment practices, particularly in industry. Indictments of Northern industrialism recurred frequently in Southern writings. *DeBow's Review*, in particular, dedicated as it was to the economic cause of the South, derided the social organization of Northern manufacturing towns and decried the exploitative practices of "Yankee Manufacturers" in innumerable articles. These practices, from dumping merchandise on the Confederate states to failing to care for employees, seemed to most Southern physicians to expose the failings of emancipation and the limitations of Reconstruction. The industrial North, the abolitionist North, did not breed freedom; rather it bred consumption.

If most Southern physicians turned the evidence of increasing consumptive mortality against the North, some—including Stanford Chaillé, professor of physiology and pathology at the University of Louisiana—applied the data to more introspective ends. In 1868, Chaillé and his colleague S. Bemiss embarked on a study of the "sanitary history and condition" of New Orleans. Chaillé's research convinced him that, much though his colleagues might protest to the contrary, New Orleans was a very unhealthy city—not just in epidemics or during the hot season or to foreigners but to all who lived in it at all times. "I have been advised that this publication would injure the sanitary reputation of this city," Chaillé wrote, but he refused "for immigrants and profit [to] suppress the truth," primarily because he believed that a close analysis of the causes of disease in New Orleans would "result eventually in rescuing annually thousands of lives from an untimely grave."[63] Chaillé's systematic review of census and other materials drew attention to "the comparatively large number of deaths by Consumption, Intemperance and casualties" that occurred in New Orleans, and he exhorted "political economists [to] reflect on this."[64] Political economists, in particular, he suggested, should turn their attention to a closer examination of the systems of habitation and employment that encouraged the development and spread of consumptive disease, especially within New Orleans.

CITY AND COUNTRY: AGRARIANISM, MASCULINITY, AND HEALTH

Chaillé's plea was that of a Southern physician who struggled to delineate his region's weaknesses and strengths in order to preserve its unique cultural identity, but in the years that followed the Civil War he was not the only physician who seized on the relationship between city life and consumptive disease. The data amassed during the middle decades of the nineteenth century—especially the mortality statistics for Massachusetts—repeatedly drew attention to the prevalence of tuberculosis in cities. In Massachusetts as a whole, tuberculous mortality began to fall after 1850. Between 1861 and 1870, the death rate from tuberculosis and other respiratory diseases fell from 365.8/100,000 to 343.3/100,000. During the two subsequent decades, it dropped again, to 308.1/100,000 in 1880 and 258.6/100,000 in 1890. Yet, despite this general decline, in Boston and other cities mortality rose to almost 400/100,000.[65] The tuberculous death rate in New York, Philadelphia, and other cities of the Eastern seaboard similarly climbed during the 1860s. Nor were American experiences singular. When the newly formed Canadian nation undertook its first national census, in 1871, it too named tuberculosis the leading cause of death and placed mortality at 183/100,000.[66] Montreal, Toronto, and the towns of the Maritimes established themselves particularly as strongholds of consumption. By 1870, mortality in these cities had risen to 200/100,000—a rate almost double that found in the countryside.[67] America and its values were rural, and as cities and TB grew side by side, disease seemed part of a more general threat to the established agrarian order. Consumption came to symbolize all that was wrong with American life. The altered means of production, the habits of city life, and the shifting relations between classes and sexes all came under scrutiny as causes of TB.

Concerns about the connection between cities and tuberculosis had their roots in Jeffersonian ideals and rhetoric.[68] "Mr. Jefferson had taught us that cities were evils," an anonymous author commented in *DeBow's Review*,[69] and Southerners, Cartwright among them, generally found much wisdom in these warnings. But the Jeffersonian idealization of the agrarian order, so sanctified in Southern writings, was also revered in the North. If Cartwright believed that "the history of the early pioneers tells how consumption may be prevented and even cured" and that this history provided clear demonstration of the advantages of industry, adventure, and love for the out-of-doors, he had learned such lessons from his teacher Rush. And if Cartwright believed that "an unprofitable life of indolence and ease, with the mind caged from the real world and fed on vain abstractions mistaken for true science, and novel reading for literature, will as certainly cause consumption and give it the character of an epidemic, as heat and miasm the intermittent fever,"[70] his disdain for city habits resonated strongly with that of Northern transcendentalists. To both Northerners and Southerners, cities represented an evil that seduced Americans away from the healthy, outdoor, independent existence their ancestors had enjoyed and rendered them consumptive.

The explanations that American physicians offered for why cities bred disease consequently began from the premise that rural locales were healthy, and they built on that premise to condemn the locations of cities. By the 1860s, American physicians generally acknowledged that physical environment played a role in the development of consumptive disease. When he presented his classic study of *Consumption in New England* (1862), Henry Ingersoll Bowditch, professor of clinical medicine at Harvard Medical School, ascribed local variations in this "scourge of the human race" to the proximity of damp, marshy areas,[71] and, taking Bowditch as their starting point, other physicians investigated the influence of variations in temperature, sunlight, and altitude. Climates "which are moist and subject to frequent laterations of cold and warmth" promote TB, classic textbooks like Flint's warned.[72]

Americans, it seemed, had too often built their cities and towns in unhealthy locales, but while many lamented the failures of urban planning, few attributed the prevalence of consumption in urban centers to geography alone. "City habits, city houses, city life, and city occupations," Frank Donaldson warned the American Public Health Association meeting of 1874, all conspired to produce consumption.[73] That conditions in cities bred disease was hardly a novel assertion, nor was it one that was specific to TB. By the 1870s Americans clearly understood that poorly ventilated, crowded, ill-heated, damp, dark dwellings acted as breeding grounds for numerous diseases. The cholera epidemics of 1832, 1849, and 1866 had demonstrated particularly dramatically how vulnerable tenement dwellers were to acute diseases, and bills of mortality regularly testified to the preponderance within a city's poorer districts of dysentery, typhoid, and more chronic infections. However, unlike cholera, TB was not simply a disease of huddled masses who lived in impoverished slums. "We may venture to assert," wrote Henry Wiley, echoing many physicians, "that the necessary privations of poverty on the one hand, and the absurd excesses of wealth on the other, tend more to the formation of tubercles of children than all other causes combined."[74]

In this sense, consumption embodied the threat of departure from an agrarian way, from the simple life lived in harmony with nature—in other words, from the rugged, masculine norm that transcendentalism set. Unlike debates over cholera and yellow fever, which linked disease with sinful behavior, mid-nineteenth-century discussions of consumption made implicit connections between disease and unmanly or unnatural behavior. "An indoor, sedentary, luxurious and artificial life," Bowditch argued in 1862, most frequently engendered consumption. But, he maintained, "an active life, spent chiefly in the open air, in healthy situations, followed by an adequate amount of sleep at night, in dry, clean and well ventilated chambers, with a sufficient supply of appropriate nourishment and clothing constitute the conditions which would most certainly guarantee against its occurrence."[75] When, almost a decade later, Bowditch polled 210 prominent New England physicians, he again found that they overwhelmingly ascribed consumption not to filth, drink, or other artifacts of urban poverty but to "overwork in trades," "over-study," and "excess."[76]

The rebukes against excess, indulgence, and luxury that had formed part of the North's claim against the South thus reemerged in the analysis of cities. Whether wealthy or poor, Donaldson explained, city dwellers led a sedentary and indoor life, got too little exercise, and partook of a poor diet characterized by foods either too meager or too rich.[77] Consumption, Flint similarly observed, was rife in cities but occurred rarely in rural, newly settled, and remote places. To explain this phenomenon, Flint proposed that "the pioneers who compose the early population in these places, are persons, generally, of sturdy, vigorous health, and the habits of life, in such a population, are protective against the disease."[78]

Tuberculosis thus seemed just punishment for deviation from the habits of rugged masculinity that mid-nineteenth-century Americans equated with health, strength, and virtue. These included habits not only of life but also of employment. If consumption evoked fears about the demise of agriculture, it also raised the specter of another threat to the American order—the rise of industry. Physicians and other writers who early in the century made implicit links between consumptive mortality and industrial growth drew the connection increasingly clearly. Shattuck, for example, exposed the ways in which in Massachusetts disease rates rose with the growth of manufacturing, and, through the era of Reconstruction, physicians commented with increasing frequency on the association between consumption and particular manufacturing trades.[79] To their general concerns about sedentary indoor occupations and occupations in trades that produced dust, they added specific reservations about millwork.

Consumption thus became associated with men who lived in cities, indulged in frivolous pastimes, and worked at indoor occupations or otherwise shunned the outdoors, but it also came to be constructed as a disease of women, who departed by definition from the male norm. Women's fashions and women's sedentary habits were obvious sources of apprehension. Flimsy dress that exposed the neck and throat, high-heeled shoes that encumbered a healthy gait, and a "natural aversion" to vigorous outdoor exercise all appeared in lists of the causes of consumption.

In an era when changing economic and gender relations intersected, female occupations also provoked concern. "The class of trades which appeared most frequently to induce phthisis," an anonymous contributor to the *Boston Medical and Surgical Journal* proposed in the 1830s, "was that in which circumstances were united of a sedentary, bent position, and great exercise of the upper extremities." These, it happened, were also the trades, like millinery, embroidery, and artificial flower-making, in which women predominated, and in the author's view those peculiarities of employment "satisfactorily accounted for the fact that phthisis occurs peculiarly among females."[80] But household work, which confined women to the indoors, also posed a threat. In his *Report*, for example, Shattuck noted that in the country TB preferentially affected women, while in cities it took its greatest toll among men.

Household work distinguished women from men and starkly delineated the masculine from the feminine, but as female employment outside the domestic sphere became more common, physicians shifted their attention away from the threat of femininity to the threat of female competition. Women's domestic duties took on new health-inducing characteristics, and their unique reproductive capacities emerged as protective. With greater frequency, physicians noted that pregnancy appeared to "suspend" or "retard" phthisis.[81] In contrast, virtually all extradomestic work appeared to compromise women's health. Even agricultural labor, presumed to be beneficial to men, had its risks. Though "the effect of outdoor farm labor on adult women appears to be favorable to health," an editorial in the *Boston Medical and Surgical Journal* cautioned, "there is a good deal of evidence . . . to show that field work demoralizes women, or at any rate girls. Woman is a domestic creature, and a mother does more service to society by tending her children and going through the details of her little household, than by mowing grass or hoeing turnips."[82] Millwork and manufacturing appeared as particular threats to woman's health. Some of the threat derived from the nature of the work itself. As Flint noted, "The disease prevails much more among those whose pursuits are sedentary than among those whose occupations involve outdoor life."[83]

Greater threat, however, derived from the new status of working women. The associations between tuberculosis and the growth of manufacturing that became so apparent to mid-nineteenth-century physicians soon led to an explicit attack on the urban working classes, as physicians and social critics identified the rush to cities, the habits of city life, and workers' powerlessness, economic insecurity, dependency and loss of autonomy as contributing causes of tuberculosis.[84] Initially insulated, the women who flocked to cities and milltowns in search of social and economic independence seemed particularly to fall prey to the influences that particularly predisposed to consumption—the tendency to work long hours in confined quarters, to skimp on meals, and to indulge in "excesses." Thus, in making the mill girl a problem, late-nineteenth-century physicians exposed dual concerns about the emergence of industry and female aspirations to a male, or public, sphere.

THE THERAPEUTIC IMPULSE TO SOCIAL REFORM

Debates over susceptibility to consumption, articulated in the years that bounded the Civil War, were consequently interwoven with disputes about the merits of various natural and social environments. The competing political and economic agendas of North and South dominated but in no way monopolized these disputes. Concerns about the emergence of cities and industries and the shifting gender of the workforce also played their part. As physicians associated consumptive disease with a changing social order, their therapeutic advice to consumptives attempted to preserve and re-create the world that they feared was slipping away. "The most probable method of curing the consumption," Rush had proposed, "is to revive in the constitution, by means of exercise or labor, that vigor which belongs to the Indians, or to mankind in their first stage of civilization."[85] By the end of the Civil War, physicians who aspired to new scientific status provided physiological justification for these prescriptions. Overindulgence and other city habits, Cartwright, Donaldson, Flint, and others of their generation explained, deprived the tissues of proper nourishment and of an adequate source of oxygen or pure air, which rendered them tuberculous.

These recommendations also acquired a therapeutic authority, and the advice that the best preventive for consumption was a forced return to the habits of pioneers became canonized in the regimen of the earliest American sanatoria. Wilderness resorts modeled after a German prototype, these early sans resembled health spas and forced a return to the habits and morals of the outdoor life. Remote, informal, and often located in the South, they enabled patients to take advantage of a healthful climate, engage in vigorous outdoor exercise, and otherwise imitate the life of the "first settlers."

The climatic or wilderness cures had joint physiological and social purposes, for if they restored the consumptive's constitution to a favored state, they also recreated a "pioneer" life. These dual purposes become evident in the experience of Edward Livingston Trudeau, a physician and consumptive who founded the Adirondack Cottage Sanitarium at Saranac Lake, New York. Son of James Trudeau—an eminent Louisianian physician and supporter of the Confederacy—and of Cephise Berger, Trudeau spent much of his early life with his divorced mother in Paris. He returned to the United States in 1865 and took up residence in New York with his grandparents. Over the course of the next several years, Trudeau spent much of his time developing a transcendentalist's love for the outdoors, hunting, fishing, and otherwise engaging in sport. After watching his brother die of tuberculosis and nursing his dying grandfather, Trudeau followed the family tradition and graduated from the College of Physicians and Surgeons of New York in 1871.

Trudeau contracted tuberculosis in 1873. Following contemporary therapeutic practice, he traveled to South Carolina, where he and his physicians hoped that warmth and energetic exercise would improve his condition. They did not. In desperation, Trudeau isolated himself at Paul Smith's wilderness camp in upstate New York. An avid sportsman and naturalist, he incorporated these loves into his therapeutic regimen. For almost seven years, he did little else but live in the wild, partake in moderation of good food, fresh air, and exercise, and hunt and fish.

Trudeau's return to the outdoors, to the life of the pioneer or early settler, so much improved his condition that upon his recovery he opened his own sanatorium. Situated in the New York wilderness, his Adirondack Cottage, which first accepted patients in 1885, was to afford to others the opportunities Trudeau himself enjoyed. Minimizing the importance of climate, Trudeau founded his san on the the dictum "that it is not so much where the consumptive lives as how he lives that is important."[86] The simple, frugal life spent in sparsely furnished cottages and in harmony with the outdoors represented the consumptive's cure, or, as a patient and practitioner at Trudeau's san later reflected, "The Daily Sanatorium Routine Was the Treatment."[87]

Cast historically as a new breed of American sanatorium, Trudeau's Adirondack Cottage nonetheless borrowed heavily from a therapeutic tradition that attempted at once to promote physical and social well-being. The classification *diathetic* that had so reconciled conflicting medical interests also served as a descriptive category that allowed physicians to blend and balance their various medical and social experiences with tuberculosis. If the classification marked consumption as a general systemic condition shaped by both the physical and moral attributes of individuals, it also provided a powerful prescriptive tool that justified both medical and social reform. As they grappled with their lack of definite knowledge about the causes of consumption and their inability to employ specific preventives and cures, antebellum physicians used the diathesis to frame measures of disease control that combined medical doctrine with exhortations to proper living. Certain that tuberculous disease was caused by poor living conditions and urban life—by both moral and physical contamination—they advocated regimens that would strengthen both body and soul. A return to the country and the life it represented was chief among these. Again and again, medical texts and advice manuals suggested that exercise, proper climate, good diet, wholesome living, general hygiene, outdoor work, and reasonable caution in regard to contact with consumptives would effectively check the spread of the disease. The influence of these measures was twofold. They created strong bodies, and they also affirmed the value of the established American order, in which cleanliness, godliness, and usefulness were at a premium. Individualist in design, the campaigns against the diathesis consequently fused physiology with ideology to counteract the evil influences of urbanization and industrialization and to create good citizens.[88]

That goal gave shape to Trudeau's and other mid-nineteenth-century campaigns against tuberculosis. It also inspired the late-nineteenth- and early-twentieth-century American program to build a combined physiological and sociological resistance to tuberculosis, colored subsequent efforts to control the disease, and shaped the responses of each successive generation of physicians to new scientific knowledge.

Coping with Koch's Challenges: Bacteria, Biologics, and the Economy of Disease, 1880–1915

Mid-nineteenth century American physicians viewed tuberculosis as a disease at once physiological and social. Confronted with tremendous clinical complexity and variation, they deemed consumption diathetic, turned for explanation to gender, race, environment, and employment, and sought therapy and prevention in the transformation of behaviors. As Robert Koch observed in 1882, "One has been accustomed until now to regard tuberculosis as the outcome of social misery, and to hope by the relief of distress to diminish the disease."[1] With his classic study of the etiology of tuberculosis, presented to the Physiological Society of Berlin in March 1882, Koch introduced a method for culturing microorganisms that elucidated their etiological and pathological roles and fundamentally and systematically challenged traditional understandings of and approaches to TB.[2]

Koch's identification of the tubercle bacillus epitomized the challenge and promise of the new science, the allure of which framed some of the most significant changes that late-Victorian North America underwent. Between 1880 and 1915 science helped give shape to a middle class order; as both the United States and Canada became increasingly industrial and professional, science prescribed new standards of knowledge, new methods and modes of production, and new norms of behavior. Experimentation and systematic inquiry came to define the bounds of both natural and social knowledge, promised to transform the world, generated tremendous wealth, and amused and engaged both young and old. The formulation of a scientific curriculum in land-grant colleges, scientific schools, and new programs of graduate study divided expert from lay person.[3] The lure of applied science and the lure of wealth became inextricably intertwined. The practice of popular science—collecting, engaging in miscroscopy, studying natural history, and astronomy—marked the gentleman and gentlewoman,[4] while the legitimacy of science led to new standards for professional conduct, state action, and social interaction. If one takes as the criteria for class formation "the modes in which 'economic' relationships become translated into 'non-economic' social structures" and "class awareness," or more specifically the binding together of a social group through "embrace of a common ideology," then these decades mark the moment during which the American middle classes were born.[5]

Koch's work captured the power and the appeal of the experimental method, both its practical import and its economic value. "In the future struggle against this dreadful plague of the human race," he boldly predicted, "one will no longer have to contend with an indefinite something, but with an actual parasite."[6] When physicians and physician historians later looked back on Koch's contributions, they portrayed them as watersheds in the history of medicine.[7] In hindsight, Koch's work seemed to demarcate a new era in disease control that offered a medical generation the opportunity to alter its professional status and redefine itself as "scientific."[8] In this sense, his identification of the tubercle bacillus contributed a coherent, unifying ideology that allowed for professional consciousness, status, and economic security. Koch was not the first to suggest that consumption might be contagious, but as George Rosen suggests, no one else had offered the means to prevent the spread of infection rationally through attacks on specific microbes and had done so "unswervingly without being sidetracked by considerations of social policy."[9] Within a decade, Koch had made good on his promise by introducing tuberculin, his "consumption cure." Koch's identification of the tubercle bacillus consequently became a symbolic event to which physicians looked for inspiration in their campaigns against infectious diseases.

Yet though physicians came to construct their professional identity around fond memories of student days, during which they had first learned the value of clinical and experimental sciences, their ambivalence toward scientific medicine, as exemplified in the reactions to Koch, was equally central. In the years that immediately followed 1882 American physicians did not embrace Koch's findings as quickly and unequivocally as memory would suggest. "It is curious," Edward Livingston Trudeau later reflected, "how slow physicians were in this country to accept Koch's discovery or realize its practical value in the detection of the disease."[10] When they became more familiar with his ideas, a significant proportion of the profession continued to resist the implications of Koch's work, and even those whom history has recognized as his early champions—Austin Flint, Hermann Biggs, and William Henry Welch—neither adopted Koch's conclusions immediately nor dispensed with the hereditarian and environmental arguments altogether.[11] Most recent history has ignored this ambivalence, emphasizing instead the linear ways in which bacteriology and the new experimental sciences consolidated the professional status of medicine.

However, the nonlinear processes by which American physicians debated Koch's findings, incorporated them into medical work, and constructed them as historic events also merit attention, and they illuminate the ways in which control of tuberculosis became one of the sites around which the American middle classes formed. Professionalism, based on expert knowledge and with practical and saleable applications, is usually seen as the promise and project of the new middle class, but scientific professionalism also fundamentally eroded the therapeutic impulse to social reform that had served both medical and emerging middle-class interests well. A therapy of social reform had provided mid-century physicians not only with a sense of professional solidarity but also with economic security, for it was this therapeutic that patients sought and most easily accepted. Reciprocally, a therapeutics of social reform enabled physicians, through medical prescriptions, to accomplish the behavioral transformations that defined the middle classes. Koch's bacteriological hypotheses eroded the old therapeutics, but in the decades that immediately followed 1882 it offered physicians little instead. The very different American and Canadian reactions to Koch—physicians' varied efforts to reconcile conflicting agendas, weigh the intellectual and economic significance of scientific theory and practice, redefine tubercular disease, and reframe programs of disease control—expose the complexity of the relationships of science, professional medicine, and middle-class status.

SCIENTIFIC KNOWLEDGE AND MEDICAL ORGANIZATION

Memory and history reshaped the American reception of Koch's work as over the course of two decades in the interest of a unified scientific profession physicians hid their initial skepticism and opposition beneath the veneer of a smooth transition and of scientific progress.[12] Within this celebratory history, any opposition that existed became the obstreperous interference of backward critics. The debates over theory, practice, and organization that circumscribed the early medical reactions to Koch's work, however, provide a more textured topography of the emerging profession and expose its fault lines. Rather than binding the profession together, Koch's bacillus exposed its varied goals and expectations.

On Sunday, May 7, 1882, the *New York Times* openly chastised the American medical profession for not "recogniz[ing] the news item of the highly important results of Professor Koch's discovery of the parasitical source of tubercular disease."[13] News of Koch's work had traveled to the United States indirectly as European reports of his work slowly made their way into the popular press.[14] During the spring and summer of 1882, major medical journals offered little comment and provided their readers with only brief, editorial commentaries culled from European journals.[15] This American reticence contrasted strikingly with European, and more significantly Canadian, reactions to Koch's work. Where Canadians quickly noted the import of Koch's discovery, Americans stood back. In its "Quarterly Report on the Progress of Medical Science" (June 1882), the *Canada Lancet* prominently recorded Koch's experiments; the *American Journal of the Medical Sciences* in its "Quarterly Summary of the Improvements and Discoveries of Medical Science" (1882–1883) did not. By July 1882, the *Canadian Medical and Surgical Journal* had published a complete translation of Koch's address,[16] but the first American translation appeared only in May 1883.[17] When the Canadian Medical Association held its annual meeting in the late summer of 1882, its Committee on the Practice of Medicine hailed Koch's experiments and the International Congress at London as "the two most remarkable events of the past year."[18] Six weeks earlier, the American Medical Association (AMA) met without formally recognizing Koch. If participants at meetings of various state medical associations debated Koch's work, those who summarized the transactions of those meetings for the *American Journal of the Medical Sciences* did not consider the discussions newsworthy. Koch did receive attention in public health circles. At the 1882 meeting of the American Public Health Association (APHA), abuzz with news of Theobald Smith's bacteriological studies and new methods of vaccination, President R. C. Kedzie delivered an address on bacteria and sanitary science. Yet though Kedzie acknowledged that "the discovery of the bacillus which is the cause of consumption by Dr. Koch of Berlin, marks an epoch in the history of medicine,"[19] his membership showed little interest in or enthusiasm for Koch.

Americans paid Koch greater attention during the year that followed, but it was by no means consistently favorable and continued to differ from that paid by Canadians in both degree and kind. Where leaders of Canadian medicine easily and publicly accepted Koch's bacillus as the specific cause of tuberculosis and quickly began to formulate programs of disease control predicated on the eradication of this bacterium, Americans felt compelled to rediscover Koch's principles for themselves. Between 1882 and 1884, when Koch published an expanded account of his investigations, the etiology of tuberculosis became a testing ground for professional standards. Much of the debate turned on intricate scientific details, but American and Canadian physicians used these details to frame distinctive relationships to European science and new standards for medical practice.

From the outset, the debate over Koch entailed questions of the applicability of experimental science to medicine. Here, the experiences of Peter Bryce, who became the first secretary of the Ontario Provincial Board of Health, and T. Mitchell Prudden, consulting pathologist to the New York City Department of Health, exemplified the range of response. Bryce and Prudden had strikingly similar careers. Bryce took his B.A. and M.A. in natural science at University College, received an M.B. from Toronto in 1880, left Canada to study in Edinburgh and Paris, then returned to Ontario in 1882 to assume charge of the province's newly founded Board of Health. Prudden also took his early degrees at home. He received his B.S. from the Sheffield Scientific School and his M.D. from Yale, then traveled to Berlin and Heidelberg to supplement his scientific education. Upon his return home, he became director of the New York City Pathological Laboratory and joined the staff of Columbia University's College of Physicians and Surgeons, where he introduced courses in bacteriology.

Despite these parallels, Bryce and Prudden responded quite differently to Koch. The British medical establishment had accepted Koch's findings with dispatch, and Bryce, the weight of the Empire behind him, willingly and immediately accepted this metropolitan knowledge at face value and applied the basic premises established in England and Europe. Indeed, by October 1882, Bryce had easily and publicly accepted Koch's bacillus as the specific cause of tuberculosis, and he had begun to formulate and implement programs of disease control predicated on the eradication of the tubercle bacillus.[20] This reaction contributed to the development of a public health apparatus that served increasingly as a testing site for foreign biomedical theories and technologies.[21]

The close ties to Britain that fledgling Canadian medicine enjoyed seemed to offer English-Canadian doctors a confidence in appropriating foreign medical ideas that their American counterparts lacked. Where Bryce had been willing to adopt Koch's bacillus on the authority of English studies and to apply this knowledge in novel ways, Prudden could not unquestioningly apply European knowledge to the solution of practical American problems. Instead, Prudden felt compelled to rediscover

Koch's principles for himself. As Americans attempted to carve out a new national style, they found the appeal of science as much in the method of inquiry as in the substance itself,[22] and Prudden typically found Koch's premises and methods as intriguing as the findings. He quickly traveled to Berlin to observe Koch's research firsthand, then returned to New York determined to repeat the investigations for himself. This was not a simple exercise in emulation. Prudden followed Koch's methodological instructions to the letter, rigorously tested Koch's premises, and judged his own work more stringently than his mentor's.

The problem was that neither Prudden nor George Sternberg—the renowned bacteriologist who later became surgeon general of the Army— nor the eminent Philadelphia physicians H. F. Formad, Horatio Wood, and James Wilson could replicate Koch's results. Instead, they found that "tubercular lesions can exist without the presence of tubercle bacilli in them."[23] Such observations increasingly divided experimentalists from clinicians and exacerbated the opposition to academic physicians who hoped to secure the authority of medicine on experimental or scientific grounds.[24] Prudden, with ardor befitting a novice experimentalist, clung to high expectations of scientific theory, which Koch dashed. Others focused less on technique than credentials; Koch, another critic colorfully objected, might claim to be a "botanist, a mycologist, or an experimentalist but he was neither clinician nor pathologist."[25]

The very basis of Koch's investigations proved most divisive. Best remembered for his elucidation of the etiology of tuberculosis, Koch had only secondary interest in the control of disease. His primary concern was with questions about the order and origins of life, and his bacteriological research developed out of an earlier fascination with natural history.[26] A student of Jakob Henle, Georg Meissner and Friedrich Wohler, Koch studied bacteria in order to determine the nature of and limits to biological species and to resolve debates over spontaneous generation and pleomorphism. Koch's earliest investigations, into the etiologies of anthrax and wound infections, represented an effort to resolve these questions. Koch was fascinated with such questions as whether microbes were the causes or concomitants of fermentive disease processes, whether they invaded from without or were generated spontaneously as the tissues putrefied, whether they existed in definite species, each corresponding to a distinct disease, or in numerous plastic and interchangeable forms—harmless bacteria becoming pathogenic in the course of disease.[27] From his perspective, the major contribution of his pure culture technique was that it made it possible to prove that diseased tissue did not either generate microbes spontaneously or transform them from a virulent to an avirulent state.

Close study of the organism's life cycle, of the conditions under which it developed, and of the role of the spore demonstrated that the characteristics of bacilli remained virtually constant over extended periods of time and under varied conditions.[28] Even though bacterial species lacked the distinct morphological markers used to classify larger organisms, Koch believed that he could delimit them on the basis of their pathogenic characteristics. Koch consequently proposed that each type of bacterium possessed the power to generate one specific disease.[29] Thus Koch was interested primarily in diseases as benchmarks for the differentiation of bacterial types, and his studies of tubercle bacilli bore the mark of his preoccupations with pleomorphism and spontaneous generation. His insistence that bacteria formed fixed, specific, universal types and that bovine and human bacilli were identical was part of a larger effort to demonstrate that diseased tissues neither generated tubercle bacilli nor transformed them from harmless to pathogenic forms.

The bounds between clinical and experimental knowledge again became an issue as Prudden and other Americans debated the relevance of Koch's inquiry, however valid from experimentalist or natural historical perspectives, to medical practice. In Toronto, Bryce had recognized Koch's interest in the origins and nature of species but paid it little attention. He adroitly summarized the arguments on both sides, and he as easily moved away from them to practical matters of disease control.[30] "Having examined some of the principal objections raised against the *Bacterium* theory" and having expressed his belief "that the great bulk of proof at present is in its favour," he emphasized the importance of "the *methods which both science and experience* teach ought to be taken towards the end of preventing these diseases."[31]

South of the border, despite Koch's best efforts, well-worn debates over the origins of microbes and their pathogenic characteristics persisted.[32] Formad, pathologist at the University of Pennsylvania, voiced the concerns most clearly. Russian-born and German-trained, Formad was an ardent student and great advocate of bacteriology and pathology. Having spent many years searching for the bacillus of diphtheria, he was open, in principle, to Koch's approach. Yet Formad became Koch's most vociferous American opponent. He accused Koch of having been so bound and "biased by the determination to find for each disease a specific fungus" that he had ignored the numerous instances in which no bacilli could be found in the sputum or tissues of consumptives.[33] Formad also feared that Koch's desire to distinguish species by the diseases they caused led to an unnecessarily narrow definition of disease and the erroneous conclusion that all diseases in which tubercle bacilli could be found were identical. Because Koch believed that the production of one specific disease was the characteristic ability of each species of pathogen, he also presumed the converse to be true—that every form of tubercular disease had as its cause the same species of tubercle bacillus.[34] But neither clinical nor pathological evidence convinced Formad that the many forms of tubercular disease—phthisis, scrofula, miliary and bovine tuberculosis among them—were one and the same.[35] Invoking the pathologist's prerogative, Formad ascribed the peculiarities of tubercular disease to variations in tissue reaction and openly defied Koch with the claim that "[t]here is a poison in tuberculosis, but it is generated by the body itself."[36]

Other eminent American physicians shared Formad's concerns. At the annual meeting of the AMA in June 1883, the chairman of the Section on Surgery and Anatomy cautioned colleagues against the "alleged tubercular relations" of Koch's bacillus. "That these peculiar micro-germs exist there can be no longer any doubt," he admitted, "but whether they are the cause of tubercle or whether the tubercle develops them, the profession has not made sufficient progress yet to justify an unequivocal statement."[37] Similarly, the chair of the Section on Practice of Medicine, John Hollister, reminded his colleagues: "One very important question arises in this connection, in fact a pivotal one upon which all others must turn. The presence of specific organisms in many forms of disease even the most skeptical must concede; but the main question is this, are they causative, or only concomitants? It certainly will not be conclusive to simply assert the presence of characteristic bacilli in the parts diseased, for in such the soil may be nourishing to one and sterilized for others, affording as many pretty examples of the survival of the fittest."[38] Ezra Hunt expressed the same sentiments in his presidential address to the APHA (1883). Like his colleagues at the AMA, Hunt willingly conceded that microbes existed, but he would not yet accept that they always entered the body from without.[39]

Thus, Koch's findings might represent "a triumph for scientific botany and mycology," but they seemed "far too one-sided to have an application to scientific medicine," and they had still less relevance to clinical practice.[40] Caught in the crossfire between experimentalists and clinicians, Prudden carefully underscored the differences between Koch's "positive, experimental studies" and the far more complex phenomena of human disease.

SEED AND SOIL: MICROBE AND PREDISPOSITION

As discussion of Koch's work continued, distinctions between experimental and clinical relevance became critical, and debate focused on the origin and significance of tubercular disease. Rooted in experimental method and definitions of causation, Koch's bacteriological revolution was essentially an intellectual revolution. Those like Prudden who could not reconcile actual experience with laboratory evidence consequently questioned the wisdom of basing clinical practice on remote experiment. Some of the concerns were again symbolic microcosms of larger debates about the origins of life and the distinctiveness of human experience. For example, Koch's seemingly incautious extrapolation from animal to human experience troubled Prudden, who could not accept the unity of human and nonhuman reactions. "Dr. Koch's experiments have not been done on man, but on the lower animals," he cautioned; "proof that the human organism reacts toward the bacilli in the same manner as that of other species has not been furnished."[41] Concerns about the uniqueness of human experience aside, however, Prudden could not easily reduce pulmonary phthisis to a simple bacterial infection. "In the prevailing furor," he cautioned, "it is important to remember that even if all that is claimed for the new bacillus should be proven true, still the morphological basis upon which the present knowledge of tuberculosis rests has not been in the least disturbed, and that even the proof that this bacterium causes all the lesions of tuberculosis does not explain either the peculiar reaction of the living organism against the parasite or the varied phenomena of the distribution of the tubercle, heredity, variations in mode of attack, etc."[42] Much as Koch might wish to define diseases by the bacteria that caused them, American physicians could not accept that tubercle bacilli were the sole cause of tuberculosis.

When Henry Ingersoll Bowditch declared that neither clinical nor experimental support for contagionism existed, he spoke with the authority of his profession. Before the 1880s few American physicians accepted either contagionism or germs as sources of the true epidemics—cholera, yellow fever, smallpox—let alone consumption.[43] Thereafter, even such ardent proponents of contagionism as Dr. W. H. Webb of Philadelphia rarely accepted a germ as the sole agent of disease, denied that other causes such as heredity and environment, played a contributing role, or dismissed the importance of the diathesis.[44]

And what was really at stake here was the diathesis, the explanatory model that had bound together physiological and social causes of disease and served as a focus for mid-century campaigns against tuberculosis. After Koch, experiment and experience continued to indicate that consumption was a diathetic disease.[45] TB continued to preferentially affect those who lived in cities, and both statistical and clinical study confirmed that occupation, gender, and race affected its distribution. Faced with the wealth of evidence for differential susceptibility, it was easy for physicians to maintain that "phthisis is not a specific infectious disease, but the individuals suffering from tubercular disease are themselves original, and form a special species of mankind."[46] It was equally easy to attribute the disease, despite the presence of germs, to "misery of life, loss of sleep, malnutrition and seclusion."[47] A diathesis, located in the anatomy of the connective tissue, seemed the real cause of tuberculosis, and it was this diathesis, they argued, that should command their attention. "In the prominence given to the doctrine of the mycotic specificity of disease," Hunt warned, "there is much danger that associated influences will be overlooked."[48]

To make his point that microbes would not grow outside of a suitable host, Hunt invoked a metaphor of seed and soil. "It cannot be said of any disease proven to be dependent upon or associated with a specific infective particle," he maintained, "that its presence or virulence is independent of person or surroundings. Even where the seed is not indigenous and the sower who goes forth to sow is unseen, yet if it falls by the beaten wayside, or where there is no depth of earth, in the unfriendly soil of a pure life or pure dwelling place it perishes as an invading army perishes without its commissariat."[49] This metaphor of seed and soil became so pervasive that, in 1884, Koch parried it alongside his opponents' technical criticisms, with an extended study of the etiology of tuberculosis.[50] Koch acknowledged "the material difference in the course taken by the disease in different individuals of the same race," but he denied that a predisposition could account for individual reactions to tubercle bacilli. Instead, he attributed these reactions to opportunities for infection, the number of infective germs to which individuals were exposed, or the more general health of the respiratory system.[51]

Few American physicians found this effort to explain away the diathesis compelling, nor did they easily discount the etiological importance of heredity, occupation, nutrition, and state of mind.[52] After 1884, American physicians more readily accepted Koch's methods and conclusions, but even as they became more convinced of Koch's findings, they continued to debate the meaning of infection and to insist that consumption had a diathetic origin.[53] For example, when the Ohio Medical Society met in June 1884, its members generally endorsed Koch's claim that tuberculosis was an infectious disease caused by the tubercle bacillus, but nonetheless they issued a caveat. "For the occurrence of tuberculosis in any given case, two factors are necessary, the proper soil and the infectious agent. The first, which we call the predisposition, is either hereditary or acquired."[54] This became a typical response in climatological and public health communities as well. "Granting, as it appears we must, that the immediate exciting cause of miliary tubercles is the invasion of the body by these organisms," B. F. Westbrook told the American Climatological Association, "we have still to consider what are the conditions which precede this invasion and render the tissues susceptible to it. The importance of examining carefully into the question of predisposition is evident, in as much as the seed can not ripen and bring forth its harvest of death, unless it falls upon a soil favorable to its development."[55] Similarly, in the paper "The Bearing of the Discovery of the Tubercle Bacillus on Public Hygiene," which he read to the 1884 meeting of the APHA, Ludwig Bremer reminded his audience that "the tuberculous virus is not an universal one like that of small-pox, syphilis, scarlet fever, measles and other infectious diseases; . . . a predisposition, i.e. a congenial soil is necessary for the development and growth of the specific tubercle germ."[56]

Such sentiments prevailed even among Koch's strongest champions. Bremer, for example, had trained in Germany before settling in St. Louis, and he was Koch's devoted supporter. He admitted without hesitation "that I am a firm believer in the doctrines of Koch, and that I subscribe from my own observations to everything he has said and written about tubercle bacillus."[57] Flint, who with Biggs and Welch is remembered as Koch's first and greatest American advocate,[58] also continued to maintain that a constitutional predisposition was a necessary cause of tuberculosis. In January 1884, Flint read a paper, "On the Pathological and Practical Relations of the Doctrine of the Bacillus Tuberculosis," to the New York County Medical Association; in it he encouraged his colleagues to accept the etiological role of tubercle bacilli and to adopt the view that TB was a contagious disease. Koch's experiments, he argued, left little doubt that the microorganism was the true and necessary cause of tuberculosis. Yet in virtually the same breath Flint added: "Pulmonary phthisis is eminently a diathetic disease." The microbe and the predisposition, he suggested, interacted "like the blades of a pair of scissors; . . . their efficacy depends on their being joined together; separated, each is powerless."[59] Flint asked, how else could one explain the fact that the vast majority of the American population was exposed to the exciting causes of consumption yet only a portion succumbed to the disease? How otherwise could one understand the predominance of disease among particular families, in certain climates, in the cities, or among those who lived in poorly ventilated houses, ate poorly, or suffered from mental depression?[60]

The advent of sputum tests, which demonstrated precisely how deep and apparently intractable the problem of tubercular infection really was, fueled this debate. Late-nineteenth-century American physicians had harbored no illusions about the magnitude of the tuberculosis problem, which records and experience alike confirmed was widespread. Nonetheless, they were unprepared for the revelations of early sputum tests. Koch had introduced these tests, based on new staining methods, in his 1884 paper and promised that they would enable physicians to identify the sick more quickly and accurately than before. The few American physicians who actually adopted this technique in the years after its earliest introduction, like Trudeau, hoped it would replace a nosology based on symptoms and signs with one predicated on the presence or absence of bacilli. New stains did make it easier to identify tubercle bacilli, and they lent themselves easily to diagnostic uses. But contrary to the hopes of the physicians who adopted them, the new stains did not immediately simplify diagnosis. Rather than narrowing the tuberculosis problem, sputum testing revealed vast, unsuspected reservoirs of infection. More important, sputum testing failed to establish a simple correlation between infection and disease; instead it highlighted the complexities and ambiguities of the disease process.

Thereafter, experimental, clinical, and epidemiological studies seemed repeatedly to confirm what early critics of Koch had anticipated—that exposure to tubercle bacilli did not necessarily result in tuberculosis. In 1884, Sternberg complicated interpretations of microbial action by demonstrating that numerous bacteria, which were neither virulent nor pathogenic, lived normally within the human body.[61] With time, it also became apparent that only a small fraction of those who tested positive for tubercle bacilli showed any signs or symptoms of tuberculosis, and an indeterminately small number of these later developed active disease.[62]

The absence of a simple link between infection and disease forced physicians to reevaluate more fundamentally the relative importance of seed and soil. These efforts became so messy that in 1886 Trudeau attempted to resolve the question experimentally. Trudeau constructed a simple exercise to test systematically the influence of seed and soil. He took fifteen healthy rabbits and divided them into three groups of five. He injected the first group with live tubercle bacilli, confined it to a small, dark cellar, and deprived it of adequate light, fresh air, and food. Trudeau placed the second group in an equally unwholesome environment; however, he did not infect it with tubercle bacilli. The third group, like the first, received injections of virulent tubercle bacilli, but Trudeau allowed these animals to roam freely and provided abundant quantities of food, sunlight, and fresh air. Three months later, when Trudeau evaluated the health of the animals, he discovered that all of the first group had developed tuberculosis and four had died. In contrast, only one of the rabbits inoculated with tubercle bacilli but allowed to roam free had contracted TB. The animals of the second group, which Trudeau had confined to poor quarters but had not infected with tubercle bacilli, all showed general signs of poor health; none, however, had developed tuberculosis.[63]

If Trudeau's work verified the essential role that tubercle bacilli played in the development of tuberculosis, it demonstrated as compellingly that the microbes on their own did little harm. That infected animals did not necessarily become tuberculous and that under the right conditions the host appeared able to resist even the most virulent of tubercle bacilli now seemed indisputable. Nonetheless, two years later, Trudeau cautiously repeated his original work. This time, the critical role of the environment emerged more clearly still, and Trudeau concluded that various studies "furnish proof that the tissues themselves can, under certain conditions, either limit the destructive action of this microbe or even entirely rid themselves of its presence."[64] This observation lent credence to what clinicians had long maintained: the physiological state of the consumptive reflected deeper social and economic decay. Crowding, hunger, dampness, and darkness weakened the host and rendered it susceptible to tubercle bacilli. The "endless rush to the cities," "centralization," and the blind love of the "average proletarian . . . for the chorus of citylife" helped to create susceptibility to TB; so, too, did powerlessness, economic insecurity, dependence, and lack of autonomy.[65]

THE CONTROL OF TUBERCULOSIS

At the 1884 AMA meeting, members reflected back on the time that had elapsed since Koch first announced his identification of the tubercle bacillus and noted that only two of those present at the meeting had actually studied Koch's bacillus in any detail.[66] Following Koch's announcement, most American physicians had not immediately come "bounding up the stairs . . . waving a newspaper . . . and crying, 'I knew it, I knew it!'"[67] Rather, they judiciously appraised Koch's conclusions. As they weighed the offerings of Koch's bacteriological revolution, many found that its intellectual content—the debates it engendered over experimental method, bacterial species, and theories of causation—engaged a medical elite, to whom it offered a privileged status based on a collective allegiance to science. However, the symbolic lure of scientific professionalism conflicted directly with the average physician's need to eke out a living. The practical implications of Koch's bacillus touched these physicians most directly and presented two interrelated but nonetheless contradictory challenges, which were most evident in their efforts to control tuberculosis: acceptance of Koch's bacillus and the methodology on which it was based might be the card to professional membership, but it eroded the therapeutic base that served at once to define medical identity, ensure economic livelihood, and shape social relations.

Koch himself understood the challenge. From Koch's perspective, the power and beauty of his work was that it disentangled the goals of social reform from the biological control of disease. Having identified microbes as the cause of TB, he logically concluded that a way would be found to control tuberculosis by isolating and eliminating tubercle bacilli. Convinced that the microbes were of one fixed kind and lived only inside the host and that they could be transmitted through only limited means, he confidently predicted that measures that destroyed the sources of infection—sputum in particular—would eradicate tuberculosis. Yet it was precisely the disassociation of the physiological from the social and the new plan of attack that it prescribed that Koch's American colleagues found so problematical. Just as a range of American physicians hesitated to adopt a simple microbial etiology, so they mistrusted preventative and therapeutic measures that focused narrowly on bacteria while ignoring the soil in which they grew. "We can but repeat the warning against the anti-parasitic treatment of phthisis," the editors of the *Philadelphia Medical Times* warned in 1884, "the adoption of which was due to a hasty and ill considered application of the new theory of the etiology of consumption."[68]

Some of the misgivings about microbe hunting were pragmatic. Laboratory studies did not necessarily translate into practical applications, as Koch himself well knew. "Up to the present time," he noted, "hygiene has been able to gain but little advantage from recent strides in our knowledge of the pathogenic organisms,"[69] and he hoped that his work would be different. It was not. Laments about the limited utility of Koch's bacterial hypothesis soon became common. "As interesting and valuable as the discovery of Koch is from a biological stand-point," Formad had objected, "its practical value is decidedly overestimated."[70] Physicians in the major medical centers readily concurred. "Has the treatment of tuberculosis been affected much by the discovery of the tubercle bacillus?" asked Eric Sattler, a member of the Cincinnati Medical Society who was a great student and translator of bacteriological classics; "the answer must be decidedly no!"[71]

Despite varied efforts to control it, Koch's bacillus proved intractable. Numerous disinfectants, including sunlight, effectively checked its growth in vitro but not in vivo. Whether inhaled, ingested, injected, or applied in suppository form, none destroyed the bacillus without also harming the host.[72] Nor did Koch's bacillus lend itself easily to immunological research. After 1882, efforts to develop an attenuated vaccine based on modified live organisms or to develop an antitoxic vaccine similarly failed.[73]

Even Koch's staunchest advocates, Bremer and Flint among them, conceded that Koch's model of microbial infection offered little of real or practical value to therapeutic or preventive campaigns against tuberculosis.[74] Prevention, Bremer regretted, "is not likely to be benefited to any great extent by the knowledge we have gained in the etiology of phthisis" and "meets under present circumstances with almost insurmountable difficulties."[75] Registration, isolation, and disinfection presented the best means for limiting the spread of the tubercle bacillus. However, mounting evidence about the extent of tuberculous infection furnished new arguments against the feasibility of such measures. "Even with the most severe laws and regulations the bacillus will not be destroyed for a long time to come," one physician charged; "there will be only too many chances to contract tuberculosis through the carelessness of consumptives or the unscrupulousness of meatdealers, farmers or dairymen, or through the bacilli that even with the best intentions on the part of everybody are likely to escape detection."[76] With time, skepticism deepened, so that even advocates of registration came to doubt whether tuberculosis could be controlled by identifying and isolating consumptives or disinfecting their sputum.[77]

Yet the challenge went further. While some physicians debated the feasibility, efficacy, and ethics of measures to limit the spread of tubercle bacilli, others continued to question the desirability of, indeed the need for, concentrating on the bacilli. Koch's bacillus cut to the core of doctrinal debates between what Trudeau termed "older clinical" views—which identified "unhygienic surroundings, malnutrition, struma, defect of anatomical structure, and heredity" as the main causes of tubercular disease— and "experimental research which favored the role of tubercle bacilli."[78] Though late-nineteenth-century American medicine is typified by a process of transformation from individualism and specificity to universalism, this transformation occurred slowly in the case of tuberculosis. Belief that gender, occupation, race, and habitat contributed to the onset of the disease persisted, as did faith in personalized regimens of wholesome outdoor living.[79] Koch's assertion that one microbe produced one disease and one germicide one cure undermined this individualism and raised in its stead a therapeutic universalism.[80] His opponents were not about to accept this conclusion silently. Identifying the predisposition as the embodiment of personal differences, they rallied to preserve it. "We must tremble," cautioned Sattler, "lest in the eager hunt for specifics and preventives we lose sight of that most important factor, the predisposition, the soil upon which the bacilli seem to flourish."[81]

Koch's arguments similarly undercut the links among filth, disease, and deviance that gave shape to American medical and public health traditions. Hence, while some American sanitarians found the germ theory appealing, others opposed it or viewed it with suspicion because it failed to take account of the ways in which civilization bred disease.[82] At the 1883 meeting of the APHA, Hunt warned that hygienists who designed campaigns against the bacterial causes of disease were likely to focus their work too narrowly.[83] Tensions between those who advocated the germ theory and those who remained loyal to older traditions complicated any attempts to do battle against tubercle bacilli. In Ontario, where the founding of the Provincial Board of Health coincided with Koch's first announcement, Bryce could adopt the germ theory and implement anti-microbial measures without having to quell the opposition of an old guard.[84] The same was not true in the United States, however, where tradition and sanitarian sentiment ran strong in established public health communities and where Koch's open and direct challenge to the link that such eminent elder statesmen as Rudolph Virchow had forged between social misery and disease could not be ignored. As Bremer suggested, "The present generation . . . is still too much imbued with the doctrine of cellular pathology, which is in principle opposed to the germ theory of disease" to uncritically accept Koch's model of bacterial infection.[85]

Critics continued to attempt to accommodate Koch's innovations to tradition. "By conceding the bacillus as a factor we are not logically required to address our treatment to this factor alone," one wrote, "but as heretofore, we must use all our means to extinguish the predisposition."[86] Another similarly offered that "tuberculosis it would seem is best prevented by measures which shall increase the vital resistance of the organs and render the tissues of the individual an unsuitable soil for the reception and development of microbes of any description."[87] By the late 1880s, sputum testing reinforced this advice by indicating beyond scientific doubt that neither consumptives nor the bacilli they harbored posed a clear threat. After 1886, even Trudeau, much though he admired Koch, shifted his own attention from the bacillus to the soil. "The best promise of success in the management of tubercular affections," he recommended, "lies not so much in the search for specific germicidal methods of treatment as in a study of all those measures which tend to increase the vital resistance of the individual."[88]

Trudeau's conclusions framed a new paradigm of treatment and prevention, one predicated on building resistance by rendering the soil inhospitable to tubercle bacilli. As hard experience highlighted the difficulties of waging wars on tubercle bacilli and as experimental, clinical, and epidemiological studies continually challenged the premises of such wars by indicating that infection did not necessarily produce disease, a range of physicians returned their attention to measures that would improve and enrich the soil or render it resistant to tubercle bacilli. These efforts, which were undertaken in a variety of forms and locations including boards of health, voluntary agencies, and sanatoria, attempted to reconcile scientific knowledge of the seed with social efforts to till the soil.

Sanatoria came to dominate the turn-of-the century medical campaign against tuberculosis, and they similarly dominated the medical effort to build resistance.[89] Prior to 1885 two sorts of sanatoria had existed in the United States. One catered exclusively to the destitute and the terminally ill;[90] the other, fashioned after German health spas and resorts, attempted to rehabilitate consumptives by removing them to the wilderness and enforcing rigorous regimens of outdoor activity.[91] In 1885, with his personal experiences with tuberculosis behind him, Trudeau opened his "new breed" of institution at Saranac Lake. Trudeau premised his model sanatorium on the notion that institutions could not provide effective treatment for TB by concentrating single-mindedly on the apparently impossible task of preventing the spread of infection. The object of the sanatorium was to build resistance to TB by showing those who were particularly susceptible to the disease how they might avoid illness. To accomplish this goal, the san needed to be more aggressive and creative in producing resistance to the bacillus; it needed to rely less on climate and more on how the patient lived. Thus, behavioral change and regimens of simple living, good food, fresh air, and moderate exercise also became important. The environment experiment conveniently provided Trudeau's novel institutional initiative with compelling scientific backing, and it allowed physicians to accommodate the traditional therapeutic impulse to social reform to changing medical knowledge.

Sanatoria attempted to build resistance in two distinct ways. The first was by a subtle shift in clientele. The new institutions that emerged during the late 1880s and early 1890s—like the Winyah Sanatorium in Asheville, North Carolina; the Sharon Sanatorium in Sharon, Massachusetts; the Loomis Sanatorium in Liberty, New York; and the White Haven Sanatorium in White Haven, Pennsylvania—accepted fewer destitute and dying patients and more early cases, whom they could prevent from developing full-blown disease. The second way they attempted to build resistance was by a different emphasis in treatment. No sanatorium physician denied the causal role played by tubercle bacilli, and instruction about sputum management formed an integral and essential part of the sanatorium routine, but the most basic object of the sanatorium was to create a soil that would resist disease. Hence sanatoria focused their efforts on measures that would countermand the influences that seemed to "pave the way for invasion of the disease germ."[92]

Here again, Trudeau's environment experiment provided the template; good food, fresh air, sunlight, and exercise became the central components of the sanatorium regimen. At Saranac Lake, Winyah, and other sanatoria patients typically slept from 9 P.M. to 7 A.M. During the early stages of their stay, they rested for much of the remainder of the day. Sans also encouraged patients to eat plenty of butter, milk, and meat. The typical diet for a sanatorium patient included "one solid meal of soup, meat, three kinds of vegetable, dessert like rice pudding or fruit and coffee at mid-day; three glasses of milk and two raw eggs for breakfast and supper; two glasses of milk and one raw egg for lunch between breakfast and dinner and for lunch between dinner and supper."[93] As the patient's health improved, cereal, fruit, and bacon (or some other meat) later supplemented breakfast; bread and butter or rice and some meat were added to supper. Situated primarily in rural and agricultural settings, sanatoria could sustain these diets relatively cheaply and simultaneously ensure the interests of farmers. But there were other justifications for diets rich in animal fats. By the late 1880s, physicians had adopted a plastic view of the interchange between heredity and environment that led them to equate the predisposition with what Karl Von Ruck, founder of the Winyah Sanatorium, described as "a departure from the physiological standard of nutritive processes tending toward, or already constituting a pathological state, . . . effecting changes in the fluids and solids of the body, favorable to the growth of pathogenic bacteria."[94] From this vantage, tuberculosis became a nutritional disorder, the onset or cure of which ultimately depended on the nutrition of the host. As Von Ruck put it, "Every remedy must stand or fall as it is useful in furthering the nutrition of the patient."[95] Proper diet thus had obvious physiological advantages. It would promote the formation of the connective tissue and enrich the blood.

The emphasis on nutrition, however, also allowed physicians a broader therapeutic license. Insufficient or inadequate foods were not the only causes of a nutritional deficiency. "Overwork and dissipation," Trudeau argued, also tended to "depreciate the nutrition of the body" and to "render the individual hitherto immune susceptible to the tubercle bacillus."[96] Trudeau consequently combined his dietary advice with prescriptions for fresh air, rest, and moderate exercise, which would improve the metabolism indirectly by stimulating appetite and directly by increasing respiration and oxygen levels. Crowding, dampness, and dark seemed also to compromise the nutritional integrity of the host. Hence, drawing on an ancient and traditional lore that found "health in a sunbeam," sanatoria advocated "heliotherapy" to reverse the damage. Sunlight, they promised, would serve as "a potent ally of therapeutics in restoring convalescents."[97]

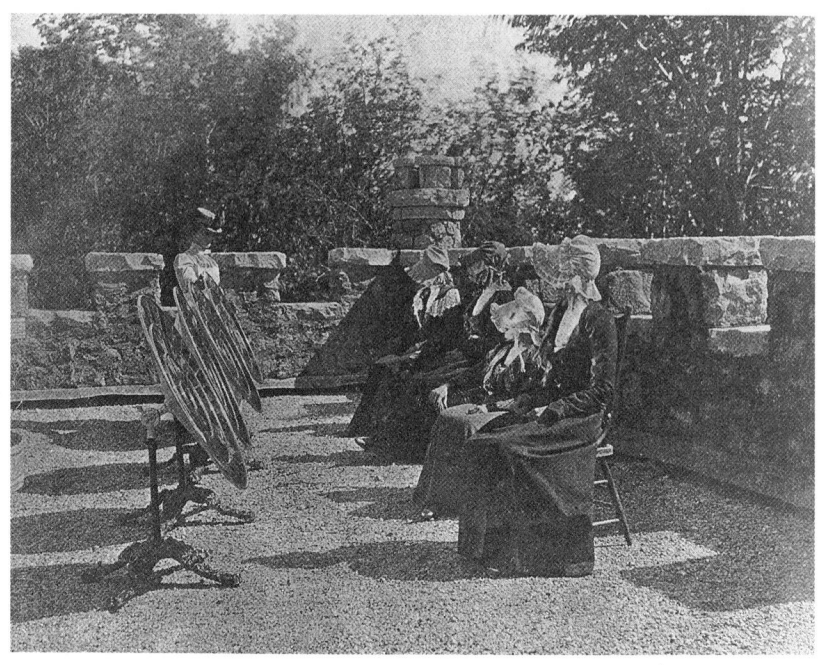

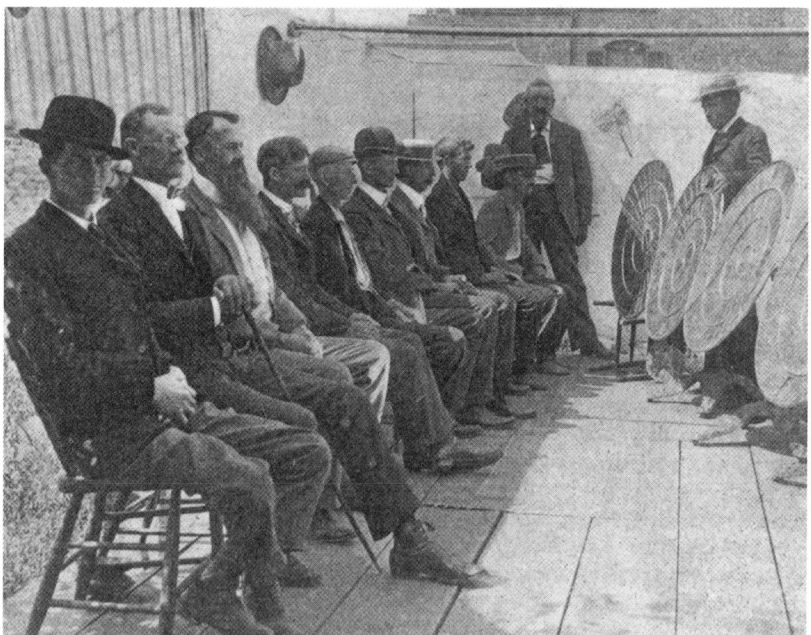

Sun Cures

Source: J. W. Kime, "The Use of Concentrated Actinic Sunlight in the Treatment of Tuberculosis," Medical Record: A Weekly Journal of Medicine and Surgery *62 (November 1, 1902): 682–683.*

With the proper precautions of smoked glass and parasols, sunbaths taken on porches, rooftops, or solaria were tonics for physiques compromised by heredity and city living. Sunlight cleansed the body of bacteria, strengthened tissues, stimulated appetite, promoted healing, increased vitality, and "restored the contagious sparkle . . . [to] the eyes and lives of young patients."[98]

Through these measures sanatorium physicians found a way to combine scientific prescriptions with exhortations to proper living and to justify social interventions on medical grounds or to justify medical interventions on social grounds. For physicians struggling to find a responsible approach to the treatment of TB, Trudeau's new sanatorium consequently provided a pragmatic solution to a problem that was at once scientifically and socially uncomfortable. After all, neither his rabbit experiment nor the therapeutic regimen that he had implemented denied the importance of the bacillus; they merely shifted attention to the conditions that allowed the bacillus to thrive and attempted to create an environment in which tubercle bacilli could do no harm. The secret of Trudeau's success is that his new institutional model undermined the fundamental importance neither of the bacillus nor of the social conditions in which the disease thrived. By following Trudeau's example and addressing social circumstance through the mediating category of a nutritional predisposition, physicians could adopt new scientific strategies against tuberculosis without breaking completely with the past.

THE INTRODUCTION OF TUBERCULIN

Regimens of diet, rest, and heliotherapy alone or in combination did much to restore the physical strength consumptives needed to resist infection, and they allowed physicians to refashion their campaigns against disease. These were, however, nonpharmaceutical products, and in an era during which the industrial manufacture of drugs and biologics came increasingly to define medical prowess, the appeal of such products gradually faded. The coincidence of Koch's identification of the tubercle bacillus with Louis Pasteur's first forays into vaccination presented the opportunity for the development of a biological preparation that would eradicate tuberculosis. In theory the combination of Koch's work with Pasteur's made it possible to render the host permanently immune. However, neither of the two distinct strategies for developing vaccines established by 1890—the "French" method of injecting into a healthy host modified organisms whose virulence had been "attenuated" by passage through serial cultures, or the "German" method, which relied on toxins produced during the microbial life cycle—initially proved successful.[99]

Koch's tuberculin, first described in August 1890, constituted one of the first serious alternatives to traditional programs of disease control. The American reaction to tuberculin reveals the complexity of the effort to build resistance, the conflicting challenges of science and social reform, and the pervasiveness of American physicians' efforts to reconcile these through a campaign that focused on the soil rather than the seed.

Tuberculin took firm hold in the United States—at least in comparison with Canada and Europe. In Europe Koch's lymph (as tuberculin was otherwise known) quickly became known as a false cure and soon lost favor, but tuberculin attracted considerably more American allegiance. Economic, institutional, and intellectual concerns all contributed to its rise and fall, but in the final analysis both the considerable success and the ultimate failure of tuberculin in the United States in the period 1890–1925 stem from the fact that physicians continued to view TB through the lens of seed and soil. Because tuberculin acted to increase the nutrition of the host, it captured an American audience that found it quite consistent with their belief in a tubercular diathesis and with the goals of their more general campaign to render that soil resistant to TB.

American researchers rarely participated in early efforts to develop a biological vaccine against or cure for tuberculosis, in part because institutional constraints prevented them from doing so. French and German investigators conducted their bacterial and immunological studies in special research institutes and state laboratories that had no North American counterpart. The laboratories of local boards of health, which later gained renown for their work on diphtheria antitoxin and other sera, did not come into existence until the 1890s; before 1902, the Hygienic Laboratory of the PHS remained a mere shell.[100] Spurred by graduates who had recently returned from study in Europe, American universities of the 1870s and 1880s had just begun to develop an interest in biomedical research, but the scope of their work was still narrow. Laboratory space and the funds needed to buy equipment were scarce.[101] An American drug industry flourished during the nineteenth century, but it had not yet followed the German lead into research. American manufacturers contentedly produced standard preparations, leaving innovation to foreign chemical companies, which then further constrained American research by retaining control of patents.[102] Hence, American public institutions, universities, and private corporations offered little incentive for or support to bacteriological and immunological research.

Yet institutional barriers did not alone inhibit the American quest for biologics against tuberculosis since those who wished to undertake bacteriological and immunological research, such as Smith and his associate

D. E. Salmon, found the means.[103] But even then, neither Smith, who had a particular interest in tuberculosis, nor Salmon nor many of the other American researchers who studied immunity seriously tried to vaccinate against tuberculosis. The peculiarities of tuberculous disease also acted as deterrents. Tuberculosis seemed to differ from other infections in that it yielded to none of the standard techniques. Trudeau, one of the few Americans who had engaged in the effort to develop a vaccine against TB, soon abandoned his quest because "[n]o immunity seems to have been conferred by a saturation of the system with the chemical substances evolved during their growth in artificial culture media, or by the production of a mild form of the disease."[104]

Tuberculin forced Trudeau to reconsider. Koch introduced tuberculin in "An Address on Bacteriologic Research," which he delivered in August 1890 to the International Medical Congress held in Berlin. In what was again primarily a discussion of new methods for studying microorganisms, Koch closed with a brief, cautious account of a "lymph," extracted from cultures of tubercle bacilli, that appeared to have diagnostic and therapeutic properties. Tentative and fundamentally disinterested in therapeutics, Koch initially said no more than that the "brownish, transparent liquid," of unknown composition, possessed the power of "preventing the growth of tubercle bacilli, not only in a test tube but in the body of an animal."[105] He guardedly and carefully restricted his claims to animals, but the public did not share his reticence. Medical and lay presses clamored for more, and their pressure compelled Koch to publish, less than three months later, a fuller account of his discovery. Koch's "Further Communication," which appeared in the *Deutsche Medizinische Wochenschrift,* again underscored his uncertainty about tuberculin.[106] Nonetheless, it elaborated the preparation's curative properties, injections of which seemed, within months of first administration, to cure tuberculosis and to cause fever, sweats, and other external symptoms of the disease to diminish or even disappear. In contrast, tuberculin had no effect on healthy individuals or on those suffering from nontubercular disease.

The news of Koch's "cure" created a worldwide stir as popular and medical presses alike heralded the end of the great white plague.[107] Only days after the *Deutsche Medizinische Wochenschrift* published Koch's "Further Communication," the *British Medical Journal* printed a full translation of that address.[108] This time Americans also followed suit. Though reports of tuberculin, like those of the tubercle bacillus, reached a fractured and potentially ambivalent American audience, the initial response was uniformly enthusiastic. The *New York Times* ran a front-page article under the headline "Koch's Great Triumph,"[109] and American and Canadian medical journals quickly commented on Koch's cure. The same Americans who had been so leery of Koch's bacillus now seemed to throw caution to the winds. Though they once again rushed to Berlin to observe Koch's work for themselves, this time they returned home to put his lessons into practice. Discussions and appraisals of Koch's lymph flooded American medical journals throughout 1891. The *Index Medicus* assigned tuberculin a special category, which included evaluations of Koch's investigations as well as reports of the numerous attempts made to verify his findings. Nor did American physicians restrict their interest in Koch's cure to academic dialogues held on paper. During 1891, tuberculin seemed to be under study and in use in virtually every state of the Union.[110] Practitioners in New York, Detroit, Cincinnati, Boston, Minneapolis, Birmingham, Nashville, Denver, and many smaller communities much further afield assessed its therapeutic worth.

Koch's cure also attracted the attention of public agencies. In late 1890, impressed with and driven by the public response to tuberculin, the Hygienic Laboratory sent a representative to Berlin to observe Koch's work. Soon thereafter Surgeon General Joseph Kinyoun ordered Dr. H. D. Geddings to begin official experiments.[111] Almost simultaneously, the Veterinary Department of the University of Pennsylvania established its own commission to evaluate the therapeutic, prophylactic, and diagnostic value of Koch's tuberculin in cases of bovine tuberculosis.[112] These independent investigations, taken together, resulted in the establishment of guidelines and standards for the use of Koch's lymph in both human and animal populations.

Once again, Americans found themselves unable to replicate Koch's findings, and once again they showed considerably more interest in method than substance. But this time, instead of abandoning Koch, they held fast to the principles on which tuberculin was based, as American physicians rushed to test tuberculin's limits. Indeed, Koch's original preparation and derivatives based on similar principles soon became the most popular and widely used remedies for tuberculosis in the United States.

This response to tuberculin differed significantly from the response in Germany, Britain, and Canada. Though fully aware of all that Koch's tuberculin might offer to their campaigns against the disease, European and Canadian physicians moved rapidly to temper the initial rush of popular enthusiasm for Koch's work by prescribing a healthy dose of caution. Nationalistic, intellectual, and clinical concerns informed the mounting opposition. Koch's discussions of tuberculin rekindled old rivalries between French and German bacteriological traditions. The address in which Koch announced his discovery of tuberculin had been less a treatise on disease prevention than a disquisition on the aims and methods of bacteriology, and it once again raised the concerns about bacterial species that had informed Koch's original research on the tubercle bacillus. The conclusions that Koch drew about the relationship of bacterial types to matters of infection, allergy, and immunity brought him into direct conflict with Pasteur, who during the 1870s and 1880s led the French school of bacteriological research. Pasteur had far less interest in the isolation and identification of bacteria or the morphological and biological characteristics of these organisms than his German counterparts. He and his students dedicated their energies to practical applications of theories of infection and immunity, and they triumphed in their studies of vaccination, most particularly vaccines based on attenuated or modified microorganisms. The fundamental premises of bacterial transformation on which Pasteur based his work were anathema to Koch. Convinced that bacterial forms remained true to type, he persistently dismissed as misguided efforts to develop preventatives or cures that took the transformation of species as their starting point.[113] "Bacteria, like the higher vegetable organisms," he informed those who heard his address to the International Congress, "form constant species though the limits of these are sometimes difficult to determine." Species of pathogenic bacteria," he further maintained, "have the tendency rather to preserve their properties rather than to change them quickly."[114]

Koch took direct aim at Pasteur's attenuation not only on grounds of species transformation but also because it seemed to him that "any view of immunity which had to deal with purely cellular processes, with a kind of struggle between the invading parasites on the one hand and the devouring phagocytes on the other, is steadily losing ground, and that here also it is most probable that chemical influences play the chief part."[115] This endorsement of research on chemical influences—of research on poisonous albumins, toxalbumins, or chemical by-products of the bacterial life cycle—was an endorsement of the research at which his colleagues in Berlin excelled and which they had found so useful in the control of anthrax, diphtheria, and tetanus.[116] In a show of solidarity with his compatriots, he insisted again and again that his tuberculin did not act directly on tubercle bacilli; rather, it was a bacterial toxin that transformed susceptible and diseased tissues and allowed them to heal, absorb any microbes still present, and resist further infections.[117]

Despite Koch's allegiances, neither the means used to prepare tuberculin nor its mode of action was as consistent with the antitoxic preparations as he would have liked his readers to believe. He had overconfidently and precipitously baptized tuberculin into the German research tradition.

Alongside the French opponents, some of his German colleagues quickly identified gaps and weaknesses in his arguments. Virchow, the elder statesman of German medicine, led the attack. In an address to the Berlin Medical Society on January 7, 1891, Virchow openly shared his doubts about tuberculin and his fears for the safety of patients submitted to Koch's treatment. Concerned that Koch could not clearly identify the precise nature of his liquid, nor with any certainty its locus of action, Virchow also charged that tuberculin therapy contradicted the tenets of his cellular pathology. Here, Virchow's opposition adumbrated the tensions between "scientific cure" and social reform that would shape the debate over tuberculin. Rather than curing tuberculosis, he suggested, tuberculin might actually cause the disease to spread and the patient to grow worse.[118]

As the debate over tuberculin took on practical therapeutic concerns, it extended beyond a French-German rivalry and drew in British opponents. John Syer Bristowe, author of the classic *Treatise on the Theory and Practice of Medicine,* who had gained fame throughout the English-speaking world for his studies of diseases of the chest, quickly allied himself with Virchow and tore into Koch's premises, methods, and conclusions. Now in the twilight of his career, Bristowe offered criticisms so harsh that he asked his audience to excuse his strong language. "It is certain that Virchow's calm, philosophical and business-like account not only gives no support to Koch's theories and holds out no hope of the successful treatment of tuberculosis by Koch's method," he wrote, "but proves beyond question that all the fears of its most skeptical opponents are more than justified."[119] Bristowe's skepticism grew as each communication on tuberculin made him increasingly sure that Koch built on shaky premises with a faulty method. Koch, it must be remembered, had little interest in clinical practice and therapeutics. The purpose of the "Address on Bacteriologic Research" had not been to unveil a newly developed cure for tuberculosis but to bolster arguments about species. His "Address" consequently provided the mere skeleton of an argument, and his "Further Communication," composed in haste to satisfy public appeals for an encore, was equally brief. Koch's vagueness did not help his cause, and it especially irked Bristowe. "I must acknowledge that the skepticism which I had hitherto entertained with respect to the efficacy of the treatment became largely increased," he wrote, "partly because of the important admission herein contained that his remedy had no direct influence on the cause of the disease, partly because his account seemed to me to imply that he had hitherto been working in the dark and was still in search of a working hypothesis."[120] The substantial differences between tuberculosis and the "self-protective" diseases exacerbated Bristowe's doubts. Unlike anthrax, diphtheria, and the other diseases for which antitoxins had seemed useful, tuberculosis was not easily cured. Nor, it seemed, did cure render the victim invulnerable to future attacks. On the contrary, Bristowe wrote, "Every new focus of disease is, as in cancer, the starting point of further infection."[121] Given these considerations, Bristowe strongly doubted that Koch would have much success.

Even those who remained more charitably inclined to Koch, like Sir Joseph Lister, harbored reservations. Lister, recently returned from a trip to Berlin, had observed Koch's work for himself and declared himself impressed with both the diagnostic and the therapeutic powers of tuberculin. Unlike Virchow, he saw no reason to doubt a priori the principles on which Koch based his remedy. He believed, moreover, that the "theoretical argument against the possible efficacy of the treatment [fell] to the ground" and was "completely refuted by experience."[122] Whereas most critics devoted their attention to Koch's claims for the therapeutic properties of his lymph, Lister focused on its preventive properties. "The immunity, gentlemen, seemed at the time a less striking thing than the cure," he argued, "[b]ut the immunity is that which we now long for."[123] Lister's greatest fear was thus that tuberculin neither would nor could produce immunity to TB, but even more he feared that his colleagues' eagerness to cure TB would overshadow any efforts to develop an effective vaccine.

Virchow's concerns about theory, Lister's about the direction of research, and Bristowe's about method all appeared in the Canadian reaction to tuberculin. An editorial in the Montreal-based *Canada Medical Record* questioned the mode of action of Koch's lymph and asked whether its worth warranted the heavy costs of preparation.[124] The Toronto-based *Canada Lancet* dissected Koch's method. Above all, the editors of both publications stressed their fears about the safety and efficacy of Koch's preparation. Though the editors of the *Lancet* expressed interest in the premises that underlay tuberculin and acknowledged that early work by Sir James Grant of Ottawa foreshadowed and supported Koch's claims for the physiological effects of bacterial by-products, they nonetheless cautioned against estimates of tuberculin's success "made rather upon a knowledge of the discoverer of the remedy than upon the results of its use."[125] Writers in Canadian medical journals warned of the experimental and tentative nature of Koch's conclusions. No physician had yet undertaken the careful studies, conducted at the bedside, needed to verify these conclusions, the Berlin correspondent of the *Canada Medical Record* reminded readers.[126] "While we are anxious to see this or any other remedy which has been vouchsafed for by a scientific observer given a fair trial," the *Canada Medical Record* advised, "and while we shall be only too happy to record its brilliant success, we fear it will hardly realize the sanguine expectations of its inventor and his followers."[127] These were not casual concerns, nor were the men who made them merely paying lip service to physicians in England and abroad who doubted Koch's work. The Canadian Medical Association took the various warnings about tuberculin to heart. It issued strict guidelines for research on Koch's lymph, and it advised that experiments with this preparation be confined to major hospitals in Montreal and Toronto.

The first American response to tuberculin was quite different and betrayed few of these concerns about the premises from which Koch had prepared tuberculin, the safety of his lymph, or its use in clinical practice. Though many American physicians had been loyal to Virchow during the earlier debates over the etiological role of tubercle bacilli, they now paid little heed to his diatribe against Koch's cure. Nor, initially, did most physicians credit Lister's apprehensions about the relative merits of cure and prevention, and they virtually ignored Bristowe's warnings about method. Debates over the advantages of attenuated preparations or antitoxins seemed of little consequence. Even Dr. Paul Gibier, director of the New York Pasteur Institute, who understood the "German" context within which Koch worked, held his own allegiances to the "French" tradition, and recognized that tuberculin bore no resemblance to the vaccines prepared by Pasteur, readily endorsed Koch's lymph.[128] Unlike their Canadian counterparts, Americans also seemed initially unconcerned that tuberculin had not been fully tested or might even be dangerous; optimism outweighed caution on both public and professional fronts.[129]

This is not to suggest that tuberculin had no American opponents. As American physicians became more conversant with Koch's tuberculin, they too began to appreciate some of the limitations of his work; yet this opposition was far more disparate, and tuberculin persisted in the United States partly because its opposition was unorganized and had little regulatory authority. By the fall of 1891, the agencies charged with investigating tuberculin—the Hygienic Laboratory of the PHS and the Veterinary Department at the University of Pennsylvania—had developed reservations about the efficacy of Koch's lymph. While two of the twelve cases Geddings treated at the Hygienic Laboratory improved, four worsened. Similarly, researchers at the University of Pennsylvania found that cattle responded to tuberculin in unpredictable and irregular ways. As Geddings and his co-workers at the Hygienic Laboratory cautiously narrowed their estimations of tuberculin,[130] the University of Pennsylvania issued a terse but clear warning about the dangers of Koch's lymph. "In none of the tuberculous animals used in the experiments," they wrote, "could the least curative effects be observed," and, moreover, "injection of the tuberculin causes the rapid distribution of the tubercle bacilli and a generalization of the disease."[131] But as the institutions mandated to test tuberculin grew increasingly aware of tuberculin's limitations, they could do little more than advise American physicians and veterinarians to use Koch's lymph cautiously. Neither institution had the legal authority to restrict or in any way prohibit the use of tuberculin, nor did it necessarily have the professional status to do so. The tuberculin research conducted in institutions might have scientific rigor, but, as had been the case in debates over the tubercle bacillus, the relationship of experimental findings to individual clinical practice remained unclear.

The independent clinicians who conducted their assessments of Koch's lymph alongside the Hygienic Laboratory and the University of Pennsylvania rarely allied themselves with the institutional authorities. Rather, like Joseph Stickler of Orange, New Jersey, they appealed to their more senior and eminent colleagues. Stickler, who had originally endorsed Koch's work and defended tuberculin against its critics,[132] grew skeptical as he became convinced for "fourteen reasons" that tuberculin was a failure. Stickler's fears mounted as he pursued his investigations, and in 1892 he believed he had reason to conclude that Koch's lymph caused some patients to grow worse and others to die.[133] Despite his extensive evidence, Stickler was unsure that his own voice would carry. To rally support, he did not invoke the authority of the governmental or educational laboratories that had organized tuberculosis research. Instead he called on and allied himself with the renowned New York pediatrician Abraham Jacobi. Yet if the opinions of Jacobi and other eminent physicians held considerable professional sway, they had no more regulatory authority than the pronouncements of governmental and educational institutions. Thus, in the United States, the ill-defined regulatory apparatus and loose professional regulatory structures so often thought to inhibit biomedical investigation seemed actually to cultivate research on tuberculin.

Tuberculin consequently retained its popularity in the United States well into the twentieth century and, like the disease it was meant to cure, established foci that were deep-rooted, persistent, and hard to disperse. Well after most physicians had dismissed Koch's original tuberculin as a false cure, staunch American supporters continued to rally in its defense. In this effort, they again took advantage of the distinction between methods and outcomes, which Koch's own work now allowed. Koch invested little intellectual capital in the tuberculin cure itself and on many occasions dismissed therapeutics as uninteresting. In his "Further Communication," he sharply distinguished the product of his research from the theory on which it was based. Whatever might come of tuberculin, Koch remained unfailingly dedicated to the principles on which tuberculin was based and the methods by which it was produced. It was to these methods that American physicians similarly remained loyal. "If [Koch] overshot the therapeutic mark," one observed in 1899, "he pointed to a target of treatment which men have since sighted with greater success. If he did not find a curative agent, he suggested a scientific method of dealing with disease in its use."[134] Hewing to a loose definition of a tuberculin—which came to refer not just to Koch's lymph but to any chemical by-product of cultures of tubercle bacilli that contained bacterial protein—Americans continued to manufacture and use these agents. Several dozen varieties of "tuberculin" were available in the United States in 1910, and by one estimate sixty-five were available in 1927.[135]

The persistence of tuberculin illustrates the conflicting professional impulses that guided American responses to Koch. Tuberculin persisted primarily in sanatoria; in fact, it inspired few more ardent supporters than those at Trudeau's Adirondack Cottage and Von Ruck's Winyah. Though they were primarily rehabilitative or care-providing institutions, by the late 1890s these sanatoria had also established research laboratories dedicated to the investigation of the etiology, treatment, and prevention of TB. These specialized labs produced the clinically oriented knowledge and materials deemed necessary for the care of consumptives. At a time when the relationship of laboratory findings to clinical practice remained unclear and clinicians such as Stickler betrayed a fundamental ambivalence about the intellectual and professional status of experimental findings generated in new, central laboratories, the experiments on tuberculin conducted in sanatoria provided the hands-on testimonials that clinicians demanded. The tuberculin research conducted in institutions like Trudeau's Saranac Laboratory consequently carried considerable professional sway.

Though Trudeau and Von Ruck shared an intense interest in tuberculin, the two physicians were strikingly different. Both held the post of chief physician on the medical staff of a sanatorium, and both established research laboratories ancillary to their sanatoria. However, Trudeau represented the medical establishment, to which he belonged, and Von Ruck the fringe. Yet tuberculin served the institutional, professional, and economic interests of both men, who used it to reconcile the appeal of science with a more nuanced and traditional therapeutic. Hence, their sanatoria continued to produce tuberculins, for therapeutic use, until as late as 1923.

The Appeal of Science: The Von Rucks

Von Ruck was possibly the quirkiest of the American supporters of tuberculin. Born in Germany, he had studied science at the University of Stuttgart and medicine at the University of Tübingen before emigrating to the United States in the early 1870s. After receiving a second M.D. from the University of Michigan (1879), he practiced medicine briefly in Ohio, then returned to Germany in 1882 to study with Koch. Six years later, he returned to Asheville, North Carolina, where with his brother Silvio he established the Winyah Sanatorium. As the climatic theory of disease gained favor during the 1860s and 1870s, Asheville became a haven for consumptives. Located in the Blue Ridge mountains and renowned for its climate, it became home to numerous residences for the sick. Winyah, only one of many cottages, was larger and more formal than most, and it sought the therapeutic edge that Von Ruck hoped tuberculin might provide.

A devoted and almost blind disciple of Koch, Von Ruck initially endorsed Koch's lymph with all the ardor national pride could instill and assumed the role of Koch's bulldog. He frequently defended tuberculin against many forms of attack. It was he who, in 1892, took on Stickler's "fourteen objections" to tuberculin with the greatest force, invoking in his defense both his clinical experience and his conviction that the principles and methods of Koch's cure were both valid and legitimate. A true experimentalist, Von Ruck nonetheless conceded the need for research that would clarify the details of the manufacture and administration of tuberculin.[136] His effort to provide this research became part of an initiative to carve out a therapeutic terrain. Unlike Stickler, Von Ruck did not attempt to rally the medical elite in his support; rather, he invoked the unassailable authority of experiments and institutions.

The Von Ruck Research Laboratory, which he opened in 1895 to produce the sera used to treat Winyah's patients, provided this authority. Between 1895 and 1900, the lab also became a testing ground for tuberculin as the Von Rucks attempted to amass the clinical and experimental evidence needed to demonstrate that their products were effective and safe. Over time, their endorsements of tuberculin grew increasingly broad and impassioned. Linking efforts with those of their students, most notably F. M. Pottenger, who had opened his own sanatorium in Monrovia, California, they established a network that consolidated and institutionalized their expertise.[137] Though they were interested primarily in tuberculin as a cure, after 1907, when the Viennese physician C. Von Pirquet introduced a new, simple, and safe method of tuberculin testing, they widened their campaign to the use of tuberculin in diagnosis. Thereafter they exploited interest in the diagnostic uses of tuberculin to further promote tuberculin's therapeutic properties.[138] Nor did the Von Rucks champion tuberculin for its therapeutic and diagnostic uses alone. Working from a loose definition of tuberculin, the Von Rucks also attempted to produce a modified extract, or tuberculin "vaccine," with preventive properties.[139]

The Von Rucks developed such an impassioned commitment to tuberculin that in 1909 a colleague from Asheville protested formally against what he perceived to be the dangers of a "second tuberculin era."[140] His fears were not unfounded. The apparent therapeutic and preventative properties of tuberculin so convinced the Von Rucks that they even brought their "vaccine" to the attention of the PHS. In October 1911, they wrote to the director of the Hygienic Laboratory with an offer to share their protective vaccine and make public the results of eight years of investigation. The PHS initially declined this appeal for external legitimacy. Though the Biologics Control Act of 1902 expanded the functions of the Hygienic Laboratory to include regulation of the production and distribution of biological products, the lab remained relatively small and unstructured. It had neither the staff nor the facilities required to follow up on the hundreds of alleged cures and preventives for tuberculosis brought to its attention, and the cost of determining the safety and efficacy of these sera was prohibitive.[141] The Von Rucks initially received a classic response: "it would be of the greatest interest to take up investigations of this character, but the labor involved necessarily limited the number that could be taken up at any one time."[142]

Not dissuaded, the Von Rucks rapidly brought popular opinion to bear. In 1903, F. Friedmann, a German physician, had introduced a vaccine against tuberculosis derived from an attenuated form of turtle tubercle bacillus. In 1910 he attempted to market this vaccine to Americans. Pursuant to the provisions of the Biologics Control Act, which governed both foreign and interstate trade in biologics, the Hygienic Laboratory had undertaken an investigation of the "Friedmann Vaccine." The Von Rucks objected and demanded to know why their own preparation was ignored. Playing cleverly on emerging nationalist sentiment, they chastised the PHS for spending time and energy on a foreign preparation while neglecting the home-grown American product. They also publicized both their case and their cure by airing their dispute with the PHS in numerous medical journals, in which they simultaneously published their findings.[143]

This pressure led in May 1913 to enactment of a Senate resolution calling for an investigation into the Von Rucks' tuberculin funded under the Sundry Civil Act. The PHS subsequently sent Surgeon A. M. Stimson to Asheville to test the Von Rucks' claims. These claims rested on both clinical and experimental trials, which allegedly proved the Von Ruck vaccine safe and effective for both animals and humans. Because he recognized that the clinical evidence would be difficult to repeat and evaluate—confounded as it was by lack of controls and by natural variations in TB—Stimson at first confined his mission to re-creation of the animal experiments, which he hoped would confirm that the Von Ruck vaccine caused the production of antibodies to the tubercle bacillus and rendered the vaccinated animals immune to a challenge dose. However, when he arrived at Winyah in June 1913, he found the laboratory conditions so horrifying that he quickly redeployed his investigation to the Hygienic Laboratory.

A heated debate between the Von Rucks and the PHS ensued, at the heart of which was the centrality of clinical and experimental authority. In a formal protest against Stimson's actions, the Von Rucks insisted that the PHS ought only to observe the investigations being conducted at Winyah. Stimson again protested the "slovenliness" of the Von Rucks' procedure, cited the independent re-creation of the Von Ruck experiments as part of his mandate, and maintained that if the Von Ruck experiments were truly scientific, a skilled investigator, working anywhere, ought to be able to repeat them.[144]

During the months that followed, Stimson challenged not only the Von Rucks' methods and facilities but also their conclusions. Stimson's careful experiments failed to replicate the Von Rucks' findings, and the guinea pigs that the staff of the Hygienic Laboratory injected with the Von Ruck serum neither developed antibodies nor resisted a challenge dose of tubercle bacilli. Without attempting to repeat the Von Rucks' clinical trials, which he recognized as "a task which under practical conditions amounts to an impossibility," Stimson questioned the design of the studies. The Von Rucks, he charged, had not controlled their experiments. They had chosen too small a sample and too short a period of investigation. They had not adequately considered the influence of differing opportunities for infection or of the "presence of factors which might influence resistance to infection." Stimson therefore deemed the Von Ruck vaccine—a tuberculin—a failure, and he proceeded to tar all tuberculins with the Von Ruck brush. "[Tuberculin], like the Von Ruck Vaccine prepared from the tubercle bacillus has been before the medical profession for something like 30 years," he wrote in the summary of his investigations, "and the opportunity of experimenting with it has been most widely indulged, and yet the indications for its use, the method of its application, and the ultimate results to be expected from it are still the subjects of controversy, and the final verdict has not been rendered save in one particular; it is generally admitted that tuberculin, except when skillfully administered, is a dangerous thing; that its injudicious use might result in catastrophe."[145] The PHS took a leaf from the Von Rucks' book and aired Stimson's findings publicly.[146]

The Von Rucks responded to the Hygienic Laboratory's rebuke by assuming the role of unappreciated scientists. Having failed to publicize their findings through the agency of the Hygienic Laboratory, in 1916 they published an extensive treatise on their "new vaccine" in which they accused their countrymen of "far-reaching therapeutic nihilism." The Von Rucks harshly criticized the conservatism and complacency of those who did not embrace the cause of science. They accused their American colleagues of failing to appreciate the power that the new sciences of bacteriology and immunology had imparted to campaigns against disease and of unfairly and unwisely resisting efforts to incorporate these sciences into programs of TB control.[147] Thus, the Von Rucks marketed tuberculin in the garb of "science," and they additionally clung to it because they believed it to be scientific. In the wake of Flexnerian reform, which restructured North American medical education to promote the authority of laboratory science, these were thinly veiled ploys for professional legitimacy.

The Von Rucks could not, however, so easily wield science to professional ends, in part because the intellectual authority of science was not the sole issue. Professional and economic concerns were also important. By the turn of the twentieth century, sanatoria had begun to lose their status as the preeminent institutions for care of consumptives. Two related developments challenged the sanatorium's status. First, by the late 1890s tuberculosis seemed indisputably an urban problem that prevailed in slums among immigrants, mill girls, and blacks. Consumption, noted S. Adolphus Knopf, an attending physician at the Riverside Hospital Sanatorium in New York City, "is most frequent among the poor, the badly housed, the underfed, the intemperate, and individuals debilitated by other excesses, disease or certain occupations." Rates in New York City, he noted, far exceeded those outside, and within the city itself mortality in the "poorest quarters" was almost double that in the more affluent. Second, some physicians came to question the adequacy of sanatorium care. Knopf, in fact, had grown particularly concerned about the urban consumptive poor, who neither could nor would be institutionalized and who seemed to him to represent vast reservoirs of infection. He appreciated that unless the needs of this sizeable population were addressed, tuberculosis could not be eradicated. Hence, he asked his colleagues to consider the prospect of treating consumptives in their homes as a strategy for reaching a wider audience more cheaply. This suggestion had clear professional and economic implications, for Knopf fully appreciated that it would transfer considerable authority to private practitioners.[148]

As the debate over whether tubercular patients might fare better in their own homes escalated, and sanatoria struggled to retain their status, tuberculin became critical to the sanatorium's self-defense. Sanatorium directors had long heeded Koch's recommendation that tuberculin not be used in general practice or in the absence of hygienic and dietetic measures. They had grasped his preparation firmly and tried their best to maintain a stranglehold on it. Now, to reassert themselves as preeminent institutions in the fight against TB, sanatorium directors invoked Koch's warning that tuberculin be used only in institutions. Von Ruck, who led the opposition, charged that outside the sanatorium tuberculin might "fail to accomplish good results, and disaster may follow its use."[149]

Others concurred, for they too found that tuberculin gave the sanatorium an edge over other institutions.[150] Thus tuberculin became an integral and standard part of the sanatorium regimen, and sans readily advertised that they employed this product. In 1909, a law passed by the Nebraska State legislature stipulated that "county authorities might treat indigent patients in institutions approved by the State Board of Health, but that such institutions must use the 'modern method of vaccine therapy.'"[151] That same year the staff at the White Haven Sanatorium of the Henry Phipps Institute in White Haven, Pennsylvania, regretted that they had not done much with tuberculin and established a committee to look further into its uses.[152]

The economic incentives for using tuberculin appeared so obvious to both sanatorium directors and their critics that the directors frequently defended themselves against charges of greed. Von Ruck, for one, felt compelled to deny even the slightest insinuation that he was mercenary. "It is perhaps unfortunate," he wrote, "that I am the director of an institution for tuberculous patients, because my motives in urging treatment of such with or without tuberculin in such establishments whenever possible, could be easily misunderstood."[153] His opponents remained unconvinced, and as they continued their assault on the sanatorium, they also took aim at tuberculin itself.

Knopf once again typified the opposition. Knopf was not a doctrinaire opponent of either the germ theory of TB or laboratory-based efforts to control the disease. Deeply impressed with Koch's bacteriological studies, he initially waxed enthusiastic about tuberculin. He had been among

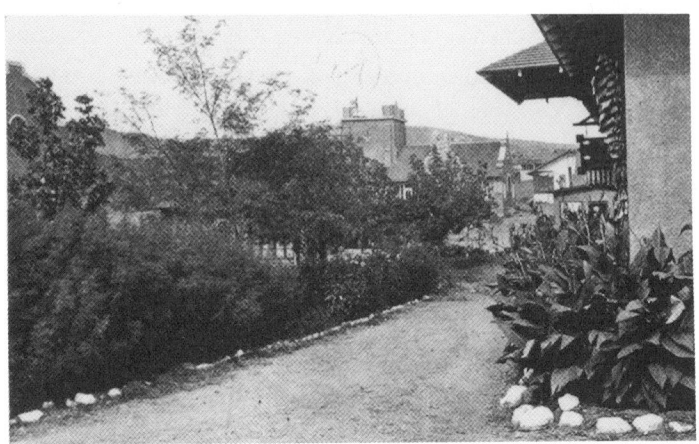

New Mexico Cottage Sanatorium

SILVER CITY, NEW MEXICO

For the Treatment of Tuberculosis

Physician-in-Chief
E. S. BULLOCK, M.D.

Manager
WAYNE MacV. WILSON

Beautiful situation in the mountains of southern New Mexico. Climatic conditions wonderfully perfect. Cool summers. Moderate winters. A flood of sunshine at all seasons. Food excellent and abundant. All the milk our patients can consume from our own dairy of selected cows. Moderate charge. Institution partly endowed. Separate cottages for patients. Complete hospital building for febrile cases. Separate amusement pavilions for men and women. Physicians in constant attendance. Livery for use of patients. Well equipped laboratory, treatment rooms, etc. All forms of tuberculosis received. Special attention to laryngeal tuberculosis. Tuberculin administered in suitable cases. One of the largest and best equipped institutions for tuberculosis in America. Patients received only through physicians.

WRITE TO THE MANAGER FOR DESCRIPTIVE BOOKLET

Ad for a Sanitorium

Source: Philip P. Jacobs, A Tuberculosis Directory *(New York: NASPT, 1911), advertisements, III.*

the many American physicians who traveled to Berlin and Vienna during the late 1880s to observe Koch's work first-hand, and upon his return he immediately began his own experiments with culture products. His initial response to tuberculin in many ways crystallized the early American reaction to the tubercle bacillus. Like Prudden, Knopf could not unquestioningly accept European wisdom or research; he was bound to rediscover the principles for himself and his reaction to tuberculin betrayed a tenacious American resistance to the blind incorporation of metropolitan knowledge. By the late 1890s, however, Knopf accepted the premises of tuberculin therapy.

Still, Knopf objected to the use of tuberculin for two distinct reasons. First, he feared that the rush to use culture products in institutions disadvantaged those clinicians outside sanatoria. To further promote the home treatment of consumptives, Knopf questioned the advantages of tuberculin. "We may employ serotherapy in acute exasperation due to an association of microbes," he mused, but "[c]an not anyone, private practitioner or sanatorium physician, report just as good or even better results, whenever the hygienic, dietetic, symptomatic and educational treatment has been carried out without the aid of any specific or antibacillary remedies?"[154] Second, beyond these allegations about the efficacy of tuberculin, Knopf charged that tuberculin was at best insufficient and at worst actually counterproductive because it inevitably focused attention on the physiological determinants of tuberculosis at the expense of the social conditions that both bred disease and demanded reform. From Knopf's perspective, tuberculin drew attention away from the many factors that predisposed to tuberculosis. He envisioned a campaign that would also wage "a vigorous war on all that is unsanitary in our cities, towns and villages."[155] Hence, he found tuberculin wanting because, though it might affect the tissue cells and the tubercle bacillus, it had no effect on the social conditions that made the host weak and did nothing to help wage "vigorous war" on urban squalor. The most powerful objection to tuberculin—even among lab-oriented physicians—was consequently that the sponsors of tuberculin focused too narrowly on creating physiological resistance when TB was a disease that had both physiological and sociological determinants.

Sanatoria had a response to these objections as well, and Trudeau played a part in framing them. As Trudeau's allegiance indicates, tuberculin was more than a scientific cure. It was a preparation that allowed American physicians to resolve the essential tension between scientific professionalism and social reform, and in the end it contributed to the campaign to build resistance.

Professional Legitimacy and Resistance: Trudeau and the Saranac Laboratory

The Von Ruck brothers, though quirky and particularly devoted and outspoken advocates, were neither the lone producers nor the lone supporters of tuberculin, and the weight of the blow that the PHS leveled against tuberculins demonstrated how extensively the "problem" extended beyond them. But the technical and structural barriers that the PHS raised did not put an end to private production or use of tuberculin. And of those who continued to use tuberculin, none was more respected than Trudeau at Saranac Lake.

Though initially doubtful that a vaccine against tuberculosis could be developed, by 1892 Trudeau had conducted his own clinical trials of Koch's lymph. These trials convinced him that Koch's method, while still ill understood and potentially dangerous, was "certainly the first thus far proposed which can be shown by clinical observation to produce a distinct and appreciable impression on the areas of diseased tissue."[156] On the strength of studies that suggested that laboratory modifications could eliminate the harmful elements while retaining the benefits, Trudeau conducted further investigations. In 1894, he established a laboratory at Saranac Lake, which, though generally dedicated to research on the etiology, treatment, and prevention of TB, soon focused on studies of tuberculins. Trudeau had not previously committed himself to any particular approach to the development of an antituberculosis vaccine, but his lab now devoted itself to "the chemical study of the subject";[157] and Trudeau temporarily narrowed his interests to two questions: whether liquid cultures of tubercle bacilli contained a "remedial element of sufficient efficacy to cure tuberculosis anywhere and in any animal" and whether "this substance is to be found in the bacilli themselves or in the culture-medium in which they have been developed."[158] During the next five years, the laboratory at Saranac Lake approached these questions through studies of Edwin Klebs's "antiphthisin" (a culture product separated from tuberculin by chemical methods and purported to have germicidal properties), Koch's "new tuberculin, T.R." (a modified form of his original lymph), and other tuberculins.[159] Each preparation seemed to pose particular problems of manufacture or clinical use, but despite these problems Trudeau remained interested in the development of a tuberculin that would "heal tuberculosis by the production of a toxine immunity."[160]

Under the direction of E. R. Baldwin, Trudeau's Saranac laboratory became a major, respected producer of tuberculins. Indeed, from 1905 onward, Baldwin received innumerable requests for tuberculin from other sanatoria, from city and state boards of health, and from drug companies. Vincent Bowditch, of the Sharon Sanatorium, Herbert King of the Loomis Sanatorium, Charles Parfitt of the Free Hospital for Poor Consumptives (in Gravenhurst, Ontario), and H. D. Pease, director of the State Hygienic Laboratory of the New York State Department of Health, all wrote to him with requests for tuberculin, and Baldwin generously granted them supplies.[161] For some, Saranac Lake was a convenient and extraordinarily cheap supplier; it refused to sell any of its products. That the lab filled its requests gratis embarrassed some of its clients. "Now that we are beginning to use the substance therapeutically in occasional cases, I do not feel it right that the sanatorium should receive so much without remuneration," Bowditch demurred in 1905.[162] Still, Bowditch did not put an end to his requests for tuberculin when Baldwin repeatedly refused to accept payment. The quality of the Saranac Lake product lay behind other requests. Trudeau and Baldwin had established themselves as cautious and well-informed producers of tuberculin, and whether it was free or not many valued their product. "It is generally conceded that the only reliable tuberculin for inoculation purposes procurable in this country comes from your laboratory," King flattered Baldwin in December 1905, and Parfitt similarly couched his request with the admission that "I certainly feel afraid of that [tuberculin] of German manufacture."[163]

The demands placed on Saranac increased further after 1907, when Von Pirquet's studies revealed the diagnostic uses of tuberculin. Both Trudeau and Baldwin had previously drawn their own conclusions on this subject. After 1897, Trudeau had employed tuberculin extensively at Saranac Lake, and these studies, along with the results of work conducted elsewhere, convinced him that tuberculin could be safely and effectively used for diagnostic purposes.[164] They also based their conclusions on work done collaboratively with Koch.[165] Hence, when Von Pirquet advocated wider use of tuberculin, those who sought information or materials naturally turned to Trudeau's lab. Small and large manufacturers of biologics, such as Kalle and Company, C. Bischoff and Company, H. M. Alexander and Company, and H. K. Mulford Company, all hoped that Baldwin would test, standardize, and endorse their products.

By January 1908, Mulford had begun to use Baldwin as an unofficial advisor. In response to requests for tuberculin, Mulford had started work on a tuberculin laboratory that would manufacture products suitable for diagnosis, prevention, and therapy. Its plans to open the laboratory were delayed, however, and, afraid that it would disappoint and lose its clients, Mulford asked Baldwin to "furnish us a supply"[166] that would be "furnished complimentary to such physicians who have made requests for supplies of the product and who are unable to wait until our laboratory is completed that our own product can be furnished."[167] Mulford then tried to cajole Saranac Lake into testing its products by combining flattery with an appeal to Baldwin's professional principles. H. K. Mulford himself wrote to Baldwin with the plea that "we are determined to use no Tuberculin preparations until we have learned from clinical tests that preparations are reliable, and to this end it is our purpose to co-operate with the foremost experts of the country. Will you test our various tuberculin preparations?"[168] Baldwin obliged the first part of the request and sent the company samples of various preparations from the Saranac Lake lab. However, he declined the honor of testing Mulford tuberculins. Unable to use the Saranac Lake lab for this purpose, H. K. Mulford Company then began to refer the inquiries about tuberculin that it received to Baldwin and Saranac Lake.[169] Between 1908 and 1912, F. E. Stewart, director of Mulford's Scientific Department, repeatedly asked Baldwin's opinion on the subject of tuberculin and tuberculin therapy. "Our correspondence files on the subject of tuberculin and bacterial vaccines within the last two years contain between fifteen and twenty thousand letters," Stewart wrote to Baldwin. He then used this evidence of overwhelming popular interest to try to convince Saranac Lake to help Mulford meet demands for supplies and to fulfill the responsibility of being "exceedingly accurate in what we say."[170]

Mulford was not the only drug company to tap Saranac Lake's expertise. In June 1908, H. M. Alexander and Company asked Baldwin and William Hallock Park—the director of laboratories at the New York City Department of Health who was esteemed for his work on diphtheria antitoxin—to cooperate in an effort to manufacture and standardize tuberculin.[171] Public agencies similarly turned to the Saranac Lake lab. The AMA Council on Pharmacy repeatedly asked Baldwin to test and evaluate various tuberculins brought to its attention.[172] When the Hygienic Laboratory was presented with tuberculins and when it considered the problem of "formulat[ing] a standard for tuberculin," it too turned to Saranac Lake.[173] Likewise, foreign institutions, the Montreal General Hospital among them, asked Baldwin's advice.[174] Indeed, Trudeau's lab retained its status as a major producer and supplier of tuberculins well into the 1920s, and the Children's Department at Johns Hopkins and the Sharon Sanatorium, among others, continued to use tuberculin prepared at Saranac Lake for both therapeutic and diagnostic purposes.[175]

Unlike the Von Rucks, who blindly and idealistically appealed to the power of experimental science, Trudeau grounded his tuberculin research in a solid economic and professional base. His lab enjoyed the respect of both pharmaceutical manufacturers and the professional elite. Moreover,

Trudeau carefully located his own efforts within the context of accepted avenues of research. By 1900, antitoxins had become the preferred American brand of biologic, as leaders of American bacteriology and immunology, Smith and Park among them, endorsed this school of research, applied it to their own studies of diphtheria, and used it to set forth their own principles of the immune response.[176] Despite early opposition and obstacles, by the early years of this century production of diphtheria antitoxin had become a respected, successful, and established enterprise in the United States.[177]

Smith and Park lent legitimacy to serum studies, and Trudeau clearly appreciated their assurance that the principles of antitoxic immunity could be applied to other diseases. "The brilliant and beneficent results which have followed the discovery and use of diphtheria and tetanus antitoxic serum," he wrote in 1898, "have stimulated similar research in many of the infectious diseases."[178] Trudeau identified tuberculin as one of the many products of that research, and he conceded both here and later that the success of efforts to develop antitoxic immunity to other diseases guided his views on tuberculin. "[I]n the light of recent contributions made by [Paul] Ehrlich, [August von] Wasserman and [Emil von] Behring to our knowledge of the mechanism of immunity and antitoxin produced in the body," he wrote, "the outlook for an efficient tuberculosis antitoxin is by no means a hopeless one."[179] Hence, Trudeau's dedication to tuberculin was neither arbitrary nor coincidental; it demonstrated his professional solidarity with the ideas and achievements of his colleagues.

Trudeau also carefully shielded his research from economic taint. When Von Ruck was charged with being mercenary, he parried with the observation that "Dr. Trudeau, of Saranac Lake, and others who have under their charge *charitable* institutions in which the number of patients is of no personal advantage to the director, have all arrived at the same conclusions, being as much in favor of the treatment in institutions as I."[180] Nor was it entirely accidental that Trudeau's lab gave its products away. By doing so, sanatorium directors maintained both institutional and professional autonomy in the face of the federal government's first efforts to regulate the production of pharmaceutical products. Congress had passed the Pure Food and Drug Act in 1906 to regulate the drug trade, especially to counter "the use of false or deceptive labelling claims concerning a product's contents, safety, or therapeutic effect."[181] Scholars have paid considerable attention to the way in which the Food and Drug Act created new ties between doctors and industry and to the debate that these ties engendered.[182] In the case of tuberculin, however, it would appear, ironically, that the Food and Drug Act allowed and actually encouraged sanatoria to continue to manufacture and use their own products free from government regulation. While the act stipulated that "manufacturers" of biologics be licensed, its definition of manufacture presupposed "sale, barter and exchange,"[183] for as a matter of settled constitutional doctrine the federal government could regulate "manufacturing" only as a form of "commercial regulation."[184] Moreover, the act applied only to interstate and foreign traffic or sale within the District of Columbia. As long as sanatoria made no effort to sell tuberculins across state lines, they apparently stood beyond the reach of the law. Hence, by producing but not selling their own tuberculins, sanatoria could avoid controversy and circumvent any involvement with drug manufacturers or federal regulatory agencies.

Tuberculin consequently allowed physicians to work out their relationships with the new experimental science and with the administrative and institutional apparatuses that emerged to regulate scientific medicine. It allowed them, as well, to retain control over their own therapies and to secure an institutional base for their efforts. However, the economic, institutional, and professional concerns that helped to prolong the life of tuberculin might as easily have been invoked to justify the use of any number of preparations against tuberculosis. For example, Friedmann's vaccine might easily have commanded an economic advantage, as might have bovo-vaccine, a preventive for tuberculosis whose development was based on the principles of Edward Jenner's cowpox and introduced in 1902 by Behring, an eminent German physician.

But tuberculin offered something that these other preparations did not. Unlike bovo-vaccine or the Friedmann vaccine, tuberculin could be shown to act on the soil rather than the seed. Moreover, tuberculin nourished that soil. Koch had insisted all along that tuberculin was not a germicide. He had made it clear that it did not kill or destroy tubercle bacilli. Arguing a general principle, Koch had explained that "it is not necessary, as has often been erroneously assumed, that the bacteria should be killed in the body; in order to make them harmless to the body it is sufficient to prevent their growth, their multiplication."[185] He had then applied the principle to his remedy, proposing that it prevented the growth of tubercle bacilli both in vitro and in vivo. Koch reiterated this point in his "Further Communication," where he proposed that "there is no question of a destruction of the tubercle bacilli in the tissues, but only that the tissue enclosing the tubercle bacilli is affected by the remedy."[186] American readers of Koch's work immediately seized on the argument that his tuberculin created an environment in which tubercle bacilli could not grow, and his claim that tuberculin acted as a fertilizer rather than as a pesticide became critical to the definition of this class of product.[187] It became particularly critical as sanatorium physicians staked their turf.

What the debate between the advocates of home care and the advocates of institutional care made clear was that it was not sufficient merely that a remedy act on the host; it had to act on the host in a particular way. Some of the conditions were physiological and once again underscored the nutritional causes of tuberculosis. Initially, Koch argued that his lymph caused necrosis of diseased tissues, which he maintained promoted healing. Both critics and supporters feared that these alleged necrotic properties would actually hasten the course of the disease,[188] and they parried Koch with the suggestion that necrosis or wasting was simply the "expression of an overdose, *i.e.*, a poisonous dose."[189] Instead, they proposed that tuberculin, when properly administered, acted as a restorative, "as a powerful upbuilding alterative to the tuberculous subject."[190] By 1893, their claims had become so compelling that Koch even reformulated his explanation for the action of tuberculin to emphasize its nutritive properties. His American audience quickly seized upon this change of heart. When given as recommended, Koch stated, tuberculin stimulated rather than eroded tissue, and as Von Ruck suggested, it accomplished this stimulation by augmenting "the local nutrition."[191] This alternate explanation allowed Von Ruck, Trudeau, and many others to locate Koch's lymph within the framework of their more general efforts to combat tuberculosis. Tuberculin, Von Ruck argued, assisted nature in repairing the damage done by microbes in much the same way as diet, fresh air, and exercise did. It exerted a "specific effect upon the local tubercular process by... leading to increased local nutrition."[192] Thus, tuberculin counteracted the influences that had rendered tissues susceptible to TB, and it prevented disease by fortifying the tissues so that they might withstand any new assault. Trudeau made the case particularly strongly. He endorsed tuberculin because it seemed to nourish and increase the vitality of the tissues in much the same way that good food and fresh air did.[193] In short, it could be used in sanatoria to build resistance.

Tuberculin could consequently be adapted to the more general American campaign against tuberculosis in a way that other preparations could not. It highlighted the complex relationship between bacillus and host and served the ends of those physicians who held on to a complex etiology in which the bacillus represented only one cause of the disease. Because it acted to nourish the soil rather than directly destroy the seed, tuberculin fit well with the prevailing view of the control of TB.

The contention that tuberculin built resistance also gave its sponsors an edge in defending their preparation against those critics, like Knopf, who warned that tuberculin (and other similar biologics) undermined the traditional hygienic and dietetic regime. Professional jealousies and rivalries played no small part in determining the fate of each newly introduced preventive or cure. Knopf had his own vested interests in a particular approach to the control of tuberculosis. So did critics, like W. L. Dunn, of Asheville, North Carolina, who as late as 1909 maintained the importance of individualized therapeutic regimens and worried that "the most dangerous and most really harmful side of tuberculin therapy has been that it encourages and favors a neglect of the necessary *régime* by both physician and patient. By the physician, although he may have been personally fitted to successfully carry out the dietetic-hygienic *régime*, because it divides his interest, calling his attention away from the individual and directing his specific efforts toward the disease itself."[194] However telling such a criticism might have been when directed at other biologics, it proved rather less damaging against tuberculin. As Trudeau, Von Ruck, and others defended tuberculin, they emphasized that this "cure" differed from others in that it did not necessarily compete with either the goals or the structure of an individualized hygienic and dietetic campaign. To the accusation that tuberculin would lead to the neglect of diet and hygiene, they responded that, on the contrary, tuberculin therapy could work together with and hence reinforce the traditional therapy.

Such assertions built on a framework that Koch himself had laid. Koch, for one, had countered his professional rivals with this concession:

> In many cases I had the decided impression that the careful nursing bestowed on the patient had a considerable influence on the result of the treatment, and I am in favour of applying the remedy in proper sanatoria, as opposed to treatment at home and in the out-patient room. How far the methods of treatment recognized as curative—such as mountain climate, fresh air treatment, special diet, etc.—may be profitably combined with the new treatment cannot yet be definitely stated, but I believe that these therapeutic methods will also be highly advantageous when combined with the new treatment in many cases.[195]

Trudeau and Baldwin, Von Ruck and Pottenger, and other American advocates of tuberculin capitalized on these predictions. All recommended tuberculin therapy as an adjunct, not an alternative, to hygienic and dietetic measures. Use of tuberculin, they argued, reinforced rather than contradicted the aims of the hygienic-dietetic regimen, as it was carried out either inside sanatoria or without. Von Ruck suggested that the traditional regimen quickened and facilitated the action of tuberculin, advised his colleagues to combine the principles of cure, and concluded that "the results must in proportion be better as we intelligently combine the various means at our disposal rather than depend upon this or the other single effort."[196] Trudeau went still further. He asserted:

The only immunity, therefore, we can invoke to protect the patient against the dangers of reinfection, while attempting to bring about, by injections of tuberculin, pathological changes tending to necrosis of tubercle, is that produced by all measures which have been found to improve nutrition. These measures consist of climate, an open-air life, hygiene, feeding and medical supervision; and although by combining with these the specific impression exercised by tuberculin on tubercle, the treatment of incipient phthisis seems at present to hold out an added promise, its success or failure will still depend in the future, as in the past, on the persistence and thoroughness of our efforts to stimulate nutrition.[197]

From Trudeau's perspective, tuberculin therapy and the broader goals of sanatorium treatment worked hand in hand.[198]

Trudeau argued the case convincingly, and he successfully persuaded many other advocates of the hygienic and dietetic regimen, who quite readily agreed to tuberculin's advantages. Thus, though sanatoria became the bastions of tuberculin therapy, they did not alienate proponents of the broader dietetic, climatic, and hygienic regimens. These regimens both allowed for and accommodated the use of tuberculin. In fact, publications like the *Transactions of the American Climatological Association* and *Colorado Medicine*, which had a vested interest in competing curative regimens, soon became forums for the advertisement of tuberculins.

With time, other physicians expanded Trudeau's argument, suggested that tuberculin and sera like it produced only an incomplete resistance, and reiterated the symbiosis of tuberculin therapy and the sanatorium regimen. Sera like tuberculin offered only a partial solution, Allen Krause of Johns Hopkins objected in 1923, for no preparation could successfully cure or prevent TB if it did not simultaneously stimulate metabolic functions and encourage patients to modify their habits and behaviors. "Of those who, *while living an active life*, relied on drugs or vapors or 'serums' or vaccines to fight their battle, few have made the journey back," Krause warned.[199] "Drugs, tuberculins . . . would not show much effect if at the same time rest was not part of the treatment, . . . that is, the patient allowed to go on his own way, with life unregulated and activities unrestrained, would in most cases 'crumble' nevertheless."[200] Convinced that any American who wished to recover or to resist the disease successfully would have to live a "well-regulated life in the open air," Krause boldly declared that "discipline, regulation of life, is really the keynote to success in treatment."[201] He incorporated this conviction into his research, his clinical practice, and his professional and popular teaching, where he exhorted physicians to pay attention to the entire organism and to adopt regimens of nutrition and rest, which would modify both the behaviors and the physiological status of patients.

In tuberculin, as in the metaphor of seed and soil, American physicians had consequently found a comfortable balance between the professional drive to science and the combined economic and therapeutic appeal of more traditional, individualized, behavioral transformation. Tuberculin enjoyed a comparatively favorable reception among American physicians because it acted to make the soil more resistant to tubercle bacillus, and these physicians' responses to tuberculin reveal how deeply committed they remained to the belief that TB was a disease of both seed and soil. Both the metaphor of seed and soil and the goals of building resistance became ubiquitous during the decades that followed Koch's identification of the tubercle bacillus, for through them a range of physicians found the means both to reconcile Koch's irrefutable microbial hypothesis with the equally undeniable evidence that infection with Koch's bacillus could not fully explain the phenomenon of tubercular disease and to accommodate Koch's new bacterial hypothesis to their desire to improve the soil. Koch himself had not anticipated this distinctively American reconciliation. He had introduced his 1882 paper by contrasting the old view of TB (which understood the disease "as an outcome of social misery") with "the future struggle" (in which it would be possible to concentrate on "an actual parasite").[202] The American interpretation of Koch's discovery was different precisely because American physicians refused to distinguish as starkly as Koch had between the past and the future, and between social misery and "actual parasites." For most Americans, in short, the beauty of Koch's discovery was that it did not force them to jettison the other considerations that they believed relevant to explaining or treating disease. That is why the metaphor of seed and soil was so well-suited to describe the American understanding of TB, and that is why it remains a useful way of understanding the strategies of disease control that followed from the discovery of Koch's bacillus. The "future struggle" in the United States did not concentrate on the newly discovered seed at the expense of the soil. It concentrated, rather, on understanding how the seed interacts with the soil, and how the soil could be improved and enriched to withstand the seed's implantation.

CHAPTER 3

Spit and Polish:
The Middle-Class Crusade to Build
Resistance, 1900–1925

"When the discovery of the tubercle bacillus was announced," Dr. Louis Warfield told the National Association for the Study and Prevention of Tuberculosis (NASPT) in 1908, "there were those who confidently predicted that another generation would see the stamping out of this most dreadful disease. It only goes to show how difficult it is to arouse to the proper pitch both physicians and laymen, when nearly forty years after this discovery we are still agitating."[1] Warfield and the other physicians who turned their attention to tuberculosis during the first quarter of the twentieth century confronted contradictory scientific and social messages. Judged in terms of the goal of eradicating TB, the precise value of the bacteriological revolution that Robert Koch had begun remained unclear. Though scientific refinements like tuberculin testing promised to clearly identify the sick, these new diagnostic agents proved both too limited and too successful. When Edward Livingston Trudeau first used tuberculin diagnostically, in 1897, he found to his dismay that many who showed no other signs or symptoms of TB tested positive.[2] Within a decade, extensive application of C. Von Pirquet's improved tuberculin test (1907) exposed the masses of apparently healthy citizens who harbored disease. Children especially, by some estimates as many as 60 percent of those who lived in urban centers, had been infected.[3]

The omnipresence of infection posed a health hazard that American physicians alternately decried and downplayed. "Not everyone who is exposed to the infection of tuberculosis—the tubercle bacillus—becomes a victim of it," a typical manual reassured, for "[t]hree quarters of us have had tuberculosis and recovered from it without knowing anything about it."[4] Tuberculosis, it seemed, preferentially affected some Americans—females, children, immigrants, and the indigent among them. Between 1900 and 1925, American physicians consequently directed their attention "to the study of every factor that makes infection disease"[5] and to the groups that seemed especially vulnerable to it.

The evolving debate over who contracted tuberculosis and why became almost circular as it returned repeatedly to seed and soil. Clarence Lucas, for example, familiarly advised the readers of his 1920 work that "[t]wo things are necessary in order to contract tuberculosis—the tubercle bacillus, or seed, and the soil."[6] But though the metaphor of seed and soil that had served to explain the course of TB to nineteenth-century physicians thus persisted, the debates about what rendered the soil receptive and what should be done to contain the seed's growth took a distinctive turn as they reflected the consciousness and objectives of an emerging middle class.

Professionalism, we saw in the previous chapter, was one project of the middle class; social reform was another. Unlike the working class, which established itself and its conflicts in terms of the relationship of labor and capital, the middle class defined itself by means of standards of conduct and appeals to the moral authorities of science and the state. Behavior was its standard, and transformative prescriptions its currency. Between 1900 and 1925, TB offered a powerful rationale for the prescriptions that gave the middle class its shape and substance. During these years, rates of tubercular infection and disease seemed to substantiate fears about gender, ethnicity, and dependency. In boards of health, sanatoria, voluntary agencies, and the popular press, American physicians reacted to those fears with a renewed therapeutic of social reform in which they once again fused the goals of medical and social improvement.

Much of their activity focused on sputum. Spit represented the microbial sources of infection, the exposure that was a necessary cause of the disease. But spit also represented the social behaviors and class divides that determined susceptibility. The antispitting campaign allowed for the control not only of public behaviors but also of what Nancy Tomes has described as the "the private side" of public health.[7] Hence, the campaign against spitting crystallized the political and social challenges of medical intervention. As it developed, it became at once an effort to control tubercle bacilli, to redefine a therapeutic of social reform, and to articulate the middle-class status of both practitioners and patients. In this effort, behavioral transformation, through education, became central.

THE CONTROL OF TUBERCULOSIS AND THE MIDDLE-CLASS STATE

The effort to control spit began in the boards of health that had already moved to safeguard the interests of the middle classes. From colonial times, publicists, politicians, and physicians agreed that health, a fundamental attribute of the American nation, was one of the characteristics of American exceptionalism. Health was a symbol of both private and public virtue, which the state had a duty to safeguard. But beyond this symbolic value, health also intersected with the social and property interests of American citizens.[8] The spread of infectious disease disrupted production, depressed consumer demand, and in other ways weakened commerce. Interventions like quarantine and vaccination ensured the public health, but they also restricted trade and commercial relations. Hence, as boards of health across the country introduced and enforced public health legislation, they fought recurring battles over economic and individual liberty. Their victories in cases like smallpox and yellow fever testified to the dangers disease posed to a middle class order and to a growing faith that state action might protect and promote middle-class life.

Tuberculosis served as one of the sites on which state institutions and middle-class interests negotiated the boundaries of public health intervention. Sheila Rothman, for one, has suggested that in the case of TB "[t]he stakes were so high as to justify the most exceptional intrusions of state authority into the life of the individual,"[9] beginning with registration measures that allowed officials to know "who the infected were"[10] and ending with proposals to incarcerate carriers. In fact, however, the very pervasiveness of TB made it more rather than less difficult to justify drastic interventions. Both the epidemiology of TB and the social experience of the illness repeatedly forced physicians to confront the differences between infection, disease, and illness. Because these were not identical, tuberculosis did not lend itself to the simple preventative or curative approaches that Rothman suggests dominated American efforts at control. "Infection, of itself is relatively unimportant," Allen Krause noted, as other physicians also did repeatedly. "The problem of preventing the outbreak of frank disease in the legions of the infected is the crux of the programme of prevention."[11] This challenge posed a series of social, medical, and legal problems that registration, notification, and other legislative interventions would not easily contain.

Early administrative efforts to control TB consequently provoked controversy. During the 1880s, Hermann Biggs of New York, Charles Chapin of Providence, Peter Bryce of Toronto, and other leaders of local boards of health first argued that tubercle bacilli posed a public nuisance that the state had an obligation to regulate. Biggs's proposals for registration and mandatory reporting, compulsory disinfection of the lodgings of the ill, and regulated inspection of milk and meat met staunch opposition. In the era of laissez-faire constitutionalism, such statist efforts to protect the public health seemed thinly disguised attempts to regulate the market, and Biggs could convince neither his colleagues nor the public that they were legitimate and necessary.[12] The balance between state responsibility and individual economic liberty, which was tenuous and delicate even in the case of clearly infectious diseases, seemed especially precarious in the case of tuberculosis, where the efficacy of preventive measures was so uncertain and the relationship between infection and disease so ambiguous.

Biggs's proposals had clear economic costs. Yet even the strongest proponents of administrative controls, William Osler among them, could not promise that they would prevent the spread of bacteria.[13] Hence, individual practitioners cautiously weighed the professional advantages they might gain from new scientific knowledge against the costs registration might levy on their practice. Biggs, Chapin, and Osler, from whose vantage the institutions of the state legitimated bacteriology, sought professional prestige in a marriage between state and scientific authority. However, rank-and-file physicians mistrusted such an alliance. An amalgam of professional and economic concerns persisted—that mandatory reporting would force physicians to "divulge of a medical secret," compromise the confidential trust between patient and physician, infringe professional autonomy, challenge medical judgment, curtail the physician's ability to prescribe an individualized therapy, and require practitioners to provide services for which they went unpaid.[14]

Throughout North America, both the scope of legislation and enforcement remained limited. Michigan's State Board of Health became the first to mandate reporting of tuberculosis in 1893. Rhode Island and Biggs's New York City followed suit in 1894, but these were exceptions. Even in New York State, most cities did not declare consumption communicable and make it reportable until after 1900.[15] North of the border, in Toronto, Bryce's efforts to translate acceptance of the microbial origins of TB into a public health effort proved similarly unsuccessful. Though Ontario's Provincial Board of Health approached Premier Oliver Mowat in 1894 with a request for legislation to require reporting of TB, notification did not become compulsory until 1912.[16] As late as the 1920s, the NASPT regretfully noted that "in a few states all phases of the tuberculosis problem are covered by some form of legislation, but that in many states the laws on this subject are still meagre,"[17] and New York City's Department of Health lamented that private physicians and laboratories were "refraining from furnishing the identifying data" for tuberculosis cases and that "there is no law which compels them to furnish this information."[18]

Where registration did not work, spit provided an alternate focus. Stymied in his original effort to have consumption included among the notifiable diseases, Biggs shifted both target and strategy. He published a circular subtitled *Rules to Be Observed for the Prevention and Spread of Consumption*.[19] This circular, which the New York City Department of Health distributed to all households in which a tuberculous death had been reported, focused on the management of sputum. Through it, the city conveyed information about the sources of infection, apprised readers of the bacterial causes of the disease, warned against infection that occurred through the passage of sputum, outlined precautions for the disposal of sputum and disinfection of linens, and proffered simple advice about personal and domestic hygiene that would prevent infection.

Biggs's informational circular, which won him acclaim as a "pioneer in health education," provided an alluringly simple and effective means of curtailing the spread of the disease.[20] It also framed a distinct and enduring strategy for public control of tuberculosis. Circulars that promoted the management of sputum became pillars of the American campaign against TB. In 1889, the Maine State Board of Health initiated its campaign against tuberculosis with the publication of *Circular #54: The Prevention of Consumption*. By 1900, twenty-one other state boards and an even larger number of local authorities had also followed New York City's example. Several states committed significant sums of money to this purpose. In 1904, Maryland allotted the State Board of Health $5,000 to issue circulars.[21]

These circulars were both useful in themselves and a means to a greater end. "If every man and woman in the United States were familiar with the main facts relating to the manner in which tuberculosis is communicated and the simple measures necessary for their protection," Trudeau suggested, then one "might reasonably expect as a direct result of this knowledge a great diminution in the death rate."[22] Beyond the intrinsic informational value of education, at least some of the anti-TB campaigners viewed education as instrumental in the development of a more ambitious public health program and as a necessary step along the path to greater state activity. Once the dangers posed by tubercle bacilli became clear, Trudeau predicted, "the people would soon demand and easily obtain effective legislation for its prevention and control."[23]

The educational efforts to contain spit circumvented some of the initial obstacles to administrative control of tuberculosis. Many might question the legitimacy of reporting, registration, and inspection, which might interfere with trade, violate doctor-patient trust, and compel physicians to render services for which they received no remuneration. But no one could deny the public's need to "understand the sources of infection and the mode in which the infecting material gains entrance to the organism,"[24] the value of educational instruments, or the state's duty to provide them.

As Trudeau predicted, educational initiatives also prepared the way for legislative control. Spit, unlike tainted milk or meat, had no commercial significance, and by pointing out broader public health issues public health reformers easily justified the need for regulations that controlled spit. First, they graphically illustrated and publicized its dangers. Second, they likened spit, a bodily discharge, to other wastes that government had established its duty to control.[25] Public health reformers spoke of spit and refuse in much the same language and allied their cause with a larger, better understood crusade against the dumping of sewage. A New York State statute, for example, prohibited the disposal of "sputum, saliva or other bodily secretion or excretion."[26] By 1911, 150 cities and three states had passed antispitting ordinances. These often linked spit to garbage and prohibited "not only spitting in public places but also the throwing away of refuse and food."[27]

Nonetheless, there were limits to both the success and the scope of the campaign against spit. Enforcement and compliance posed the first obstacles. Local officials upheld antispitting ordinances with varying degrees of rigor. Though New York City took its task seriously and launched "periodic raids," to ensure a "complete prohibition of promiscuous spitting in public,"[28] other jurisdictions treated legislation more casually. Even in municipalities where antispitting regulations were enforced, public violations remained numerous.

Noncompliance and other legal obstacles also returned attention to the complexities of the tuberculosis problem, its broader social origins, and the fundamental distinctions between spit and spitting, the behavior that spread it. Spit, like the fly as polio vector, was a "dread specter" of both disease and social degeneration.[29] It was itself a noxious substance with base associations to dirt, squalor, and ignorance. But it was distributed through obnoxious habits that were far more difficult to regulate than spit itself. The language of New York State's 1908 antispitting law captured the dilemma; it identified the improper disposal of sputum as a "danger" and a "nuisance" and an "offense." If New York capitalized on the ambiguity of the infraction to empower health officers to take nuisance complaints seriously and to act to "remove all reasonable cause of offense or danger,"[30] other jurisdictions acted more cautiously. Offensive as the habit of spitting might be, it was common and not confined to any particular class. The spittoon, like the cigar, was an emblem of refined masculinity, and, positioned beside the potted palm, it enjoyed pride of place in public areas. The lace-edged linen handkerchief, which so discreetly preserved tubercle bacilli, was an equally powerful emblem of genteel femininity. Virginia's General Assembly grappled with the problem in 1906, by at once prohibiting "expectorating or spitting in public places, buildings, theatres, steamboats, railways and street cars and other public conveyances" and requiring "a sufficient number of spittoons or cuspidors to be provided in smoking compartments and smoking cars."[31] Fall River, Massachusetts, similarly required employers "to furnish spittoons, which are of cheap material, so that they may be destroyed every week."[32]

Besieged from both above and below, the antispitting campaign shifted attention to "careless consumptives"—those Americans who failed to dispose responsibly of the bacilli that they harbored in their sputum. The specter of the careless consumptive was a powerful one, its most graphic image being the misanthrope who spat willfully, consciously, indiscriminately, and "promiscuously." Thus portrayed, careless consumptives had little in common with responsible Americans who deserved protection. Having failed to act as dutiful adults or citizens, they were threats and pariahs who contravened the rules of health, posed a public nuisance, and compromised their natural rights. But while such images justified extreme state interventions, neither this portrayal of careless consumptives nor the measures imposed to contain them were the norm. Careless consumptives were not just reckless spitters whom the state had to confine. More troublesome still were undetected cases, who spread disease unknowingly, and the ignorant, who, though aware that they were ill, did not understand the actual processes of infection. Then there were the poor. During the first decade of the twentieth century, as social reformers took to the streets and saw the toll that tuberculosis took in tenement houses and slums, they underscored the connections among squalor, lack of opportunity, and the spread of disease.

The regulation of deviants would not readily resolve these problems. Spitting was not an essential attribute of the individual, nor were spitters incorrigible. Rather, it was typically a behavior born of ignorance, lack of opportunity, or lack of control. This construction of the problem renewed the demand for a therapeutic of social reform or for measures that both provided information and promoted self control. Hence, as the campaign against spitting narrowed to expose the public hazards that careless consumptives posed, it simultaneously widened to target both the bacillus and the behaviors that encouraged its spread. It demanded measures that *"would have the emphasis laid on the behavior of the human being and not on the bacillus."*[33] And as it widened, it trod the fine line between public and private.

Boards of health rose to the challenge of this reconstructed mandate not with further regulation but with modified circulars. The second generation of circulars continued to provide information about the spread of the tubercle bacillus and sputum management but also confronted the private side of spitting. The public actions of the careless consumptive were most easily identified, publicized, and discountenanced, but private behaviors were also hazardous. Common domestic activities—such as sweeping, washing, and kissing—spread spit. Though these habits were hidden from public view and were apparently confined, physicians came to believe that they posed a far greater potential danger than public spitting, for they were widespread and they disproportionately infected the innocent and unsuspecting. Tuberculosis, one physician reflected, "is a house disease; . . . it is practically never contracted out of doors."[34] With advice about proper methods for washing, sweeping, and cleaning, and with the invitation to "consult physicians about the social relations of persons suffering from suspected consumption,"[35] circulars attempted to address these additional social and domestic threats. The evolving campaign, directed primarily to the working classes, played on factory workers' aspirations to respectability, and nationality and class intersected in the effort to promote clean habits that were at once American and genteel.

Further educational initiatives consisted of classes, exhibitions, movies, and special lectures. In 1907, the California legislature appropriated $2,000 for the dissemination of knowledge to prevent the spread of tuberculosis; two years later, it granted the State Board of Health an additional $2,000 for the same purpose. In 1909, the Kansas State Legislature appropriated $20,000 for a statewide educational campaign, almost half the sum that two years later it allocated to a state sanatorium. The Iowa State Board of Health reported in 1908 that it "did a large amount of educational work."[36] The Illinois Board of Health similarly compiled and distributed a considerable body of literature on the prevention of tuberculosis, as did state boards of health in Indiana, Massachusetts, and North Dakota. In 1909, the North Carolina State Text Book Commission included a chapter on consumption in all textbooks on physiology, while Missouri required "special instruction as to tuberculosis, its nature and prevention to be given in all public schools of the state." Michigan and Massachusetts were also among the states that required compulsory instruction on the transmission of "dangerous communicable diseases," especially tuberculosis.[37] Rather than expending money on textbooks or in-class instruction, Alabama, Iowa, and Minnesota set aside funds for official tuberculosis lecturers, whom they hired to head statewide educational programs.[38] Nor were these efforts simply symbolic. Between 1906 and 1911, nine states expended close to $100,000 on educational initiatives.[39]

By informing citizens of the dangers of tubercle bacilli, the state-sponsored campaign against spitting aimed to break the chain of infection. By publicizing the dangers of infection, it legitimated intervention. By focusing on spitting, it underscored the links between behavior and disease. By resorting to education, it united the methods of social and health reform. Education was central to early-twentieth century reform efforts, which "predicated the rise of America and each citizen upon an emancipating discipline of spiritual and physical truths."[40] Education was consequently an accepted function of the state that presented a pointed alternative to more intrusive forms of legal intervention. Thus, the educational campaign against spit and spitting provided common ground for opponents and proponents of state intervention. As S. Adolphus Knopf put it, the most effective measures against tuberculosis were those that succeeded by "educating (not frightening) the masses into obedience to sanitary regulations."[41]

Despite Knopf's optimism, educational circulars, lectures, and films had limited impact on the behaviors and environments that bred tuberculosis. After 1906, the numbers of infected Americans and the asymmetry between infection and disease repeatedly reminded physicians and legislators that "the prevention of tuberculosis is for the most part a prevention, not of infection, but of manifest disease."[42] The desire to prevent "manifest disease" drew medical scrutiny back to the determinants of biological and social susceptibility to tubercle bacilli. And as physicians attempted to prevent disease rather than infection, they shifted their efforts accordingly, away from spit to "polish"—to the promotion of those public and private behaviors that enabled the host to resist disease. The desire to combat overwork, alcoholism, worry, poor diet, and bad habits again became part of their therapeutic agenda.

The shifting boundaries of medical practice, with its appeal to the ostensibly apolitical authority of science, made many physicians increasingly uncomfortable with these new efforts to practice a therapeutic of social reform. But their discomfort did not deter them. Most turn-of-the-century physicians recognized that "[t]he solution of the tuberculosis problem" required more than medical intervention and was "partly dependent on the removal of other evils and inequalities which constitute, no doubt, a more fundamental social problem than does tuberculosis itself."[43] Employing colorful political rhetoric, they rallied round the Progressive cause and demanded initiatives that would make for "equality of opportunity, intellectual and material," and "bring home to the people how inevitably is tuberculosis the child of their dirt and darkness and deprivation of the comforts of life, all this after individual responsibility is given its place."[44] Through creative alliances with other institutions of the middle-class state—sanatoria, voluntary agencies, and the press—physicians also intervened directly to fight both the bacterial and behavioral causes of TB.

SANATORIA AND THE MIDDLE-CLASS ORDER: HEALTH INSTRUCTION, MORAL GUIDANCE, AND OCCUPATIONAL TRAINING

The sanatoria that served alongside boards of health in the campaign to control spit, Bolivar Jones Lloyd observed in 1919, "serve[d] the double purpose of removing the open case and making it harmless and of benefiting the individual."[45] Sanatorium physicians capitalized on this dual role. Few portrayed their institutions as either strictly preventive or strictly curative. They extolled the virtues of remote rural settings, which did isolate the infectious from civil society, but not as the san's raison d'etre. Similarly, though historians like Barbara Bates and Sheila Rothman have presented sanatoria as precursors of modern hospitals, which eventually developed scientifically based cures, discussions of and ads for sanatoria more often emphasized rehabilitation.[46] Sanatorium directors distinguished their institutions both implicitly and explicitly from hospitals and allied them instead with asylums or reformatories. "[N]o measure can be effective in arresting the progress of the disease, until one has first gained control of the patient's mind and mental processes—in short his habits," one physician observed. "This means re-education along health lines." Thus, from his perspective, "[e]mphasis must be placed on complete control of the patient and not upon the virtues of air, climate, medicines, etc. . . . The big question is 'what is the patient going to do for himself' rather than 'what am I going to give or do for the patient?'"[47] Trudeau himself stated the goal succinctly: "Within a few months limited stay 'favorable cases' could be taught to live with their tuberculosis."[48] Graduates, like the physicians Krause and Julius Wilson, described sans as "educational center[s]" or "abodes for reconstruction, education and rehabilitation."[49] The regimen of sanatoria demonstrated how much more than microbes they hoped to control, and as a debate over public funding for sanatoria developed, this regimen demarcated the bounds of state intervention.

At the heart of sanatorium care was a form of active therapy, which combined health instruction, moral guidance, and occupational training. Instruction focused most basically on sputum management. Placards, lectures, and individualized lessons replicated the message of the public health circulars. They advised patients that tubercle bacilli caused TB and outlined the course of infection. But sans also reinforced information with behavioral modification. Daily regimens slowly eroded bad habits, as they required patients to cover their mouths, dispose hygienically of sputum, and cleanse soiled utensils and linens. The material conditions of the san, the ready supply of paper products and disinfectant, made such behavioral changes possible.

Sputum management was only a part of the san regimen however. Trudeau, the father of the American sanatorium movement, had emphasized the rehabilitative rather than the curative aspects of sanatorium care. From his perspective, rehabilitation had two components. Patients needed to learn to manage spit and live with infection, and they needed as well to return to normal life. Afraid that discharged patients would once again succumb to the hardships and temptations that had originally made them susceptible, he called for a form of moral education that would supplement instruction about sputum management and transform unhealthy behaviors. Building on this premise, he sharpened the prescriptive edge of the lessons taught within his sanatorium in order to promote the personal characteristics that would enable individuals to battle disadvantages. These characteristics included cheerfulness, self-reliance, frugality, temperance, and, above all, discipline. The daily sanatorium routine, reminisced Wilson, who had taken his cure at the Adirondack Cottage, itself became the treatment as sanatorium staff attempted to guide the patients "into the path of morality and self discipline."[50]

Trudeau's san accomplished rehabilitation through individualized regimens of diet, exercise, and personal hygiene. Predicated on the values of an agrarian order and rugged outdoorsmanship, the Adirondack Cottage encouraged its patients to re-create the outdoor life. Later sans, such as Lawrence Flick's White Haven, responded to the challenges of an industrial order with a somewhat different rehabilitative agenda, as described below. But, whether agrarian or industrial, these sanatoria shared a commitment to a twofold program. Their goals were to break the chain of infection and to restore the patient to a condition where "he could go home and resume his regular life, earning his own livelihood or even supporting a family without difficulty."[51] Hence, sanatoria taught incipient consumptives the knowledge and skills needed to resist both illness and disease.

The regimen adopted at the White Haven Sanatorium, a part of the

Free Hospital for Poor Consumptives at White Haven, Pennsylvania, offers a striking example of the way in which physicians attempted to rehabilitate their patients both physiologically and socially.[52] Flick had established White Haven in 1895. A Catholic doctor who stood at the fringe of Philadelphia's established medical community but very much at the center of both the local and the national campaigns against TB, Flick, like Trudeau, did not attempt to control tuberculosis "unswervingly, without being sidetracked by considerations of social policy." Long interested in the links between TB and poverty, he championed voluntary campaigns against the disease, and he established White Haven expressly to meet the needs of Philadelphia's consumptive poor. Like many others, Flick believed that the sanatorium should not treat the acutely ill but should be dedicated to the rehabilitation of ambulatory cases. Thus White Haven only accepted patients in the early stages of disease whose health, the admitting staff believed, would improve within six months.

White Haven, Bates has argued, typified the sanatorium effort to isolate the sick and teach them how to recognize, avoid, and manage bacteria. Yet Bates less fully appreciates the extent to which therapies offered at sans like White Haven moved beyond spit to polish, to measures that would fortify the human soil against infection. While they addressed the dangers of tubercle bacilli, White Haven's instructional materials also outlined the health hazards that overwork, a poor diet, inadequate sunlight, and overcrowding posed. Like the Adirondack Cottage and other sans, White Haven employed a dietetic-hygienic regimen rich in milk, eggs, and fresh air to improve the physiology of the host. "Rest, regular life, fresh air and . . . a diet generous, nourishing and easily digestible," Flick's medical staff promised, would increase vitality and "build the patient up to a perfect state of physical health," so that he could reenter city life.[53]

But while Flick attempted to create the necessary conditions for physical rehabilitation through diet, rest, and heliotherapy, he also stressed the need for social, moral, and economic improvement. He consequently cultivated self-reliance through a form of moral education in which patients learned that they must take responsibility for themselves and that continued progress toward good health depended on discipline and independence.[54] To this end, White Haven's staff discouraged frivolous pastimes, such as novel reading and card games, which unproductively dissipated strength. They taught patients to develop regular habits, obey orders, and practice frugality. And they waged battle against intemperance, which distracted patients from work or led them to work overzealously. At White Haven as at the Adirondack Cottage, discipline and self-reliance became the keys to successful recovery. The rules distributed to entering patients stated the san's underlying premise explicitly and plainly: "The arrest of consumption cannot be accomplished without discipline."[55] These goals seem also to have distinguished American sanatoria from their Canadian counterparts, which focused far more narrowly on the physical restoration of consumptives. Patients in Canadian sanatoria were frequently confined to bed, where it was hoped that rest and nourishing meals would restore their strength. These sanatoria taught rules of sputum management but little else.[56]

White Haven did not stop with the rhetoric of rehabilitation and independence. As patients grew stronger, its staff gradually assigned them some of the burden of running the sanatorium and caring for others. Staff tailored chores around the sanatorium to fit each patient's case, trained the ill for suitable work, and guided them toward jobs they could perform without jeopardizing their health.[57] Demonstrating their lack of concern about infection, they encouraged patients who still had bacilli in their sputum to perform simple duties such as "prepar[ing] strawberries, salt and sugar, and vinegar containers." Stronger patients cleaned, carried and prepared food, did clerical work, and at the extreme performed heavy outdoor labor.[58]

These work regimens clearly served institutional ends. By 1905, White Haven could no longer sustain the costs of free care, and it was beset by serious economic difficulties. At its April meeting, the board had revised the criteria for admission to restrict entry to those who could pay for part of their cure.[59] If money was an issue, payment could be made in kind, through labor. The board assumed that average patients would contribute four hours of work per day, but according to ability and need patients might work as few as one hour or as many as eight.[60] Nor did White Haven limit this cost-cutting strategy to patients. Whether because tuberculosis nursing was, as Flick suggested, "difficult and fraught with unpleasant features"[61] or because the conditions of work at the san were miserable and the pay pitiful, nurses refused to come. White Haven had endless staffing problems, and Flick was well aware that "[w]e will have to do something to get more nurses and better organization of our nursing forces." Consequently, in 1903 he began a training school for tuberculosis nursing. Six of its first graduates immediately joined the sanatorium staff. The practical component of the training course, which consisted of a two-year apprenticeship, also provided a ready and cheap source of labor. The trainee nurses received no remuneration during their first two probationary months; thereafter, for working eight hours a day, they received room, board, laundry, and ten dollars per month. This program dramatically reduced White Haven's operating costs at precisely the moment that these costs had begun to skyrocket.[62] Five years later, the sanatorium staff moved to offer other kinds of "employment to a certain number of cured patients."[63]

Once again, the therapeutic value of work was a significant consideration. While the labor that patients and cured patients performed helped to ensure the solvency and survival of his sanatorium, Flick offered a less self-interested justification for his therapeutic and hiring practices. Apparently convinced that the best forms of relief gave work and decent wages, he believed that sanatoria could break the cycle of poverty by providing occupational therapy, encouraging patients to take increased responsibility for themselves, and teaching them how to work without overtaxing their strength. The motto "Work persistently and hard, but do not become overtired" figured repeatedly in White Haven's literature and appeared on placards posted throughout the sanatorium.[64]

Thus Flick's decision to prescribe large doses of labor and employ cured patients was not simply self-serving. Rather, it can be understood as part of a larger therapeutic strategy—mediated by both moral education and job training—to help the victims of TB achieve economic independence. These objectives were particularly apparent in Flick's efforts to rehabilitate tuberculous women. Just as nineteenth-century physicians had been acutely aware of the gendered distribution of the disease, collected gender-specific data, and prescribed gender-specific therapies, so Flick appreciated women's special vulnerability to TB. White Haven's work regimen was fundamentally gendered; women prepared food, cleaned, and sewed; men cut wood, did the books, and tended the garden. This careful division of labor prepared Flick's patients to resume life outside the sanatorium. It taught them socially appropriate skills and trained them to perform them without further compromising their health.

There was, however, a category of patient for whom the outside world had no regular place: the single female. By 1900 the transmission of tuberculosis within households, whether by heredity or habit, was sufficiently well documented to have generated considerable debate and a sizeable medical corpus on the advisability of a consumptive's marrying. The possibility that infection might be transmitted through breast milk or infant feeding further rendered the consumptive woman a questionable candidate for motherhood. Stripped of her maternal birthright, the consumptive female also represented a potential hazard in the workplace. After 1900 a series of state and municipal laws prohibited consumptives from working as teachers, domestics, or bakers or in other trades where they might infect their unsuspecting clients.[65] Discouraged from marrying, barred from teaching and domestic service, scared away from sewing, millinery, millwork, and other trades alleged to predispose to TB, single tuberculous women had few traditional options for supporting themselves. Denied a steady income, they faced constant danger of relapse.

Such women posed a threefold threat—as patients, females, and potential paupers—that Flick appreciated fully. Though by 1900 the female tuberculous death rate had fallen and in some instances was well below the male rate, physicians and the general public continued to view women as particularly vulnerable. Left unattended or, worse still, unreformed, tuberculous women presented a combined medical and social menace. Like Typhoid Mary, they might disrupt the fabric of society and home by unwittingly or willfully spreading death. But the challenge of the tuberculous female went further. If their warnings against marriage and childbearing were issued in seriousness, then physicians and legislators forced female consumptives into an unfeminine role. In Flick's experience, these women already had a tendency to deviate from appropriate behaviors. Miss McFarlane, Miss Ewing, and many of the other previously tuberculous nursing students at White Haven seemed ever guilty of "indiscretions," which included staying out after hours, "inattention, smoking, drinking, and carrying on with interns."[66]

Finally, the single tuberculous female bore testimony to the inextricable connections between tuberculosis and poverty. Though poverty was an undeniable cause of TB, Flick, like many other middle class reformers, understood also that the disease created dependency and poverty. Moreover, he ascribed poverty and dependency to irregular or inappropriate employment. Work too great or too little, overstrain, and anxiety taxed physical health, caused illness, and prevented recovery. The sick, after all, could not hold a job that would pay for food and rent, and thus a vicious cycle began in which individuals could neither care for themselves nor become well. Flick's decision to establish training schools for nurses consequently served a secondary purpose. In addition to providing cheap ward labor, the school offered a particularly ingenious strategy for rehabilitating and maintaining the single tuberculous woman.[67] Here, the two components of Flick's rehabilitative campaign—the physiological and the sociological—dovetailed neatly.

Flick's training schools, at both White Haven and the Phipps Institute and at a similar school at the Philadelphia Hospital, accepted women of "at least twenty" but no more than thirty-five years of age who were "free from physical defects other than tuberculosis."[68] He expected candidates to possess "good moral character . . . common school education, viz arithmetic, penmanship, spelling, composition, history and geography." These characteristics were essential, for once accepted the nurse trainees studied for two hours of the day and worked for eight. Their education consisted of "lectures in anatomy and physiology, therapeutics, general medicine, minor emergency, hygiene, dietetics and gynecology"; it was later expanded to include lectures "on general medical subjects, hydrotherapy, . . . bandaging [and] elements of surgical nursing." Instructional materials included "readings from Clara Meeks' *On Nursing*, Isabel Hampton's *Principles of Practical Nursing*, Hutchinsons's and Kiber's *Anatomy and Physiology*, Gray's *Anatomy*, Martin's *The Human Body*, Wood's *Therapeutics*, and Dock's *Materia Medica*." Students also received classes in "cooking" and "special training both theoretical and practical in the nursing and care of pulmonary tuberculosis."[69]

Bacteriology, however, was conspicuously missing from the lecture schedule and readings. Instruction seemed to focus less on the tubercle bacillus itself than on the determinants of susceptibility. The first question on the examination for first-year students was, "What conditions predispose a person to the development of tuberculosis?"[70] It only then went on to inquire about measures for the care and management of sputum. In the absence of student answers or the instructor's key, a circular of information written by Joseph Walsh, the director of Flick's medical staff at White Haven, provides some clue as to what students might have been expected to answer: "The majority of people in good health are not, under ordinary conditions, susceptible. Anything tending to lower vitality improves the soil for development of this little vegetable organism. Therefore, poor and insufficient food, overwork, alcoholism, worry, dissipation, surroundings—like a damp, dark or over heated dwelling— . . . all tend to make a person susceptible."[71] The moral education nurses received reinforced this answer. Circulars of information prescribed standards of conduct in class and on the wards. Nurses were expected to work hard, be honest, and respect superiors. They were to look their part and "dress in plain wash dress, with an apron of sheeting, and a two-inch straight white linen collar." Many of these requirements were standard institutional fare, but Flick's training school also tailored its rules to consumptives. Recognizing the frailty of their health, it required the trainees to sleep a full eight hours at night and rest for an additional three to four hours daily. Finally, the training program attempted to inculcate the diligence, temperance, and discipline that would allow prospective nurses both to overcome their own illness and to take their place in the wards. Nurses were to keep their rooms in order, act responsibly, and avoid "obscene and profane language," smoking, card playing, and above all alcoholic and sexual intemperance.[72]

Flick's training program consequently addressed the manifold problems that female consumptives posed. It taught them how to care for themselves and thus break the chain of infection and disease. The program of moral instruction and reform socialized the women into appropriate middle-class gender roles by teaching them to be gentle, obedient, subservient, and responsible. Both patients and sanatorium staff reinforced the lessons. Neither those above nor those below tolerated deviation from the straight and narrow. Complaints against the "scandalous affairs" of nurses, often initiated by "a patient who could not keep silent any longer" were common at White Haven.[73] If good behavior was a necessary precondition for health and social well-being, it was also essential to the economy of medical work. On the wards, the nurses, who had been hired, schooled, even created to assist White Haven's physicians, learned to "be gentle with patients, deliver diets, accompany patients on rounds." By showing constant deference to the physician's guidance, working industriously but with due concern for their own limitations, and remaining "patient, cheerful and hopeful," they would cure by precept and example.[74]

The investigation into the behavior of Miss Heibel, a nurse instructor at White Haven, demonstrates how powerfully the sanatorium's moral and medical prescriptions intertwined. The inquiry into Miss Heibel's conduct began in 1909, in response to complaints from both patients and physicians. The litany of charges against her included "contradicting" or "changing" the superintendent's and physicians' orders, failing "to report drunken behavior on the part of patients," and "giving permission for patients to visit on and off wards." Miss Heibel apparently neglected both the patients and the trainee nurses for whom she had responsibility. She allowed the nurses to "go driving with male patients" and stay out late, and she did not take proper care of their health. Such derelictions of professional duty seemed clear reflections of Miss Heibel's character. The charges against her also included taking her meals in bed, dismissing her classes so that "she could go to a moving picture show in town," and having a "friend who went walking in the mountains with a male patient." These intersections between the personal and professional appeared most clearly in allegations of "inappropriate etiquette." Flick's behavioral prescriptions taught the tuberculous nurse deference to males and expected her to cure by caring, proffering dietary advice, practicing good housekeeping, and setting a sound moral example. By calling physicians and other staff "to task, in front of patients," Miss Heibel had overstepped the bounds of both woman and nurse.[75]

Nursing consequently cost the trainee much freedom, but it also afforded her unique autonomy. As one patient wrote to Walsh, on the matter of Miss Ewing, who had been "asked to resign because of an indiscretion,"

Miss Ewing "is entirely dependent upon herself for her livelihood as she has neither parents nor brothers, and also that she is far from well and on this account could hardly do anything except nursing in an institution similar to this."[76] Flick shared the sentiment. "The organization of the class which has just been graduated was a work of necessity," he remarked on the occasion of the first training-school graduation; "we could not find suitable occupations for patients who were cured."[77] A circular of information similarly advised that the training course "intended to afford an opportunity for self support and useful career to women who have had tuberculosis," for this seemed "the most favorable kind of occupation for such patients who must earn their own living."[78]

White Haven's ambitious educational effort to equalize opportunity by arming incipient consumptives with knowledge about the dangers they faced and the skills they needed to battle disadvantage was not exceptional. Sanatoria proliferated after 1900; almost 300 new institutions opened during the decade 1900–1910.[79] Like Flick's White Haven, many of the new institutions catered primarily to consumptives with limited means, and many advertised themselves as educational institutions. These sanatoria routinely provided occupational training, which they advertised in their promotional literature. A bulletin from the Rocky Mountain Industrial Sanatorium in Denver noted, for example, that "*the entire institution will be united upon one broad plane of usefulness*; . . . the industrial, educational and co-operative features will be utilized to the end that economy, sanitation and comfort will be the attraction for patients."[80] With time, labor and occupational training became increasingly important components of the sanatorium regimen. "Many of our more progressive sanatoria resort to occupation therapy as a means of strengthening and improving the patient's health," Knopf wrote in 1913. "Graduated labor is, to my mind, one of the most valuable adjuvants we have in the hygienic and dietetic treatment of the tuberculous patient."[81]

Despite this evident expansion in numbers, the sanatorium remained a relatively limited and elite option. It catered primarily to the small population that could and would be institutionalized. White Haven, one of the larger institutions, had only 216 beds; the more typical Adirondack Cottage contained only 110. Beyond this, the sanatorium remained a costly option. When doctors' fees were added to the normal weekly charges, the cost of a week's stay often reached $100, which only the wealthiest could be expected to pay. Hence, institutions like White Haven that catered to the needs of poor consumptives found themselves in almost constant financial difficulty.

Responses to the ever-present budgetary problems that plagued sana-

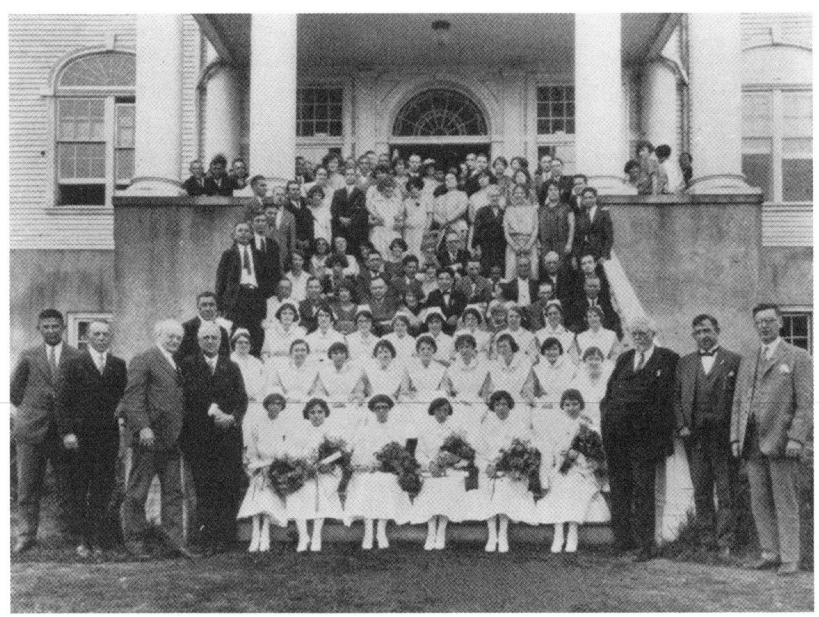

"Graduation Day—Class of 1925."
Frank A. Craig, M.D., The Story of the White Haven Sanatorium—A Memorial to Dr. Lawrence F. Flick, *47, CPP.*

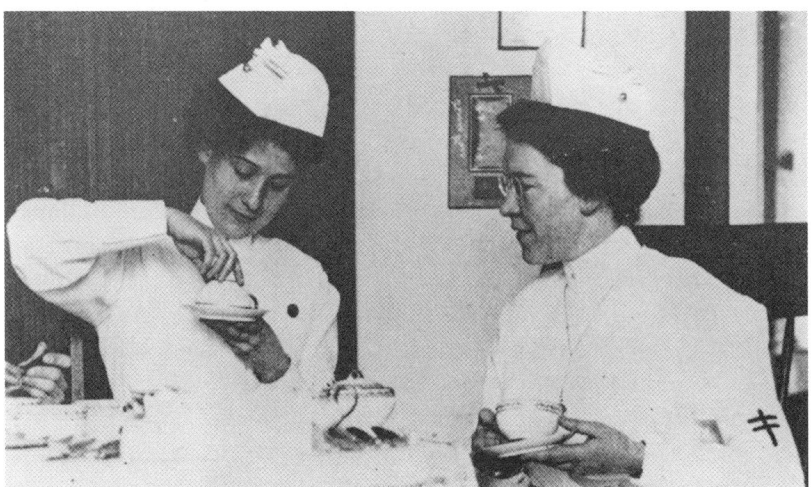

Nurses Taking Tea.
Frank A. Craig, M.D., The Story of the White Haven Sanatorium—A Memorial to Dr. Lawrence F. Flick, *50, CPP.*

toria varied. Some sanatorium directors confronted economic crises by revising their criteria for admission, emphasizing the scientific edge that tuberculin therapy lent, and restricting entry to those who could pay for at least part of the cure. Others, recognizing the magnitude of the tuberculosis problem, the links between TB and poverty, and the inability of many consumptives to pay their own way, appealed to private donors for funding. Still others urged the state to assume greater and more direct responsibility for TB control by establishing state-funded and even state-run sanatoria.

FROM CARELESS CONSUMPTIVE TO CURED CONSUMPTIVE: RHETORICS OF REHABILITATION AND REFORM

The appeal for public funding for sanatoria underscored the need for and crystallized the dilemma of extensive state intervention into the tuberculosis problem. Private sanatoria were struggling financially, and after 1906 the evidence was clear that tuberculous infection was far more widespread than anticipated. Programs that targeted a larger community were clearly necessary. But despite the apparent need state governments could not readily or easily fund sanatoria. The state's jurisdiction over the tuberculosis problem was still unresolved and entangled in a cumbersome historical tradition.

The debate over publicly funded sanatoria, although on a different level than the earlier debate over registration, engaged similar concerns about the scope of the state's police power. When sanatorium directors made their plea for funds to secure the future of existing sanatoria and to open additional institutions, some state legislatures questioned the legitimacy of public funding for tuberculosis control. Others accepted that public sanatoria were necessary but refused responsibility for treating indigent TB patients, especially those who moved easily across state lines and seemed the rightful responsibility of the federal government. Still others pleaded poverty.[82]

Requests for public funding faced yet another kind of opposition—from those who wondered whether sanatoria could do enough. In 1908, the NTA sponsored a symposium, "With a State Sanatorium Secured, What Next?", which brought to light the range of reservations to sanatorium care. The symposium participants were charity workers and physicians from major Eastern and Midwestern cities, who had different experiences with the control of tuberculosis. Though the title of the symposium suggested that the need for publicly funded sanatoria was a given, its participants were more equivocal. Both Christopher Easton of St. Paul and H. Wirt Steele of Baltimore questioned the premise that securing a state sanatorium was the "first duty" or "first step in a State anti-tuberculosis campaign." From Easton's perspective, this was "a mistaken notion," or as Steele put it, those who adopted this position "made a serious mistake; have, in fact, begun at the wrong end of the fight."[83] Neither Easton nor Steele nor any of the other participants questioned the value of the sanatorium regimen, but they equally strongly agreed that founding public sanatoria was neither a first nor a sufficient step. "With a sanatorium secured," A. E. Kepford of Des Moines asserted, "our 'what next' has been an increase in work rather than a decrease."[84] This "what next," most participants agreed, should be agitation "for a general educational campaign with the enlightenment of the community as its main object."[85]

Sanatorium directors boldly and creatively defended themselves against these varied attacks with affirmations of their institutions' educational value. In response to the argument that the state could not legitimately dispense funds to sanatoria, an astute sanatorium supporter replied that "[a] sanitorium is an educational institution, which the state has the same right to establish as to found a state university or an agricultural experiment station."[86] And if legislators questioned the benefits to be gained from their subventions, the proponents of sanatorium care responded that the state's investment would be repaid many times over because the influence of these institutions extended well beyond their walls.

Like asylums, schools, and correctional institutions, sanatoria would "serve not only as educators of individuals but as educators of communities as well,"[87] for discharged patients, who had been strengthened by their term of residence and reformed by the lessons they had learned, became the pillars of the communities to which they returned. "The knowledge [obtained within a sanitorium] is a benefit to the citizens of the whole state," one classic statement read. "People are now infected by consumption through ignorance on the part of those who give and receive infection. Each man whose habits have been corrected, even by a short residence in a sanatorium will neither do nor willingly permit to be done by others acts which before would have seemed perfectly natural."[88] Actively and by example, these enlightened patients would attack the conditions and behaviors that allowed tubercle bacilli to grow and to spread. They not only would be resistant to TB themselves but would ensure that others became resistant as well.

In the ensuing battle to secure public funding for sanatoria, the discharged patient—or cured consumptive—acquired rhetorical and even mythical significance. Sanatorium directors neither could nor regularly did claim that their institutions completely cured tuberculosis. More often, they described discharged patients as those who had learned to live with their disease. But in the face of mounting financial difficulty, cured consumptives justified both the san's existence and its appeal for support. Hence, in 1906, as he attempted to justify his training school for tuberculosis nurses and to combat White Haven's financial difficulties, Flick spoke openly of cure. Though he reluctantly noted that cure produced only a limited immunity, Flick did not let this limitation diminish the significance of the cured consumptive. Instead, he held out the cured consumptive's ability to resist relapse. "The knowledge that she had been cured before, . . . could be cured again if she suffered a relapse, . . . and will not again fall a victim to the disease," Flick maintained, filled the discharged consumptive with confidence. Thus, cured consumptives demonstrated the importance and value of teaching those with tuberculosis how to live, lent credence to Trudeau's maxim that "how" the consumptive lived was more important than "where,"[89] offered proof that TB was containable, and increased the san's sphere of influence by spreading its gospel to the communities from which patients came.

These celebrations of cured consumptives were to some degree self-serving. The mythical qualities of the discharged patient justified the path taken by Krause, Trudeau, and other medical leaders of the American antituberculosis campaign who had themselves suffered from tuberculosis. Recovery was testimony to their personal and professional successes. In prescriptions and prognoses that reflected their own experiences, hopes, and aspirations, they applauded the behaviors and conditions that assured their own health, and they used their own experience to lure others to the sanatorium way. "Among our graduates the ones who have done the best work and gone furthest in the field of tuberculosis are those who have had the disease themselves," Baldwin later wrote of his medical training program.[90] But alongside these economic and psychological contributions cured consumptives united the medical and sociological arms of the campaign against TB. They explained the physician's personal experience and justified his actions. When he assessed the campaign's needs at the 1908 NTA symposium, Warfield called for both sanatorium "care of the early causes" and "education of the public by the missionary work of the cured sanatorium cases."[91] And these defenses worked. By the end of 1910, almost 400 sanatoria, with a total of 22,838 beds, were in operation in the United States. Local or state authorities operated approximately one-third of these. Ninety percent of the institutions catered to those in the incipient or early stages of disease, and over 50 percent of their beds were free or subsidized.[92]

Nonetheless, sanatoria could not reach all who were in need either directly or through the missionary work of their former patients. Moreover, cured consumptives were amateurs in an age when Americans came to put a premium on professional expertise. As Americans came to attach increased value to professional training and sent armies of experts into the domestic sphere to promote scientific management of bedroom, nursery, and kitchen,[93] so came the call for more "specialized" and "professional" instruction about tuberculosis, which would also reach a larger population.

The writings of physician-patients provided one vehicle for disseminating expert instruction, and these writings became an increasingly frequent part of the medical armamentarium. In pocket-sized books with titles like *Rules for Recovery from Tuberculosis* and *Rest and Other Things: A Little Book of Plain Talks on Tuberculosis Problems,* Lawrason Brown, Krause, and other recovered physicians spread the rules of the cure.[94] They warned against the conditions that had made them ill, outlined the dangers of sputum, spoke of their own recovery in the san, and prescribed the rest, perseverance, and "other things" that had made them well. These tracts extended the san's sphere of influence and brought expert advice to a noninstitutionalized population.

When he wrote to Walsh, the medical director of White Haven, in 1908, William Charles White praised the care offered in sanatoria and the contributions these institutions had made to the conquest of tuberculosis. Yet White, medical director of the Pittsburgh sanatorium, was restless. Neither the san nor its missionaries seemed to reach those in greatest need— the ignorant and the poor. "With so many of the poor class of cases we come in contact with," he wrote, "I feel more and more the necessity of doing the educational work in the home and handling them in the form of classes through the dispensary."[95]

The dispensary did indeed provide state and local boards of health with the opportunity to broaden and professionalize their campaigns to build resistance. Dispensaries, with their extensive history, differed from the tuberculosis clinics the New York City Department of Health opened in 1905. These clinics, which shared characteristics with clinics for venereal disease and other specialty diseases, existed "for the treatment and supervision of patients not under care of a private physician."[96] Dispensaries, which had long linked the goals of medicine, public health, and social reform, brought outpatient care to the urban poor. In their twentieth-century form, they emphasized rehabilitation through education. Physicians stressed the educational motif as they repeatedly spoke of dispensaries as offering "home treatment in small classes under the supervision of doctors and nurses."[97] After 1910, dispensaries effectively became head-quarters for state-sponsored educational programs, and their numbers proliferated.[98]

State and local boards of health also expanded their sphere of influence by sending nurses into tuberculous homes. By 1915, armies of visiting nurses formed an integral component of the crusade against TB. The sanatorium regimen had combined sputum management with a biosocial rehabilitation; visiting nurses waged a similarly multifaceted campaign against spit, this time directed primarily at immigrants and the poor. They too began their work with instruction about the control of sputum and the best means to prevent the spread of infection. "Better knowledge in regard to the transmission of tuberculosis, the causes, and especially the dangers of insanitary practices," the New York City Department of Health proclaimed, "[is] always reflected in lower morbidity and mortality."[99] However, visiting nurses did not restrict their efforts to sanitary instruction. "Public Health nursing," the New York City Department of Health reassured physicians, who feared an invasion of their turf, "is, to a large extent, the teaching of hygiene in the home."[100]

This effort to teach hygiene in the home allowed the nurse to combine sanitary instruction with home improvement; she became, in the words of one physician, "a kind of home missionary."[101] In this role, the visiting public health nurse shared much with the sanatorium nurse or the discharged patient. Her lessons about cleanliness, like their lessons about sputum management, had a more ambitious and directive mission. These lessons promoted the skills—scientific management of bedroom, nursery, and kitchen—that women needed to do their work efficiently and well. But, as was the case at the sanatorium, the visiting nurse's lessons also included a healthy dose of moralism. In the interests of controlling tuberculosis, she closely monitored and commented on domestic relations. She too attempted to rehabilitate her charges with assistance that would help them adjust to both "social and economic problems."[102]

POVERTY, DEGENERACY, AND THE JURISDICTION OF THE STATE

The expansion of state activity against tuberculosis into dispensaries and public health nursing reflected a growing demand for measures that would combat the social dimensions of the disease. By 1915, medical reformers repeatedly argued that it was useless to treat tuberculosis independently of poverty. Like White, first director of the Medical Research Committee of the National Tuberculosis Association (NTA), and subsequently director of tuberculosis research at the Hygienic Laboratory, they maintained that "tuberculosis is closely associated with all the social problems of housing, food, wages, rest, clothing, and insurance and can in no way be separated from them."[103]

The evolving debate on how to combat both the disease and the social conditions that bred it turned on two interrelated questions: what constituted poverty and who had responsibility for it. In the era of the First World War, American discussions of poverty were powerfully mediated by the threat of degeneracy and the agenda of Progressivism. As a result concern about tuberculosis intersected with new fears about ethnicity, gender, and dependency. TB symbolized the imminent demise of the American nation.

Americans articulated these fears in several ways. Some looked outward to the experiences of war-torn Europe and scapegoated the European immigrants who sought refuge in American cities. Graphic evidence of the toll that overwork, poor housing, and malnutrition exacted fed self-congratulation about American exceptionalism. It also fueled warnings about the importation of disease.[104] The Framingham demonstration, an extensive community survey begun in December 1916 under the auspices of the NTA, indicated that rates of tuberculous infection among Italian, Irish, Jewish, and "other" nationalities were often twice the rate for "Americans."[105]

Imported deviance offered a familiar and ready explanation for American illness, but the causes of tuberculosis also appeared closer to home in such by-products of urbanization as physical and mental overstrain and "dissipation." Poor housing conditions and new patterns of work seemed disproportionately to affect mothers and children, whom refined methods of sputum testing and roentgenography, along with tuberculin testing, repeatedly identified as populations at special risk. A Von Pirquet survey of children aged one to seven, conducted during the summer of 1917 as part of the Framingham demonstration, indicated that from the time they entered school girls had a far greater incidence of tuberculosis; "33% of the males [aged 6–7] were found to be positive and 55% of females."[106] The First World War reinforced fears about the impact of American ways on the health of youth; the selective service draft found that "latent tubercular disease" left almost 5.4 percent of recruits ineligible for service in the armed forces.[107]

Responses to disease among immigrants, women, and children varied. Eugenics circumscribed the views of those to whom increases in the number of tuberculous Americans bespoke the costs of unwise population and immigration policies. After 1912, when Karl Pearson, Francis Galton's champion and successor, proposed that tuberculosis was a "family disease,"[108] the American Charles Davenport repeatedly marshaled evidence collected at his Eugenics Record Office to make the case that TB ran in families.[109] For advocates of this hereditarian position, the solution to the tuberculosis problem was simple: careful selective breeding.[110] Through the early 1920s, the Eugenics Record Office issued a steady stream of memos and bulletins that warned against the droves of immigrants who imported both TB and the tubercular predisposition into the United States, and it issued proposals to restrict the immigration of consumptives.[111] Because so many consumptives and incipient consumptives already lived in the United States, some eugenists viewed immigration restriction as only a partial solution and further endorsed the sterilization of consumptives or legal sanctions to prevent them from marrying.

Eugenic interpretations of tuberculosis were common, but few Americans adopted narrow eugenic solutions. Much as eugenists might wish to invoke "purely biological causes, such as the development of immunity and resistance by heredity and natural selection,"[112] neither logic nor epidemiological evidence supported the hereditarian argument. Natural selection could not explain why tuberculosis prevailed in cities, among women, or among those in particular occupations. "Heredity requires generations to accomplish changes like this," one particularly outspoken critic argued, "but environmental conditions can bring them about in a few years and almost in months."[113] Hence, many of the physicians who picked up on the degeneracy question in the early 1920s had little desire to paint the alternatives starkly or reduce the debate to a form of "zero sum" explanation in which either heredity or environment became cause and cure of the tuberculosis problem. They recognized a midpoint between the two extremes and linked TB with degeneracy, but they attributed degeneracy at least in part to environmental and social circumstances that acted with heredity to create a predisposition. As Krause noted, the control of tuberculosis depended on the avoidance of "over-strain, . . . mental and physical," and "dissipation," "not *because it laid [people] open to infection but because it supplied the oil to a wick that was already present.*"[114] Perfectly consistent with contemporary embryology and genetics, this accommodation also justified the campaign's focus on the "tubercular soil."

Krause saw the imperative clearly. In his classic essay *Environment and Resistance in Tuberculosis*, he stressed the importance of looking closely at the environmental causes of TB, which in his view included "the cities, the streets, the houses and backyards, the rooms in which we live and move, the baths, the windows, the stoves, the furniture, the clothing, the space, air and sunlight which people may or may not have."[115] He advocated further environmental reforms, which moved beyond these physical conditions. He urged his colleagues to look as well to "an environment of occupation" and a "social and political environment—which will allow the greatest freedom and play of individuality."[116] Thus, Krause fundamentally linked the challenge of eradicating tuberculosis to reformist campaigns to reduce poverty and increase opportunity. "More or less poverty in a community," he wrote, "will mean more or less tuberculosis, so will more or less crowding and improper housing, more or less unhygienic occupations and industry."[117]

There were several ways to meet the challenge that physicians like Krause identified. His own solution was to "contribute to the attainment of civic decency and cleanliness; of light, space and food enough for all; of a rational proportion of working and leisure hours for those who cannot dispose of their own time; and the reduction of preventable infections to a minimum."[118] But the task of altering these physical and social environments was complex; it reflected the broad objectives of Progressive social reform and underscored the need for federal intervention. White, who had long linked tuberculosis control and poor relief, spoke forcefully of this "[f]ederal duty to the tuberculosis problem." There was no greater concern to the "welfare of the whole people" than health in general and tuberculosis in particular, White insisted.[119] The proliferation of institutions and cures required a form of standardization that only federal institutions could provide. Moreover, as indigent consumptives traveled in search of the ideal cure, they invariably crossed state lines. Animal disease, hidden disease, and interstate, intercity, or international transfer of disease blurred jurisdictional boundaries.

These calls for federal control of tuberculosis coincided with other debates over state-sponsored medical and social relief. Those intersections were clear in the legislation that made its way to the floor of Congress. In 1914 and 1916, the House and Senate introduced, side by side, bills to "standardize the treatment of tuberculosis" and "provide state support for indigent consumptives." Other initiatives, like the Kent Bill (1917), incorporated the call for tuberculosis-control measures into debates over broader medical and social reforms, such as the demand for welfare and a national health service.[120] Throughout, physicians, social workers, and public health authorities agreed that TB reflected a "social problem as much as one of medicine and public health,"[121] and this insistence on the need to fully connect medical and social reform efforts helped to forestall the larger campaign for national health insurance.

The overlapping debates over governmental responsibility for tuberculosis and for national health and insurance systems did not simplify the effort to expand the state's jurisdiction over tuberculosis. If tuberculosis was essentially an outcome of poverty, then Americans could argue interminably over which level of government should assume responsibility for relief. Proposals for action consequently fell headlong into what White described as "that slippery chute, called 'States Rights' on which our ablest agents of government start their downward course to oblivion."[122] Peculiarly American concerns about welfare further exacerbated the conflict and acted as a powerful constraint on the reformist agenda.[123] If more frequent appeals to an activist state characterized the rhetoric of turn-of-the-century American reform, so did classic American fears about dependency and state intervention into commercial, private, or moral matters. Like those who preceded them, the new generation of reformers feared "barren relief system[s]" that would "destroy incentive" or stifle the independence of individuals. They demanded instead initiatives that would create a fair environment or "increase incentive by more nearly equalizing opportunity."[124]

These concerns surfaced in the debate over tuberculosis control, especially in a forum on governmental responsibility for the prevention of tuberculosis that the NTA sponsored in 1919. This forum brought together hygienic, medical, and industrial interests. Among those who spoke were the Progressive physicians Lloyd, Eugene Kelley, and Gordon Dickinson, as well as the labor arbitrator John Lapp. These participants agreed on the need for sanatoria, educational initiatives, and measures to prevent bovine tuberculosis. They further agreed about the need for "[b]etter living conditions, more and better food and clothing for the poor, better housing and working conditions, closer supervision of the lives of the working classes by persons competent to advise and help, particularly by physicians, nurses and social workers, . . . [and rehabilitation] of the indigent and partially dependent tuberculosis victim."[125] Lloyd and Dickinson spoke passionately for centralized, governmental efforts to ensure that these changes would occur. Lloyd argued particularly strongly for the creation of a Division of Tuberculosis within the PHS. Subtly conflating concerns about state's rights, jurisdiction, and democracy, Kelley equally passionately decried "complete self-functioning Federal or state systems of tuberculosis control," which then directed "the ultimate social units in which the consumptives live to open their civic mouths and swallow such systems ready made." To Kelley, the recommendations for centralized control smelled of "autocratic," "Prussian" methods, which would suffocate the "social soul inspiring our tuberculosis movement," and he advocated a very different type of reform. He insisted that it "must rest upon the fundamental concept that the state should do only such things as will assist local communities to perform better the antituberculosis functions and obligations that rest upon them." Lapp added another dimension. The need for federal intervention, he argued, was inextricably tied to the need for universal social and health insurance.[126]

In his comments on Lapp's paper, Dr. C. V. Craster integrated the varied arguments in favor of broad, governmental intervention. Ninty-five percent of tuberculous cases were indigents who bore no blame for either their poverty or their illness. The "tuberculosis case is not due to any fault of the patient," Craster argued, "but is a direct blot upon our community living methods which allowed a citizen to contract a disabling and frequently fatal disease."[127] Honest, upstanding, and hard-working Americans fell ill because they could not afford decent homes, food, and clothing. Once ill, they were bankrupted by the expenses of sanatorium treatment. From Craster's perspective, the interrelated medical and sociological demands of tuberculosis not only justified but necessitated state intervention. "[I]t is along the social help lines that our anti-tuberculosis work has been weakest," he argued; the indigent consumptive "needs assistance from the state as much as he needs medicine and open air."[128]

These debates over governmental control of tuberculosis turned on questions of the relief of poverty—the remedy of the inequality or dependency that already existed. As such, they ran up against jurisdictional, monetary, and ideological objections. Measures that prevented poverty presented what seemed a simpler and more attractive alternative. A campaign to improve the health of children, launched through the joint action of the state and voluntary agencies, offered this alternative.

VOLUNTARISM, THE PRESS, AND THE DOMESTIC ECONOMY

"Let us ask ourselves the question—What is the tuberculosis problem?" Lloyd challenged his colleagues in 1919. "Reduced to the lowest terms [the factors in the spread of this disease] are these: the tubercle bacillus on the one hand and the newborn baby on the other."[129] Having identified these two targets, Lloyd and others focused their attention on the children.[130] Their efforts to make children grow strong and tall merged the efforts of the state, voluntary agencies, and the press and fully melded the goals of medical and social reform.

Since at least the time of Tocqueville, voluntary associations have been extolled as one of the defining characteristics of American exceptionalism; their role in the anti-TB crusade was part of this legacy. By 1904, when the NASPT amalgamated their efforts, a multitude of local voluntary associations for the study and prevention of TB had emerged. Some, like the Pennsylvania Society for the Prevention of Tuberculosis, formed part of a venerable tradition that marshaled private energy and funds for poor relief. Others, like the Henry Phipps Institute for the Study and Prevention of Tuberculosis, represented a new effort to channel industrial wealth into biomedical research.

After 1900 state and local boards of health came increasingly to cooperate and join forces with these voluntary agencies in their campaigns against TB. Whereas under Biggs's direction the New York City Department of Health had acted alone, by the turn of the century it had linked up with the Charity Organization Society of New York to publish and disseminate flyers, pamphlets, and placards that again combined information and moral exhortation.[131] Nor was this an isolated example. In almost every major city cooperative ventures of some sort were undertaken, and the product typically involved this layering on of behavioral, prescriptive advice. The alliance between boards of health and voluntary agencies developed because the voluntary agencies offered the state several commodities in otherwise short supply: expertise, free and enthusiastic manpower, and a legitimate vehicle for achieving its goals when blunt state action might have appeared too intrusive. More important, however, the alliance between boards of health and voluntary agencies flourished because the two acted synergistically to promote a therapeutic of social reform. This synergism was most apparent in the campaign to promote the health of children.

The campaign to prevent the spread of tuberculosis among children began with the legislative and behavioral efforts to curb the spread of spit and, particularly, to prevent the infection of children. The needs of the innocent and unprotected child justified a range of interventions, from those that sanitized the home to those that prohibited public spitting. Could anyone, Dr. David Lyman asked, argue that the adult's right to do as he pleased was "greater than the right possessed by every child that is helpless to . . . determine its own surroundings—the right to receive from the community every reasonable chance to bring to its later tasks of life a sane mind in a healthy body?"[132]

The effort to prevent tuberculosis in children also expanded rapidly beyond the bacillus to become "essentially one for improving nutrition by food and personal hygiene."[133] Metabolic research conducted during the 1910s and 1920s, confirmed what the experiences of war-torn Europe had suggested. In Europe, the declines in tuberculosis mortality that began during the late nineteenth century seemed to reverse steadily as war depleted food supplies. In American labs, diets deficient in fat-soluble vitamins predisposed animals to TB.[134] Interest in the therapeutic properties of sunlight further stimulated nutritional research. By the 1920s many Americans understood that sunlight acted as an aid to digestion, and articles in both technical and popular journals advised that children, like plants, needed sunshine to grow. As one popular writer phrased it, "Every scrap of our food is canned sunshine."[135] Other research pointed to the ways in which "exhaustion and malnutrition in the host contribute to disease."[136] Though poor nutrition threatened their physical health, Americans, unlike Europeans, could not complain of an inadequate food supply. Even during the war, they had been blessed with cheap and abundant food. Thus, Americans' dietary deficiencies seemed consequences of ignorance and poor behaviors rather than material deprivation. Diets heavy in coffee, sweets, white bread, and meat spawned a generally malnourished youth.

Physician reformers once again carved out a range of responses to malor undernourishment. The Sheppard-Towner Act, which provided support to mothers and children, represented the most pointed intervention.[137] However, just as they had questioned the wisdom of other welfare schemes, so some physicians doubted that supplemental food allowances would remedy the ignorance and lack of opportunity that seemed to them to underlie the problem fundamentally. In the Lane Lectures, which he delivered at Stanford University in December 1921, Luther Emmett Holt spelled out the problem. Professor of the diseases of children at Columbia University and president of the Child Health Organization, Holt had conducted one of the first large-scale studies of tuberculin tests in American youth. In books and lectures, he publicized the effects of malnourishment on health and applauded recent reductions in tuberculous mortality, which he attributed to improved food, better personal hygiene, and supplementary treatments. But, Holt warned, "[n]ot much of this had been accomplished by legislative means; most of it is the result of educational measures."[138]

This appeal to education led to the voluntary agencies, which, despite their differing agendas, agreed on the centrality of using education to eliminate tuberculosis among children. Through a series of pamphlets and books the NTA taught children the regular habits that would minimize contact with tubercle bacilli, foster good personal hygiene, and promote general strength. It made a special effort to relay these messages in ways that children might find particularly appealing, and the exhortations of "Tommy Tubercle" and "Huber the Tuber" became an especially popular instructional device.

Voluntary associations also allowed for more creative and active interventions. In 1917, Charles DeForest launched his Modern Health Crusade.

DeForest, a field secretary for the NTA, had begun his career in charity work. He envisioned the crusade as part of a broader plan to "bring anew to the world a vital interest in the chivalry of health."[139] The crusade would contribute more generally to the creation of a strong and healthy race, DeForest and his disciples argued, by teaching children to recognize the sources of infection, by imparting the physical and moral strength they needed to battle disease, and by inspiring interest in "the laws of the community at large which bear on public health."[140]

The crusade took the form of a game in which youngsters "jousted for honors" and received points, titles, and medals as rewards for their chivalry. It employed literature, posters, and rule books to teach children the gospel of health. These lessons instructed children to play outdoors; eat wholesome food; avoid sugar, stimulants, and tobacco; dress tidily and properly; and visit their doctor and dentist regularly.[141] To spread the crusade's benefits to the larger community, children assumed the role of health police. One of the crusade's challenges had the players survey their neighborhoods and mark the "unhygienic" homes on a map.

The focus on children reminded some physicians, like Knopf, that children formed part of a household economy in which women, especially mothers, played a defining and even determining role. Knopf's first objective was to prevent infection in infancy and childhood. Hence, he dwelt on those measures that would increase the resistance of the host, which included practices that would combat other childhood diseases and included also, of course, heliotherapy, nutrition, and education. "The child of today is the man and the citizen of tomorrow," he maintained. To ensure that these citizens-in-training grew up healthy and strong, he drew attention to the home environment. Knopf initially proposed that children born to tuberculous parents be placed in the custody of healthy foster mothers through institutions like Biggs's Foster Parents Health Club. Under such care, they would be kept out of the way of infecting microbes and also would be rendered more resistant. "During the day proper food, rest, fresh air, sun and medical treatment are given to the club's tiny members," he quoted, "their play is directed and health, hygiene and right habits are taught."[142]

In addition to measures that removed children from tuberculous homes, Knopf recognized the need to retrain "the prospective mothers of the race."[143] His concern with women differed from earlier efforts. Turn-of-the-century American concerns about the preponderance of tuberculosis among young women had exposed dual fears: about the emergence of industry and about female aspirations to a male, or public, sphere. Unhealthy city habits seemed not only to leave girls easy prey to tubercle bacilli but also to violate the norms of acceptable female behavior, and alongside apprehensions about the stamina of the mill girl grew fears about morals and about the impact that TB might have on working women's abilities to fulfill their lives as good wives and mothers. By the 1920s, American physicians articulated their apprehensions about female competition and female emancipation increasingly clearly. Haunted by the specter of degeneracy, they subtly shifted target and chastised "modern women" for departing from traditional roles with the suggestion that modernity—or, more particularly, women's entry into the public sphere—created an environment in which tuberculosis flourished. In December 1928, the surgeon general of the PHS bemoaned the stresses that women were subjected to as they tried to take on the multiple roles of student, employee, mother, and wife. Women's desire to work "while still being a lady" and while striving for slimness and education would compromise their health he warned.[144]

Knopf provided the clearest statement of these fears when, in his essay "Tuberculosis among Young Women," he proposed that one could trace morbidity and mortality to young women's "insane desire . . . [t]o attain a boyish appearance." The quest for androgyny, he lamented, led many "hard working employees in factories, workshops or offices" to "voluntarily submit themselves to undernourishment." Though particularly sensitive to the threat that working women posed, Knopf did not restrict his criticisms to the laboring classes. He targeted as well women at the other end of the spectrum who, under their flimsy dresses, donned "the tightly laced brassiere or wide elastic band, tightly adjusted over the breasts to increase the boyish appearance" and who assumed the "stooping posture" so characteristic of educated girls. Both sets of women, Knopf charged, shirked their duties to the race. Their frivolous quests for a better figure and more amusing life not only compromised their own health but also sped the racial tumble into oblivion, for it led women to ignore the well-being of their children.[145]

In the wake of pronouncements like Knopf's, the imminent threat of tuberculosis became a vehicle for inculcating appropriate middle-class female behavior and for targeting women's fraught relationships with dress, sexuality, and food. Romanticized in literature as pallid, languishing, and virginal, the incipient consumptive more often conjured images of a female scantily clad, driven, and oversexed.[146] Knopf's rebuke of flappers, who, clad in "decollete" and "extremely short" dresses, chilled themselves by donning "thin silk stockings and low shoes" in even the coldest weathers, was typical. The "narrow skirt and the absurdly small but very high heel on the otherwise low shoes," which attracted undue attention,

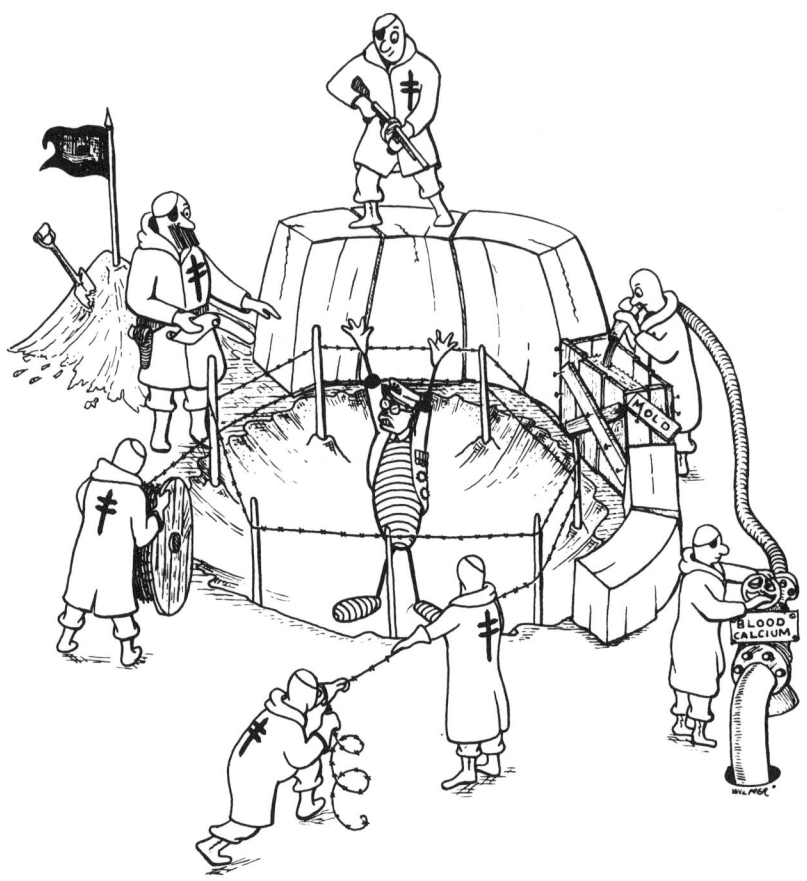

The National Tuberculosis Association capitalized on mythical battles to rally children. Following the First World War, the symbolism of St. George and his struggle against the dragon dominated the crusade. By the Second World War, the battle against tuberculosis was compared to battles against German and Japanese enemies.
Source: Harry A. Wilmer, M.D., The Lives and Loves of Huber the Tuber (New York, NTA, 1942), 63.

intensified women's sexuality, and inhibited the development of a healthy stride or gait, also provoked his physicians' wrath.

When physicians assessed the factors that made women susceptible, however, dress and even sex seemed secondary to food. Having identified poor diet as one cause of TB and having attributed inadequate nutrition to behavior rather than opportunity, physicians had little difficulty finding fault with women's eating habits. "In order to lose or not put on any

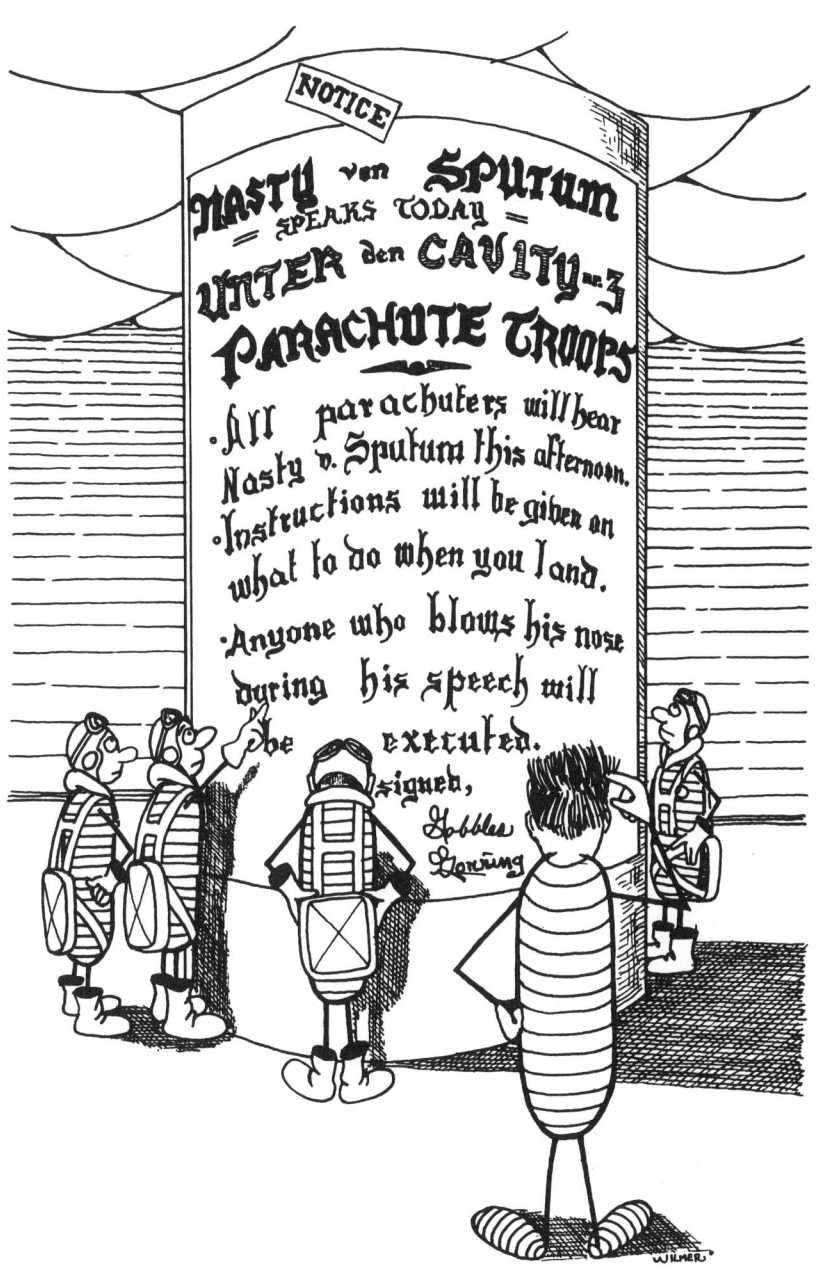

Source: Harry A. Wilmer, M.D., The Lives and Loves of Huber the Tuber *(New York, NTA, 1942), 65.*

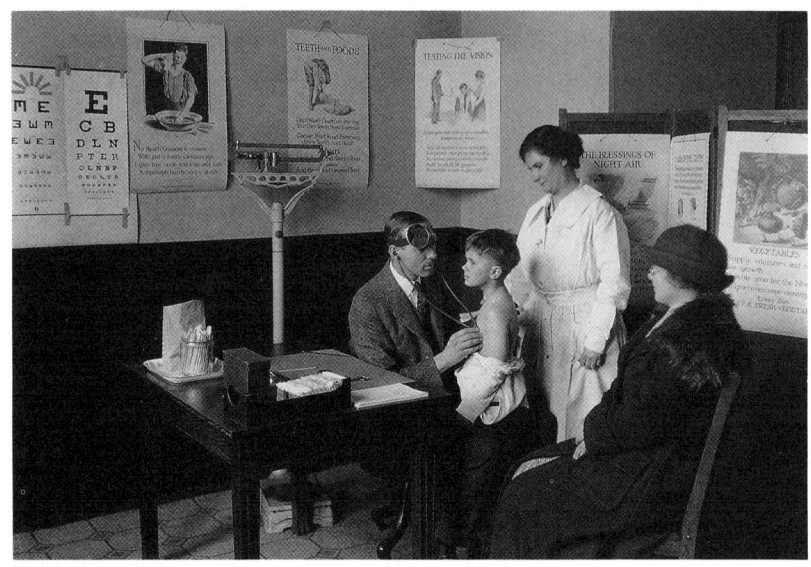

Finding TB among the city's poor: chest exam at a city dispensary, Toronto, 1923.
Source: City of Toronto Archives RG 8-32-682.

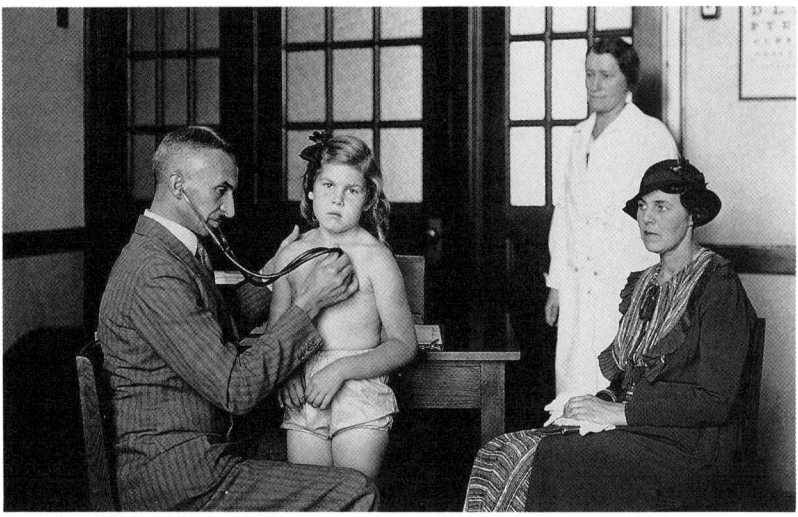

Preventing disease in the mothers of tomorrow: chest exam at a public school in an upper middle class community, Toronto, 1919.
Source: City of Toronto Archives RG 8-32-852.

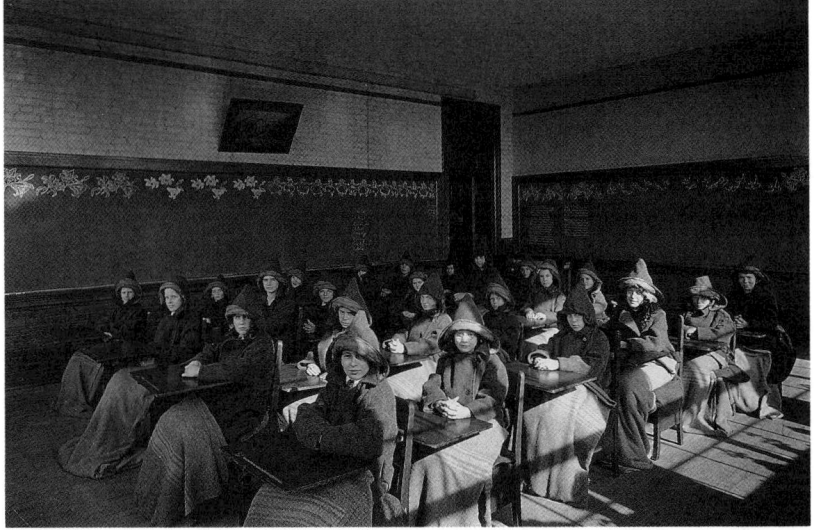

Learning to live with TB: The Orde Street Open Air School, Toronto, 1919.
Source: City of Toronto Archives RG 8-32-613.

weight," Knopf charged, too many working women "content themselves with an ice cream cone, a cup of coffee or a sandwich at luncheon time, hastily swallowed," with the result that they soon became tuberculous.[147] Yet if dieting actually predisposed young women to infection, the fad for pallor and thinness seemed also to disguise their symptoms. Eagerly active women of the twenties often hid or ignored their illness.

Here, Eleanor Roosevelt proved typical. In 1919, while traveling in France, Roosevelt became ill with the tuberculous lesion that ultimately caused her death. Physicians warned her, at the time, that her illness might be tuberculosis, but she glibly waved them aside. "They were simply unused to my pink and white English complexion," she wrote in the first edition of her autobiography.[148] Soon after her return to North America, in the aftermath of her husband's affair with Lucy Mercer, Roosevelt developed what her biographer Blanche Cook has labeled anorexia; she stopped eating and grew exceptionally thin.[149] Whether Roosevelt actually became anorexic or whether these were undiagnosed signs of her tuberculosis remains unclear. Regardless, the ambiguity of Roosevelt's symptoms speaks to the complexity of women's experience with tuberculosis. If women hid their disease, fashion also allowed it to go undetected. "Rouge and lipstick," Knopf warned, too often "hide the anemic condition [until] the cough cannot be suppressed, the loss of weight becomes emaciation, and other symptoms make a serious state of health evident to family and friends."[150]

The campaign to convince young women that it was better to be overweight than underweight and healthier to have a good appetite formed only one part of the reform agenda. In the Lane Lectures, Holt also characterized women's preparation of food as a problem within the domestic economy. Holt typified the physicians who identified uneducated mothers as a chief cause of the malnourishment of youth in the United States. He consequently exhorted his colleagues to use their professional standing, clinics, and dispensaries to teach young mothers the scientific principles of sound diet. Holt also challenged his colleagues to inculcate the regular, disciplined habits that would compel women to practice the sound nutritional lessons they had learned. Classes and public lectures in domestic hygiene facilitated these behavioral transformations, but once again they reached only select audiences.[151]

Sensitive to the power and appeal of the media, other physicians chose not to use the clinic as intermediary and issued their prescriptions instead via the popular press.[152] Through the 1920s, Dr. S. Josephine Baker (director of New York City's Bureau of Child Hygiene), Dr. Logan Clendening (professor of medicine at the University of Kansas and popularizer of medical knowledge), Dr. Josephine Hemenway Kinyoun, and other notable physicians contributed regular columns to such magazines as *Good Housekeeping, Saturday Evening Post,* and *Ladies' Home Journal.* Their articles extolled the benefits of sound diet, sunshine, fresh air, and wholesome living.[153] They also chastised "modern women" for departing from traditional roles, jeopardizing their own health, and compromising the country's future. And they attempted, through both gentle persuasion and harsh rebuke, to lure the wayward wife back into her kitchen.

In a typical piece, Clendening commended his country's efforts to reduce tuberculous mortality by ensuring its citizens a cheap and abundant supply of food. Yet, he lamented, young American women threw away all the advantages that science and industrialization had to offer by "reach[ing] for a cigarette instead of a banana."[154] Clendening's essay, entitled "Breakfastless Children, Tuberculous Youth," offered a scathing indictment of the urban woman, who in her frivolous quest for a better figure and more amusing life ignored the health of her children. He condemned the lazy and selfish mother, who compromised the future of the race by allowing her offspring to imitate her own bad habits. "Poor breakfastless children," Clendening wrote, "Mother is still in bed during the breakfast hour and father has gone to work. Or mother and father have gone to work. Or mother has gone to a lecture on the multilateral treaty, or on Is Progress Real—or Ain't It? Or best joke of all, she has gone to the baby clinic. Mother is weighing babies and the kitchen looks sort of messy and unappetizing. It has become an unfrequented spot. So we'll just bolt a little cold breakfast food, or half a glass of milk and get started. We can buy a pickle at the delicatessen on the way to school."[155] Clendening's rhetoric was particularly colorful, but at base his solution was a quite typical one from those who, touched by the eugenic argument, rested hope for control of TB on educated motherhood. An advocate of educational efforts that taught mothers better habits and reminded them that their public and private duties were inseparable, he exemplified the medical drive to create a healthy home environment.

Historians have written much about the broader, maternalist campaign of which Clendening formed a part. They have described it in the language of social control, demonstrating the ways in which the premium placed on specialized, professional knowledge devalued informal ways of knowing and justified professional intrusion into the domestic sphere. They have also reinterpreted the processes of domination to assign women agency and accord them a more activist role.[156] Both analytical traditions might be applied to the campaign to educate mothers about tuberculosis. If male physicians, who used their professional standing to regulate women's behavior, provided much of the impetus, so did Baker, Kinyoun, other women physicians, and armies of public health nurses and social workers who promoted scientific management of bedroom, nursery, and kitchen. The strong voluntary component also ensured women a place in the antituberculosis campaign. As club women and philanthropists, they too prescribed measures that reinforced standards of female conduct. What united their disparate efforts and bridged the professional/nonprofessional, male/female, and public/private divides was the effort to define the characteristics not just of female but of middle-class life. As Florence Deakins Becker, an active participant in local and international antituberculosis clubs, demonstrated, the crusade against tuberculosis equated the healthful with the genteel, and it encouraged women to aspire to a personal and domestic norm that was both. Moreover, the crusade became a vehicle for women's action and organizing that harnessed women's energies both inside and outside the home.[157]

The efforts to combat tuberculosis and define the middle classes intersected at more than a behavioral level. Clendening's advice did much to promote proper domestic activity. Good for children, good for women, good for the American middle class, his consignment of women to the kitchen was also good for the cereal, flour, and baking powder producers who often backed him financially. If physicians and club women spoke with the voice of moral certainty, corporations saw the economic advantages to be gained from the antituberculosis campaign. Thus, as middle-class cooking came to define what was at once healthful, wholesome, socially commendable, and economically lucrative, corporations increasingly promoted the medical advantages of their products and employed physicians to provide endorsements.

The intersections between moral regulation and financial gain became particularly clear as physicians extended their investigation of the domestic causes of tuberculosis beyond food to housekeeping. For decades, physicians had maintained that TB germs did not themselves pose a threat but the imprudent or slovenly housekeeper possessed the power to transform them into a menace. Poorly washed drinking cups and improperly laundered linens became potential vehicles for the spread of disease. So did damp and dark rooms. Nothing, however, carried greater liability than dust. Medical and popular manuals of the early twentieth century repeatedly warned that dried sputum, which lived in dust, was the greatest source of infection. Hence, they frequently issued instructions about the proper method of sweeping floors. As an adulation of the outdoor life once again shaped standards of health and conduct, physicians advised women to open their windows and let in cleansing sun. By the 1920s, however, corporatism outweighed environmentalism. If the dutiful woman could protect her family by first wetting the floor and ensuring that the area she intended to sweep was well-ventilated, or by letting sunshine sanitize her home, she could protect it still more with "sunlight powder" soaps or, better still, a vacuum cleaner.

EDUCATION AS THERAPY

Between 1900 and 1930, then, American physicians formulated a coherent therapeutic of social reform against tuberculosis that attempted on the one hand to control spit and on the other to discourage the physical and social conditions that made it a problem. In sanatoria, boards of health, and voluntary agencies, they grafted principles of hygiene to educational strategies in order to transform the behaviors that left women, children, and immigrants vulnerable to tubercle bacilli.

This strategy represented a diplomatic response to a situation at once scientifically and socially uncomfortable. Despite his promises, Koch's identification of the tubercle bacillus yielded few practical solutions. Through the first decades of the twentieth century, the relationship between infection and disease remained uncertain, and while few American physicians doubted the etiological role of Koch's bacillus, equally few accepted it as

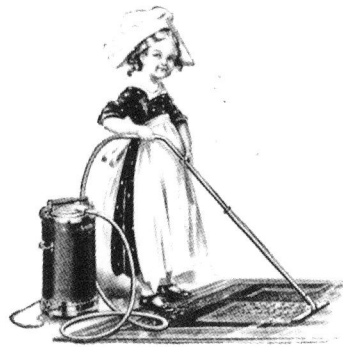
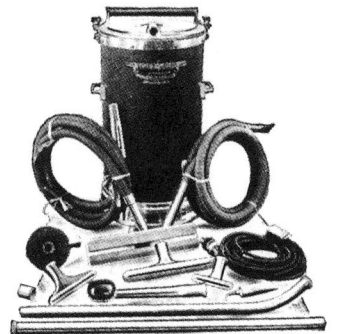
Ad for a Vacuum Cleaner.

Source: Philip P. Jacobs, A Tuberculosis Directory *(New York: NASPT, 1911), advertisements, XII.*

the single or sole cause of tuberculosis. In the absence of a neat one-to-one correlation between infection and disease, physicians could not ignore the importance of the conditions in which the susceptible host lived. And lacking either the ability to destroy the microbe or the certainty that infection led necessarily to disease, they focused their efforts instead on the creation of those conditions that would prevent the bacillus from doing any harm. As Krause had put it, they called for measures that *"would have the emphasis laid on the behavior of the human being and not on the bacillus."*[158]

The campaign's direction should not be dismissed as a last resort, a compromise course of action, or even a simple program of social control. In the campaign to limit spit and spread polish, reformer physicians had discovered a way of simultaneously fighting disease and inculcating middle class values. They demonstrated that those who worked steadily, cared for their health, shunned self-indulgence, valued self-discipline, and took pride in maintaining their independence and self-sufficiency were less susceptible to tuberculosis than those who did not. Their efforts to control bacilli and behaviors, particularly when brought outside of institutions and disseminated by trained armies of experts, served the needs of an emerging middle class bent on reforming society in its image.

This campaign drew strength from its similarity to and association with social reform; most significantly, it captured both the hopes and fears of the emerging Progressive movement. In the decades straddling the turn of the century, TB continued to serve as a metaphor for the ills of urban-industrial society, and so it dovetailed especially neatly with the Progressives' larger critique of American society. In few other diseases did the ill effects of crowding, overwork, malnutrition, ignorance, and lost opportunity, or the threat that these posed to the health of American society, emerge more clearly.

Ideological in its ends, the American campaign against TB turned to ideological means of education. As physicians came to understand TB as a social disease, they were forced to confront the dilemmas that bedeviled broader efforts at social reform. And as they did so, they turned to education to provide an effective and legitimate thrust to their anti-TB campaigns. Like the larger movements of social reform that rose to prominence at the turn of the century, the anti-TB campaign sought to inspire and empower citizens to preserve their own health by resisting the forces of corruption. In keeping with the Progressive view that enlightenment was the precondition for progress, the campaign reassured Americans that TB could be conquered. No goal was more sacrosanct than the self-reliant individual citizen; no instrument was more consistent with American cultural norms than education; and no institutions were more appropriate to direct these efforts than private sanatoria and voluntary agencies.

Contrary to what some historians have suggested, the educational and sociological concerns that motivated many of the TB crusaders were neither confined to social workers and reformers nor consigned to the flank of the American campaign against tuberculosis. The choice of education was not half-hearted, adopted only as an alternative when other more promising strategies were foreclosed, unsuccessful, or abandoned. Among anti-TB campaigners, education was not a second-best instrument. Instead, they embraced it, believed in it, defended it, and raised it as the standard against which all other preventives and therapies should be measured. It was precisely the device needed to root out what they believed to be the cause of TB—namely, "ignorance on the part of those who give and receive the infection."[159]

Education appealed to a range of physicians for a variety of reasons. Education of the people, some suggested, would in turn educate the state.[160] Even those who feared that more intrusive measures were both inappropriate and illegitimate state activities found a program based on education irreproachable. In boards of health, sanatoria, and voluntary agencies, physicians underscored the centrality of education to their tuberculosis-control efforts. For example, the Henry Phipps Institute, a voluntary agency that promoted tuberculosis research, prided itself on its educational initiatives. Initially an outgrowth of the Pennsylvania Society, designed to unite sociological with medical concerns, Phipps turned increasingly to laboratory and clinical investigations after 1905. By 1910 the institute had become the preeminent center for TB research in the United States. Still, it continued to devote 10 per cent of its budget to educational programs. While this represented less than half the amount allotted to research, it went a long way toward the maintenance of a strong presence in the area of education.[161] The NTA also underscored the centrality of education in its own crusade against TB. The association's by-laws both acknowledged education as a necessary and legitimate function and made formal provision for educational work. Moreover, at the association's first annual meeting, newly elected president Trudeau conspicuously emphasized the association's commitment to education with the assertion that "the first and greatest need is education."[162]

Trudeau's testimony is especially significant, for in a very real way he may be said to personify the complexity of the turn-of-the-century American campaign to control TB. At the apogee of his career as throughout it, Trudeau—the great supporter of Koch, advocate of thoroughgoing measures of administrative control, sanatorium director, and researcher—continued like so many others to believe that education had a special place and a peculiar importance in the fight against TB. Nor was Trudeau singular. Clinicians, pathologists, and bacteriologists became some of the most forceful and significant proponents of education, and, like Krause, those who advocated education and those who turned to the laboratory were often the same. When Charles Chapin reflected in 1900 on the progress that had been made against tuberculosis, he observed that a "great deal has been done, during the past ten years, to educate the public to a knowledge of the contagiousness of tuberculosis. A large part of this work of education has been carried on by public health officials, particularly those engaged in laboratory work."[163] The experience of the Phipps Institute further suggests that many of the physicians who used the laboratory to build resistance also turned to education. Biggs himself initiated the Foster Parent's Health Club in order to teach young children the proper habits of "health, hygiene and play."[164]

Appreciation of just how deeply the therapeutic of social reform took root and how pervasively education came to be viewed as an indispensable tool in the struggle against TB is critical to the understanding of what came later. As we will see in the next chapter, the goals of producing a combined physiological and sociological resistance to TB informed the efforts of those who turned to the laboratory for answers to the TB problem. More important, even there the dietetic-hygienic-educational campaign remained the template against which they judged their efforts and against which their efforts were judged.

Medicine, Science, and the National Interest: American Responses to the BCG Vaccine in the 1920s

The laboratory became one of the icons of early twentieth-century medical practice as physicians dreamt of productive unions among scientific, economic, and political authority. After 1900, labs raised hope for the conquest of disease with the production of diagnostics, preventives, and cures for the major infections. However, those engaged in the control of tuberculosis found few immediate answers in the lab. Rather than sharpening and simplifying the tuberculosis problem, the introduction of each new diagnostic tool demonstrated both how intractable and how unpredictable tuberculous infection was. And, initially, laboratory science delivered none of the therapies or preventives that so profitably and effectively controlled smallpox, diphtheria, and other major infections. Shortly before he died, Edward Livingston Trudeau observed that if immunity meant "that after the disease has been entirely cured, any amount of exposure to the infection will not reproduce it," then "I know such an immunity is not attainable experimentally in tuberculosis," and, he predicted, "I don't think it will ever be attained."[1]

Trudeau's pessimism was not entirely warranted. When careful readers of the *New York Times* opened their paper on June 26, 1924, they learned that twenty years of research at the Pasteur Institute in Lille had produced an attenuated tuberculosis vaccine. Based on a bovine tubercle bacillus, the vaccine was named Bacillus Calmette Guérin, or BCG, after Albert Calmette, medical director of the Lille Institute, and his coinvestigator, the veterinary surgeon Camille Guérin.[2] Touted from the first as an alternative rather than a complement to existing campaigns, BCG held out promise of being an immunological preventative that was fully consistent with the goals of the new bacteriological era. The *Times* Paris correspondent deemed it of "great importance to the human race."[3]

By 1924, when the *Times* offered its assessment and Americans entered the debate, much of the world had accepted BCG vaccination as an integral component of the campaign against TB. Calmette and Guérin first began to develop BCG in 1906, and they presented a brief résumé of their research to the Sixth International Congress on Tuberculosis, held in Washington in 1908.[4] Some Europeans and Asians began to test the vaccine immediately thereafter. By 1921 Calmette's work had been praised in major international journals, and physicians in France, Holland, Belgium, and the Soviet Union had begun experimental studies. Canadian researchers also began to test BCG in 1921,[5] and three years later the NRCC established an Associate Committee on Tuberculosis Research (ACTR) to more fully appraise the vaccine.

In stark contrast to both the worldwide response and their earlier enthusiastic reception of Robert Koch's tuberculin, American physicians did not immediately embrace BCG. The medical establishment first stood back, then cautiously evaluated the vaccine's safety and efficacy. Like the response to tuberculin, their discussion of BCG was imbedded in concerns over live vaccines and limits to species. These scientific and technical issues again demarcated American and Canadian reactions. Once more, however, the scientific debates were further enmeshed in social responses to tuberculosis and to scientific medicine itself. And the very different American and Canadian reactions to BCG—physicians' varied efforts to weigh the social and economic significance of scientific theory and practice and to restructure programs of disease control—expose the complex relationships of science, professional medicine, and the emerging middle classes.

VACCINATION AND AMERICAN SCIENCE

The medical and popular presses played an important role in shaping American reactions to tuberculin and pushed physicians into action with their allegations that the medical profession had ignored the importance of Koch's achievement. They might equally well have chided the medical establishment for ignoring BCG. Between 1906 and 1924, the journals that filled their columns with accounts of late-nineteenth- and early-twentieth-century antituberculosis preparations paid Calmette's vaccination studies little attention. The *Journal of the American Medical Association* and the *American Review of Tuberculosis* reported Calmette and Guérin's research only briefly in their foreign news sections; some major publications, such as the *American Journal of Medical Sciences* and the *Boston Medical and Surgical Journal,* virtually ignored the development of BCG. This time, the popular press did not force the issue. The same New York papers that heralded Koch's tuberculin passed BCG by. The *Times* story was singular, and even it did not deem Calmette's work important enough to warrant front-page billing; it buried its initial account on page 25.

Moreover, as it appraised BCG, the press deferred to the authority of and took its cues from medical experts. When first asked for comment, some of New York's most eminent physicians, like William Hallock Park—the director of research at the Vaccine and Chemical Laboratories of the New York City Department of Health, who was famed for his studies of diphtheria antitoxin—seemed unfamiliar with Calmette's work. Park demurred with the observations that Calmette was a "great expert," but "[i]t is hard to judge from the article to the *Times,* as lengthy as it is, how far he has developed the vaccine." Hence, he did not wish to comment on Calmette's research "until we have had an opportunity to see a protocol on the subject." S. Adolphus Knopf, who was unsure of the evidence provided and of the premises on which BCG vaccination was based, would offer no opinion until further testing had established BCG's safety, mode of action, and efficacy.[6] Dr. Maurice Fishberg, professor of medicine at New York's Bellevue Medical College, tuberculosis expert, and chief consultant to the Bedford Hills Sanitarium, was "skeptical concerning the value of Professor Calmette's discovery" and warned readers not to "hurry to Paris expecting to be cured."[7] The *Times* heeded these warnings and quickly altered the tone of its coverage. Within a day, a cautious assessment of BCG that lacked the enthusiasm characteristic of the earlier reports of tuberculin showed beneath the initial optimistic veneer. Calmette's vaccine was "not the long-waited remedy for tuberculosis," the *Times* Paris correspondent warned, and "Professor Calmette does not desire to raise premature and exaggerated hopes."[8]

Medical commentaries reiterated and underscored this cautionary advice. In September 1924, as Europeans advocated greater use of BCG, Allen Krause issued a thinly veiled warning in an editorial for the *American Review of Tuberculosis.* "No one, who is at all familiar with the literature of the past on preventive inoculation against tuberculosis," Krause observed, "will rush in to render a final opinion on the efficacy and practicability of any new method until this method has had trial in many hands, in many lands, in many subjects; . . . until Calmette's methods have had similar scrutiny the merits of his BCG must remain *sub judice.*"[9] American medicine had become both increasingly scientific and more institutionalized in the thirty years that separated tuberculin from BCG. Between

1924 and the Second World War, new alliances among physicians, pharmaceutical manufacturers, and the federal government entrenched the economic and intellectual authority of biomedicine still further. The reaction to BCG—Americans' determination to test it for themselves, by their own standards and at their own pace—reflected physicians' efforts to carve out a research style that would mold institutionalized medical science to both national and middle-class interests.

Longstanding disagreements about the ways in which research on antituberculosis vaccines should be conducted underlay the earliest medical response to BCG. After 1882, researchers had tried unsuccessfully to develop an attenuated or antitoxic vaccine against tuberculosis. American participation in this effort was limited, but a general preference for tuberculins and antitoxins guided that which existed. Killed vaccines, organisms from other species, and attenuated preparations (live organisms with reduced virulence) offered alternatives. But in the years before 1924 these did not seem to show as good results as tuberculins. The long and troubled history of vaccines and treatments against TB both shaped American views on appropriate research problems and colored their reception of BCG.

The legacies of Koch and Theobald Smith proved particularly important. In 1902, Koch's disciple Emil von Behring raised then dashed hopes with his "bovo-vaccine." Behring believed that the ingestion of bovine tubercle bacilli was the primary cause of both childhood and adult forms of human pulmonary TB. He consequently sought measures that would prevent contaminated milk, among these a vaccine against bovine tuberculosis. Reversing the logic that Edward Jenner had used when he took cowpox as the base of a vaccine against the human disease smallpox, Behring began instead with a human tubercle bacillus that he attenuated to produce a vaccine for cattle.[10] Having categorized TB as a "parasitic disease," Behring hoped the continued presence of avirulent live organisms within the host would create immunity through a form of parasitic symbiosis.[11]

At the Sixth International Congress, E. R. Baldwin of Saranac Lake warned that the protection that bovo-vaccine and other preparations like it offered was short-lived. The vaccine might produce immunity for a period that ranged from six months to two years, but, Baldwin warned, "unfortunately, exposure to natural infection or to inoculation with bovine virus after this period has resulted disastrously."[12]

Stronger opposition still came from Smith, director of the pathological laboratory in the U.S. Bureau of Animal Industry and professor of bacteriology at Columbian University in Missouri. With his associate D. E.

Salmon, Smith had investigated the use of "ptomaines," or poisons extracted from sterilized bacterial cultures, to produce immunity to typhoid, hog cholera, and other bacterial infections.[13] Smith, who later moved to Cornell, was among the most renowned American experimentalists, and in 1896 he changed the course of both American public policy and experimental science away from the control of bovine tuberculosis.[14] With a bold refutation of Koch's claims for the unity of human and bovine disease, Smith dismissed the dangers that bovine bacilli posed to humans and shifted attention to sputum. Hence, Smith discounted Behring's hypothesis of the bovine origins of adult tuberculosis, and he questioned the very premises of this research. He doubted in principle that a bovo-vaccine would do humans much good; with time, he became sure that it could do considerable harm.[15] "The Von Behring method," Smith later wrote, "brought to light a serious practical objection to the use of living cultures." When "implanted in the body," he warned, live bacilli acted unpredictably; "they persist for many months in some organ or tissue, . . . may multiply and produce definite lesions. . . . These results do not encourage the use of living cultures."[16] Smith's objections set the stage for opposition as subsequent attempts to repeat Behring's work and to vaccinate cattle with attenuated cultures of human bacilli similarly revealed that vaccination might "arrest tuberculosis but not rid the body of living bacilli"[17] or worse still might cause progressive disease.

Experiences with bovo-vaccine made American researchers leery of any antituberculosis vaccine. "The situation," Baldwin observed, "is, therefore, at present not encouraging for the establishment of a long-continued immunity by any method, either in cattle or man."[18] It left them especially wary of live vaccines. In 1910, when Gerald Webb and W.W. Williams of Colorado Springs attempted to vaccinate human infants with gradually increasing doses of live, virulent bacilli, their experiment caused progressive tuberculosis.[19] A strain of reptilian tubercle bacillus, which F. Friedmann derived from sea turtles, also caused active cases of disease when it was used as a human antituberculosis vaccine.[20]

William Charles White later summarized the scientific opposition. White, director of tuberculosis research at the Hygienic Laboratory, formerly research director of the R. Mellon Laboratory at the University of Pittsburgh, and first director of the Medical Research Committee of the NTA, was a great proponent of scientific research. Nonetheless he fundamentally mistrusted antituberculosis vaccines. First, White, like Trudeau and Baldwin, doubted that it was possible to produce immunity to tuberculosis; it was possible, he argued, only to increase resistance to natural or artificial infection. The solution to the tuberculosis problem, White suggested, would come only "through a knowledge of what occurs in the natural healing of the great majority of mankind."[21] Second, White argued his case against all vaccines on the grounds that "[t]he very essence of therapy has always been chemical." This intellectual commitment to a "chemical" interpretation of tubercular pathology predisposed him to favor chemical treatments as complex as the "gold cure," sanocrysin, or as simple as cod liver oil over vaccination. Tuberculin was the only biologic in which he had any faith.[22]

BCG particularly provoked White. Calmette had virtually thumbed his nose at the American research tradition when he took Behring's work as the starting point of his own efforts. Though he understood and appreciated the American arguments against live vaccines generally and bovovaccine in particular, Calmette nonetheless believed that Behring had correctly identified the root causes of human infection and that extensive clinical and epidemiological evidence supported his claim. With Guérin, Calmette had tested the hypothesis that infected milk transmitted tuberculosis, and at the 1908 International Congress he presented his evidence that "infection by the digestive route is by far the most important and most frequent."[23]

There were flaws to Calmette's argument, which delegates to the congress recognized. Chief among these was that bacteria retrieved from the humans whom Calmette believed had reactivated tuberculosis were rarely of the bovine form. Calmette remained unperturbed. He defended his position and further antagonized his audience by resurrecting the doctrine of pleomorphism and the age-old debates over the limits to species. In language that bore marked resemblance to that which his mentor Louis Pasteur used in his own debates with Koch, Calmette dismissed Koch's views on bovine bacilli as "too stringent." Like other forms of tubercle bacilli, he argued, digested bovine bacilli could easily change their form. "Prolonged sojourn" in the human species, he proposed, transformed the bovine into the human form.[24]

As American researchers reviewed Calmette's work, they found the species questions imbedded in it troubling. The study of various strains of tubercle bacilli, their morphological and chemical characteristics, and the conditions under which they became virulent defined an important strand of American tuberculosis research.[25] Hence, Calmette's interpretation of the relationships between human and bovine infection and his subsequent efforts to attenuate a bovine bacillus left the research community distinctly uncomfortable.

Calmette and Guérin's goal was to create artificially a "race of tubercle bacillus, stripped of virulence for all species of animals, that would serve as a vaccine like those of Pasteur, that is to say, its characteristics would be hereditarily fixed."[26] This transformed bacillus would become a "parasite" that would live symbiotically with its host, and it would succeed where all other attempts had failed. When primary infection with tubercle bacilli occurred naturally, Calmette argued, neither the number nor the virulence of the infecting bacilli was consistent enough to produce immunity. Moreover, natural infections did not generate the parasitic state that he, like Behring, believed essential to immunity. Trained initially as a naval physician, Calmette had studied parasites while serving a tour of duty in French Indochina with the eminent parasitologist Patrik Manson. He later completed a doctoral thesis on *filaria sanguinis humanis,* human bloodflukes, at the University of Paris, then took a three-month training course in bacteriology and microbiology with Emil Roux. During a subsequent term as director of the Pasteur Research Center in Saigon, Calmette distinguished himself by adapting smallpox vaccine to Asian needs and developing a serum against snakebites. These experiences convinced Calmette that TB more closely resembled syphilis and other protozoan diseases than the general infections. Immunity to general infections constituted a reaction to a specific microbe or its toxins; in protozoan diseases, immunity existed only as long as the organism harbored some element of the parasite.[27]

Calmette consequently postulated that immunity to tuberculosis might depend on the survival of a few mildly virulent bacilli within the infected organism.[28] His research problem was therefore to control the primary infection—the number and virulence of the infecting microbes—for he had no doubt that when a carefully measured and regulated dose of attenuated bovine bacilli mimicked the process of natural infection, immunity would follow.[29]

Calmette fully appreciated the controversial nature of his research agenda. If Pasteur's successes with vaccines had affirmed the possibilities of attenuation and diffused some of the friction between him and Koch, the question of the extent to which tubercle bacilli could be transformed remained. All attempts to modify the microbe's virulence or to interchange species and host had seemed to fail, and real fears of infection persisted. Hence, Calmette and Guérin proceeded cautiously. They began work in 1906 and over the course of fourteen years, interrupted only during the German occupation of Lille, carefully attenuated a particularly virulent strain of bovine tubercle bacillus.[30] Only in 1920 did they deem the attenuation fixed, and they then renamed the bacillus Bacillus Calmette Guérin, or BCG.

Vaccination trials, begun immediately on rabbits, guinea pigs, and other small rodents, confirmed that BCG was completely fixed, had lost all ability to produce tubercles, and was otherwise innocuous.[31] Trials on cattle, conducted during the following year, suggested that BCG vaccinated cows successfully resisted a challenge dose of live, virulent tubercle bacilli. One year after infection, no virulent bacilli, tubercular lesions, or other signs of active disease could be found in the test animals, but they were found in the controls. Animal experiments convinced Calmette and Guérin that BCG would safely and effectively prevent tuberculosis in cattle.

The success of these early trials awakened international interest in BCG. In Canada, where bovine and avian tuberculosis plagued farmers, the NRCC repeatedly reminded Parliament of the threats that tuberculous milk and meat posed to the Canadian economy and trade. As animal disease rivaled human infection, the Federal Department of Agriculture, which held jurisdiction over veterinary affairs, could no longer contain the problem. In this context BCG elicited a favorable response from Canadian public and private sectors. Calmette's vaccine, prominent members of the medical and scientific communities quickly agreed, "is of great scientific importance and practical interest."[32] Thus, as early as 1921 individual researchers—E. A. Watson, the Department of Agriculture's chief pathologist, and A. C. Rankin, director of Alberta's Provincial Laboratory and dean of medicine at the University of Alberta—began to test the validity of Calmette's claims.

The American response, which Strasheimer Alburtus Petroff exemplified in a 1929 review, was quite different in its emphasis on the dangers of bovine infection and bacterial transformation. Americans had slowly followed the French and Canadian leads and, under the auspices of agricultural colleges like Cornell, began their own trials of BCG. These trials suggested that BCG worked, and Petroff grudgingly conceded that BCG conferred some protection; however, he nonetheless continued to find the French BCG studies unconvincing.[33] Because of his position as director of medical research at Trudeau's Saranac laboratory and respect for his studies of TB immunity, Petroff's reservations carried some weight. He consequently spoke to and for many Americans, and the echoes of his arguments reverberated through analyses of BCG for years.

Like Smith, Petroff challenged the claim that bovine infection resulted in human disease. He acknowledged that, in countries that did not take proper precautions to safeguard cattle, milk, and meat, the ingestion of large quantities of tubercle bacilli during childhood might pose a threat. Smugly confident of American public health controls, Petroff conceded that French experience might justify Calmette's approach, but he doubted that intestinal infections—transmitted through milk—posed much danger to Americans.

Petroff's greater concern was with the safety of BCG, and as he made clear, his misgivings derived from old debates about bacterial transformation. Calmette's comments to the Eighth International Congress suggested that he was a neo-Lamarckian. He often and provocatively proposed that "by adaptation in a different environment the microorganism can mutate"[34] and that human and bovine forms of tubercle bacilli differed from one another because "they have more or less adapted themselves through a series of cultural generations to a human or bovine environment."[35] Because he believed that tubercle bacilli were pleomorphic, Calmette also believed that his BCG had been so attenuated, or transformed, that it no longer produced progressive disease. But he also maintained that this environmentally induced loss of virulence had become hereditary so that his bacterium could neither regain its pathogenic characteristics nor lose its ability to produce an immune response. He further insisted that BCG would pass its benign characteristics on to its offspring.

Petroff found Calmette's suggestion that environmental influences could act selectively on heritable characteristics unbelievable. If virulence or the lack of it could be inherited, he asked, how could Calmette argue that environmental circumstance could modify it? And if environmental influences could and did modify what Gregor Mendel had designated unit factors, why should they act in only one direction or abruptly cease to act? "Calmette admits that environment plays a very important part and that such conditions influence the virulence of the microorganism," he wrote. "But we cannot see why BCG should be an exception."[36] Though he was willing to accept that existing strains of BCG had relatively low virulence, Petroff would not rule out the possibility that with time they might become increasingly pathogenic. "We believe in the evolution and mutation of all microorganisms," he wrote, "and for this reason are strongly opposed to any method of prophylactic immunization that uses a living microorganism."[37]

Petroff did not fabricate his fears out of a wholly theoretical cloth. Calmette's assurances to the contrary, a small number of researchers had observed "definite tuberculous changes" and even progressive TB in BCG-inoculated guinea pigs. Moreover, they had been able to "pass the disease from animal to animal and by such passage to increase its virulence."[38] Some of the cattle that Calmette himself vaccinated later developed tuberculous infections. At the Department of Agriculture in Ottawa, Watson also found that, in some cases, substrains of Calmette's cultures apparently regained virulence.[39]

Calmette, Watson, and Petroff disagreed about the source and magnitude of the problem. Calmette explained reversion away with the suggestion that cultures had become contaminated. Watson proposed that the early BCG strain "was still in the process of attenuation, . . . still retained a low, uncertain and potential virulence [and] that its properties were not then completely and hereditarily fixed."[40] Petroff found these explanations lame. Morphological analyses of tubercle bacilli, which he and other Americans undertook, convinced him that Calmette's views on the nature and limits to species of tubercle bacilli were altogether too casual.[41] At Saranac Lake, Petroff had dissociated into two types BCG cultures that he obtained from Watson, from the Pasteur Institute via his colleague Lawrason Brown, and directly from Calmette. These differed fundamentally in their chemical composition, the colonies they formed, and their virulence. In Petroff's estimation, Calmette and Guérin had selectively bred nonvirulent bacilli, but the more virulent type nonetheless persisted in the BCG strain, and their presence, he maintained, showed that BCG could revert to virulence. If Calmette admitted that "by adaptation in a different environment the microorganism can mutate," Petroff taunted, how could he deny the possibility of such transformation?[42]

American anxieties about safety and efficacy mounted as Calmette shifted his attention from cattle to children. If, as he and Guérin proposed, the ingestion of bovine bacilli was the primary source of human disease, then a vaccine that effectively eliminated bovine infection had indirect benefits for humans. However, such indirect benefits seemed increasingly inadequate. Tuberculosis morbidity and mortality soared so dramatically in France during and after World War I that it drew international attention. By 1920, the Rockefeller Foundation's International Health Board had established a Commission for the Prevention of Tuberculosis in France, and American volunteers flocked overseas to assist in its work.[43] Tuberculosis took its greatest toll among infants. Calmette himself estimated that 57 percent of French children were infected with TB by the time they reached their first birthday.[44] Data from his home city, Lille, as well as more general European data, similarly identified children under one year as the most vulnerable to TB.[45]

These pressing problems of human disease impressed Calmette and Guérin with the need for more direct forms of intervention. Consequently, in 1921, after issuing preliminary reports of their animal trials, they began to vaccinate human infants.[46] Calmette justified this decision on both epidemiological and physiological grounds. Infants seemed to him to live in a highly infectious environment in which hands, mouth, and milk constantly spread bacteria. However, Calmette also believed the newborn's gut to be particularly permeable to microbes.[47] This permeability left infants vulnerable, but Calmette believed that it also made them especially receptive to toxalbumins and antitoxins. Hence, the combined environmental and physiological characteristics that placed newborns at risk also made them the optimal candidates for a vaccination trial.

The earliest human trials of BCG began in Paris under the direction of B. Weill-Hallé and R. Turpin, physicians associated with La Charité hospital. In their experimental trials, Calmette and Guérin had employed both subcutaneous and intravenous injections of BCG, but humans rarely absorbed massive doses of bacilli through their skin or blood. Hence, researchers were unsure that injection would produce the "lesions of resistance" that were characteristic of natural disease and necessary for immunity.[48] Because the gut was the usual channel of infection, Weill-Hallé and Turpin administered BCG orally in an effort to simulate more closely the course of natural infection. They tested an oral dose of BCG on one infant in July 1921. Satisfied that this procedure had been effective, they moved to a larger population of newborns.

Calmette, who had the respect of Pasteur, Eli Metchnikoff, and other renowned bacteriologists and immunologists, easily secured populations for study. The international reputation and reach of the Pasteur Institute further ensured that BCG was tested widely. Extensive trials began immediately in France, in Indochina and other French colonies, in allied nations served by the Institute (such as Belgium), and in Romania, Greece, Algeria, Ukraine and points further afield.

After 1921, the results began to flow in. The preliminary trial that Weill-Hallé and Turpin conducted between July 1921 and June 1922 suggested that infants tolerated an initial small dose well. Though only 80 of 120 vaccinated children could later be called back, these all proved to be in good health.[49] In July 1922, Weill-Hallé and Turpin increased the dosage and administered a larger quantity of vaccine orally to 469 infants. In order to test the "power of BCG in both healthy and infected environments,"[50] they chose the infants from both households in which a real danger of infection existed and those apparently free of disease. Ninety-two subjects were lost from the study, and nineteen died, but among the remaining vaccinees, mortality was low. Estimates of tuberculous mortality in Paris during the first year of life ranged from 13/100 to 28/100;[51] among the sixty-seven vaccinees born to tuberculous mothers only one— or 1.5/100—had died of TB.[52] Hence, at the June 1924 meeting of the Academy of Medicine of Paris, Calmette and Guérin presented an optimistic report of their findings and concluded that BCG had proven to be innocuous and of "practical value."[53] The evidence of the worldwide trials further justified their enthusiasm.[54]

Investigations conducted between July 1924 and January 1927 lent BCG vaccination additional support. A study of 21,000 French children, drawn exclusively from families in which at least one active case of TB existed and then divided into subclasses based on the risk of infection, suggested that after a period of two years vaccination reduced tuberculous mortality by a factor of twenty-six.[55] The independent statistical analyses of Dr. Y. Biraud, chief of the Statistical Service of the Institut d'Hygiene, at the Faculty of Medicine of Paris, also indicated that BCG worked. Biraud had studied 1,877 BCG-vaccinated infants, of whom 1,050 were raised in a tuberculous household and of whom 487 had a tubercular mother. Under normal circumstances, mortality from all causes would be high in the latter two groups; however, among the BCG-vaccinated populations he found both tubercular and general mortality reduced.[56] "If one compares general mortality among exposed, but vaccinated infants," Calmette concluded, "with that of the non-vaccinated population at large, one sees that mortality among the vaccinees is much lower."[57] And if BCG reduced mortality in groups so obviously prone to disease, he asked, would it not be even more effective in populations at less risk?

As testing continued, study after study seemed to confirm BCG's safety, efficacy, and practicality. The Health Department of the Lower-Seine demonstrated that it was both possible and practical to implement long-term, large-scale preventative vaccination programs.[58] An extension of the Weill-Hallé and Turpin trial indicated that BCG offered protection that lasted at least four years.[59] In Indochina, 20,000 infants vaccinated after 1921 resisted TB and showed no adverse effects. Vaccinations of 776 Senegalese children proved equally successful. Hence, by 1927 Calmette was convinced of BCG's usefulness. He could point to twenty-eight countries, including France's Far Eastern colonies, Belgium, Holland, Norway, Romania, Poland, Greece, Algeria, and Ukraine that produced and distributed BCG and successfully used it to reduce mortality.[60] In the March issue of the *Annales de l'Institut Pasteur* (1927), which was devoted to papers on BCG, and in a detailed book, he summarized his research and conclusions.

Calmette was the medical director of the Pasteur Institute in Lille, a protégé of Pasteur and Metchnikoff, and an internationally recognized researcher. He presented and published his findings in respectable settings—among these the Academy of Medicine in Paris, the International Congress of Tuberculosis, and the *Annales* of the Pasteur Institute. These credentials helped convince numerous European, Asian, and Latin American nations to adopt BCG as a preventive against both human and bovine tuberculosis, and they also impressed Canadians. Still, American physicians doubted Calmette.

Despite the mounting evidence, Americans continued to question the safety of live vaccines. In 1925, the editors of the *Journal of the American Medical Association* issued a general warning in which they reminded readers of early disasters and concluded that "the use of living tubercle bacilli as immunizing agents is dangerous."[61] American researchers took these warnings seriously. "Use of the vaccine in children," White observed in 1926, "does not . . . appeal to physicians with whom I have discussed it in this country."[62] In 1927, the *Journal* underscored its earlier concerns and applied them directly to Calmette, thereby muting the American response. BCG, the *Journal*'s editors cautioned, was a live vaccine, which, though attenuated, might well revert to virulence. Hence they believed the administration of massive oral doses to newborns to be risky.[63] Thus, those Americans who decided to proceed with the vaccine, such as Eugene Opie and his colleagues at the Henry Phipps Institute, moved slowly and cautiously, and they continually assessed the alternative of a killed vaccine. In New York, Park considered a long-term human vaccination trial, but before he began to vaccinate children, he felt obliged to conduct morphological and experimental tests to determine that the BCG culture was stable and fully attenuated.[64]

Fears that BCG might be harmful were hardly peculiar to Americans.[65] Still, Americans became unusually and particularly preoccupied with the safety of BCG, in large measure because the safety issue did not stand alone but was connected to and fueled by related considerations of nationalism and the socioeconomic authority of science. The discussion of the alleged shortcomings of the trials helped Americans evaluate Calmette's claims, but they additionally served the needs of a community struggling to establish national standards of scientific rigor. When push came to shove, Americans would not accept Calmette's results until they had tested his vaccine for and by themselves.

NATIONALISM AND THE INSTITUTIONALIZATION OF AMERICAN RESEARCH

The staunchest American opposition to BCG came from leaders of the American research community, like White, Krause, and Petroff. To these eminent physicians, Calmette's work seemed to issue a dual challenge: it demanded that Americans both verify his results for themselves and surpass his standards. Krause laid out the issues as he asked Americans "to hope fervently that there may be devised some plan whereby Calmette's BCG will be given the most thorough trial . . . under auspices that are beyond cavil in the United States."[66] The wording of this appeal differed markedly from that of non-American researchers. For example, Dr. J. G. Fitzgerald, director of the Connaught Research Laboratory at the University of Toronto, also warned his Canadian colleagues that BCG had not been tested widely enough and advised them to ensure that "BCG is no longer able to give rise to tuberculous lesions, . . . unable to stimulate tubercle formation while retaining its power to give rise to an active immunity."[67] But where Fitzgerald called generally for studies to confirm the vaccine's safety, Krause demanded more American research. "[O]f all countries," Krause proposed, the United States "with its favored economic and scientific outlook and its warm appreciation of the author's place in the world, is the place to have a large share in proving the value of Calmette's method."[68]

White rallied Americans most forcefully. Born in Woodstock, Ontario, White had taken his M.B. and M.D. degrees at the University of Toronto and had done postgraduate study in Leipzig and Heidelberg. He consequently had ample foreign experience, which apparently left him dubious of all but American research. Like Krause, White mistrusted both the scientific principles upon which Calmette based his research and the "foreign" evidence for its success. The question of BCG's worth, he concluded, could be resolved only when American researchers submitted the vaccine to extensive investigations, and he counseled his colleagues "to hold in check uncontrolled enthusiasm for use of [BCG vaccine] until those charged with the responsibility of safeguarding the public have carefully proved that the methods and premises are sound."[69] As part of his duties as head of tuberculosis research at the Hygienic Laboratory, White traveled to Europe in 1927 to observe Calmette's work firsthand. He began this visit convinced that "little justification" existed "for experimentation on man with vaccination of either living or dead organisms."[70] He returned home no more convinced. "It will be necessary for each country, through those specially charged with the responsibility for approving or recommending such a vaccine to develop its own policy in connection with it," he advised.[71]

Krause's and White's demands for American research formed part of a larger agenda. During the last decades of the nineteenth century and the first of the twentieth, Yankee ingenuity and Yankee science seemed inextricably linked with progress as Americans developed their own scientific style to solve their own problems and secure their own futures.[72] The assumption that only American science could resolve American problems held as true for bacteriology and medicine as any other field.

However, though the imperatives of scientific nationalism provided the perfect pretext for extensive testing of BCG, equally powerful institutional obstacles made such testing difficult. American state agencies were ill-equipped to undertake the sort of investigations that Krause and White advocated, and their leaders apparently lacked the interest or will to pursue the matter. Krause himself recognized the contradictions. "Extraordinarily ample though the resources for scientific investigation may be in the United States, and blessed above all countries though she is in foundations and institutes for research," he wrote, "not one of the latter could be expected to repeat Calmette's work if this meant a decade and more spent in the preparation of material."[73]

Unlike Europeans, Americans had no preestablished formal research program. The development of tuberculin represented the high-water mark in efforts to create a biological, lab-based means of controlling TB. Before the First World War, leaders of the American medical and scientific communities sometimes exhorted physicians to pursue laboratory studies in order to gain a better understanding of the relation between bacteria and disease, but their exhortations usually took the form of ceremonial rhetoric that was hard to escape but easy to ignore.[74] Laboratory research typically occupied a secondary place compared with education and other resistance-building programs; sanatoria, voluntary agencies, and boards of health directed the bulk of their money and energy to those programs. In 1921, the resurrection of the Medical Research Committee (MRC) of the NTA ascribed new importance to lab-based research but did little to shift the direction of the antituberculosis campaign. American physicians continued to assign diet and heliotherapy pride of place. "The emphasis on research during this period," Esmond Long, director of the Phipps Institute, later reflected, "was in the last analysis a sort of physiological study of tuberculosis, rather than a chemical or pathological, and least of all was it a therapeutic study."[75] The MRC consequently used its new mandate and budget to promote research on the factors that elicited physiological changes in the host—food and sunshine chief among them.[76] Thus in the period leading up to the discovery of BCG, prominent agencies like the NASPT spent relatively little money or effort on laboratory studies (especially immunological studies) of tuberculosis, and American physicians generally remained profoundly ambivalent about vaccines and sera against TB.

The introduction of BCG might have reversed this tide, as it did in Canada. There, the problems of tuberculosis generally, and of BCG in particular, created the impetus for a national research program. At the time of the First World War, as tuberculous mortality and morbidity among Canadian civilian and military populations rose and as rates of infection among native peoples raised the public profile of tuberculosis, Canadians became increasingly aware of the economic costs of the disease.[77] In Canada, as elsewhere, TB predominated in urban, industrial environments, where it preferentially affected the critical populations that formed the workforce. Canadian physicians, industrialists, and parliamentarians alike feared the toll the disease took on the Canadian economy and made pleas for intervention and research. "To put the [tuberculosis] problem on no higher plane than that of financial values," one physician suggested, "apart altogether from the untold suffering and misery directly attributable to the ravages of this disease among humans, there is each year an appalling economic loss rising from the illness of those suffering from it and through the premature death of thousands of the most desirable type of citizens."[78] The control of tuberculosis was consequently viewed as related to economic and industrial policy issues that Canadians, unlike Americans, had already linked formally to the agenda of national research.

In response to the trade imbalance and other economic problems that arose from the war effort, Parliament established an Honorary Advisory Council for Scientific and Industrial Research. Though more concerned with the physical problems of production, the Advisory Council also established a Committee on Industrial Fatigue to assess human factors. Industrial fatigue, it reported in 1920, was "associated very intimately with the health and diet of the worker and hygienic conditions or otherwise of his environment, not only during his working hours but also his life outside the factory or workshop."[79] Thus, the Advisory Council attempted to expand its jurisdiction into these areas.

That expansion was not simply accomplished. The British North America Act (1867), like the American Constitution, made little formal provision for disease control; the responsibilities that it did recognize it assigned to the provinces. A strong tradition of judicially supported provincial rights had persisted since the time of Confederation, and indeed during the 1920s the Judicial Committee of the Privy Council struck down several national regulatory schemes.[80] By 1924, as interest in BCG and concern about tuberculosis grew alongside demands for an umbrella organization to coordinate and evaluate various vaccination trials, jurisdictional battles with other Federal agencies—the Dominion Departments of Health and Agriculture—also emerged.[81]

The NRCC, which supplanted the Advisory Council, circumvented these turf disputes by focusing on the issues of economic production and trade and by divorcing the technical pursuit of scientific knowledge from the provision of health care. In 1923, it established the ACTR, which later metamorphosed into the Medical Research Council of Canada.[82] The

ACTR was the largest national body organized to conduct research on BCG. In keeping with its research mandate, the ACTR drew its membership from among veterinarians, biologists, and physicians who worked in university and governmental laboratories across Canada. Between 1924 and 1938 it collected and interpreted existing data, and it funded its own experimental and clinical vaccination trials on cattle, children, and Canadian Indians.

No American equivalent of the Canadian ACTR emerged. Only the Hygienic Laboratory conducted or promoted research at the national level. State and city departments of health, voluntary agencies, and especially sanatoria acted instead as the foci of research activity. The politics of funding, lack of coordination, and statutory limitations to jurisdiction constrained these various bodies. In the case of sanatoria, conflicts within the institutions themselves compounded the problem. As the MRC later reflected, sanatoria turned out to be less than ideal homes for medical research because they could not devote themselves single-mindedly and freely to scientific investigation. On the one hand, sanatorium physicians found themselves torn between conflicting obligations to the clinic, administration, and research. On the other, the MRC realized that clinical and institutional interests could too easily coopt the sanatorium laboratory.[83] These conflicting priorities jostled uncomfortably and particularly obviously where vaccine research was concerned. As the Von Ruck episode demonstrated, outsiders often suspected sanatorium directors of having mercenary motives, and they suspected that sanatoria, after all, had little incentive to develop preventatives that might put them out of business.

Recognition of the need for standardized tuberculosis treatments also generated discussion about the merits of establishing a special tuberculosis-control division or commission within the PHS. However, as we saw in the previous chapter, this debate became a pawn to larger questions of jurisdiction and demonstrated how controversial and politically charged discussions of education, poor relief, and social services were. Administrative and policy questions overshadowed the scientific and technical needs of tuberculosis control in the United States in a way they did not in Canada. As the debate dragged on, it ensured that no public machinery was formed to test BCG, and as a result private agencies, such as Phipps and the NTA, bore the brunt of the research effort.

The formal jurisdictional boundaries of public health activity, White's individual preferences for the design of tuberculosis research projects, and the relationships between medical research and pharmaceutical manufacturing further encumbered the debate. Between 1924 and 1944, the PHS had little formal jurisdiction over tuberculosis control.[84] The Hygienic Laboratory, thanks to White, initiated some investigations, but these were extremely limited and rarely engaged questions of vaccination.[85] For example, in 1922, when White pushed the Hygienic Laboratory to expand its research on tuberculosis and develop greater ties with voluntary agencies and drug companies, he initiated a cooperative research venture on nutrition rather than on vaccination.[86] The editors of the *Journal of the American Medical Association* commented on a range of other antituberculosis preparations, such as A. Jousset's and P. Dryer's "vaccine therapies" or H. Mollgaard's sanocrysin, but not on BCG.[87] Similarly, in February 1925, the *American Journal of Public Health* printed an editorial on "Sanocrysin—A Gold Cure for Tuberculosis" but overlooked BCG.

The absence of a committee like the Canadian ACTR left the PHS and the Hygienic Laboratory without an autonomous research mandate. As a result, the commercial interests of drug companies and other private manufacturers limited and defined the PHS's role. The financial interests of these manufacturers shaped American tuberculosis research generally and the response to BCG specifically. Between 1924 and 1927, the PHS and the Hygienic Laboratory served primarily as clearinghouses for information about BCG. Despite official opposition, reports of "Calmette's triumph" filtered into the popular press, and letters home from volunteers like Florence Deakins Becker, who had traveled to France to assist the Rockefeller Foundation in its campaign against TB, excited popular interest.[88] The PHS attempted to contain the public response and regularly replied to the local physicians who approached it for advice. For example, in November 1928, Samuel English, superintendent of the New Jersey Sanatorium for Tuberculous Diseases, consulted the PHS about how to respond to "considerable propaganda again in favor of the vaccine method of treatment of tuberculosis known as the Calmette method of infant vaccination." Aware that BCG had not been endorsed by the scientific community, English wrote, "It was my opinion that this method of treatment had not as yet been placed upon sound scientific basis, in this country at least. May I be advised?" Five days later, the PHS sent a typical response. "It is the judgment of this office, that the Calmette method of infant vaccination is in a purely experimental state. It can scarcely be said to be on a sound scientific basis."[89]

The PHS twice sent researchers to France to evaluate BCG and with the Hygienic Laboratory freely disseminated information that advised against its use. Yet neither the PHS nor the Hygienic Laboratory launched a full-scale inquiry of the kind that Krause and White called for or of the sort conducted on the Von Ruck serum. More striking, during the period when it chose not to conduct research on BCG, the PHS sponsored with the Hygienic Laboratory a long-term study of sanocrysin, which seemed by all accounts to be a dead end.[90]

A comparison of responses to BCG and sanocrysin illustrates the crucial role that pharmaceutical manufacturers played in defining the American research agenda. Mollgaard's sanocrysin was based on use of a gold salt—AuO_3S_2—and a serum from immunized calves or horses. The preparation, which Mollgaard claimed to have used successfully in Northern Europe, quickly interested American manufacturers. Despite disagreement over its exact nature and mode of action, Parke-Davis Company applied in 1924 for rights to market it. Claims for sanocrysin ultimately emphasized its chemical properties, but the treatment also involved use of a biologic. Hence, under the terms of the 1906 Food and Drug Act, Parke-Davis could not begin production without a license from the Hygienic Laboratory.

Parke-Davis's application for a license obliged the PHS to immediately evaluate sanocrysin.[91] G. W. McCoy, director of the Hygienic Laboratory, began by reviewing existing data and performing preliminary animal experiments.[92] On February 11, 1925, he summarized his findings for E. M. Houghton, a medical researcher at Parke-Davis. He had given the existing literature on sanocrysin much thought, McCoy explained to Houghton, and he had carefully examined with White the premises and findings of Mollgaard's study. In addition, he had presented the manuscript to "three thoroughly competent men working independently." The analyses of these "independent experts" confirmed his doubts about safety and reliability, and convinced him to withhold his endorsement. McCoy quoted extensively from the experts' reports to explain and justify his decision. He indicated that, like those who investigated the Von Ruck serum, the assessors of sanocrysin found fault with Mollgaard's clinical data. One wrote that it was difficult to judge efficacy or proceed seriously with human trials because "of the indefinite character of some of this data and because the reports are furnished by several observers whose measuring rods are different. . . . It seems to me that if clinical work is proceeded with on the data at hand that the severest criticism could justifiably be brought against those who undertake it." This assessor also feared that sanocrysin would prove dangerous. "The now available or proposed method of using it is too dangerous and the curative effects that can be attributed to it are too doubtful," he wrote, "to justify its use in the treatment of human tuberculosis."[93] Another assessor, indicated to be H.R.M. Landis of the Henry Phipps Institute, concurred. He too believed that the dangers of sanocrysin outweighed its potential benefits and hence that the product ought not be tested on human subjects.[94]

These objections were similar to those that had been or would be made against BCG, but despite them Parke-Davis continued to press for a license. It thus forced the PHS to conduct clinical trials of sanocrysin. Houghton did not find the PHS's case against sanocrysin convincing, and in April 1925 he so informed McCoy. Like the Von Rucks before him, Houghton accused the PHS of failing to follow established protocol; he argued that it had not replicated Mollgaard's findings because it had not reproduced his procedures exactly.[95] Two days later, O. W. Smith, the president of Parke-Davis, attempted to exert his influence and lend weight to his laboratory's conclusions by invoking the authority of international allies. British trials of sanocrysin, he informed McCoy, had proven successful, and the British Medical Research Council endorsed clinical testing of the product.[96]

McCoy stood firm, but the conflict with Parke-Davis that ensued placed the Hygienic Laboratory on the defensive. Sanocrysin had gained substantial popular and medical support, and McCoy recognized that his refusal to endorse it would provoke controversy. He consequently summarized his objections and results and sought support from those higher in command. McCoy submitted this summary to Assistant Surgeon General A. M. Stimson. In July 1925, Stimson returned the manuscript to McCoy with the following comment: "I believe that publication of this report might prove embarrassing. At any rate, I should rather await the development of the European experience for a while. The data is admittedly valuable, but there is considerable lack of unity and the form is not creditable. I prefer to file the report for future use in case of administrative activity concerning sanocrysin."[97] Caught in a bind, the same service that doubted the validity of the French BCG trials and refused to defer to British authority on sanocrysin shifted its burden overseas.

Despite these efforts to hedge, Parke-Davis's persistent interest in sanocrysin compelled the PHS to proceed with clinical and experimental trials, which the Hygienic Laboratory was to sponsor. White directed these trials until 1930, when mounting evidence that sanocrysin was neither safe nor effective finally convinced Parke-Davis to withdraw its application for a license.[98]

In light of these efforts to push sanocrysin, it is striking that Parke-Davis and other drug companies showed no similar interest in BCG. Moreover, pharmaceutical manufacturers did not just ignore the vaccine, they actively avoided it. During the early days of the sanocrysin affair, McCoy had tried to reduce some of the tension by redirecting Parke-Davis's interests. On June 11, 1925, he had tried to prod the company's president toward BCG. As reports filtered in from Europe, McCoy wrote again, on

July 30, to inquire whether Smith might be willing to drop the research on sanocrysin and take up BCG instead. Smith responded with a clear and unequivocal no in which he explained that "Parke-Davis and Company would be very cautious about advocating a living vaccine of this nature without very convincing evidence as to its definite value."[99]

Other American drug companies shared Smith's doubts and hesitancy. Though the Connaught Laboratories of the University of Toronto, which became an independent, licensed manufacturer of biologics in 1923, began BCG research in 1924,[100] American drug companies steered clear of the Calmette vaccine throughout the 1920s and the early 1930s. Their disinterest crippled American BCG research. In 1931, when McCoy reflected on the question of why American researchers had shown so little interest in BCG, he attributed it at least in part to the interests of drug manufacturers. Shrewdly summarizing the interests of both drug manufacturers and the PHS, he explained, "It is believed that a large element in the reluctance of American manufacturers to undertake the marketing of the preparation is to be laid to the knowledge that the Public Health Service desires some substantial evidence of value of biological products designed for the treatment or prevention of tuberculosis before it is willing to seriously consider the licensing of a preparation."[101] McCoy's opinion that regulatory barriers and scientific standards discouraged drug manufacturers is all very well; but had Parke-Davis really wanted to test BCG—as it had sanocrysin—it might easily have succeeded. After all, in 1925 McCoy had actually asked Smith to apply for a license for BCG. Hence, it is not enough to say that drug companies calculated that it was not in their interest to pursue the vaccine or that the PHS's caution reflected knee-jerk nationalism.

LÜBECK AND THE QUESTION OF SAFETY

When American physicians who practiced in the thirties are asked to reflect on the BCG question, they often invoke the the Lübeck Tragedy and turn the discussion back to safety.[102] In 1927, the town of Lübeck in Germany instituted a comprehensive campaign against tuberculosis that relied primarily on the use of BCG. Midwives routinely vaccinated newborns with much the same ease that they administered silver nitrate eyedrops to protect against venereal infections. Between 1927 and 1929, 250 infants received BCG and suffered no serious side effects, but during the summer of 1929 these vaccinated children began to develop active tuberculosis. By the summer of 1930, 71 of the 250 vaccinated children had died.

Lübeck impressed itself deeply on the minds of BCG's opponents, who years later routinely resurrected the incident to support their misgivings about BCG's safety. At the time, however, the events at Lübeck did not seem to unnerve BCG researchers. By 1929, concerns about safety had begun to diminish. Park, who monitored the physical characteristics of BCG cultures over the course of a year, had found that they remained constant. He had further found that the administration of varying doses of bacilli to monkeys and other laboratory animals did not produce the tubercles characteristic of a virulent infection and that he could not associate a single case of active disease with the oral vaccination of newborns.[103] Watson, in Ottawa, similarly found evidence to allay his doubts.[104] Even Petroff laid his misgivings to rest and conceded reluctantly that the vaccine was innocuous.[105]

Rather than reviving fears, Lübeck represented a turning point in the American debate over BCG because the tragedy forced American researchers to confront the question of safety directly. Once they did so, they ultimately laid that question to rest. In August 1930, the Seventh Conference of the International Union against Tuberculosis met in Oslo. The program, set well beforehand, had already identified BCG as a subject worthy of examination, and the coincidence of the events at Lübeck provided an ideal opportunity for evaluating the vaccine. As BCG's proponents and opponents organized their lines of defense, they might easily have marshaled the Lübeck disaster as ammunition. They did not. "No speaker touched the recent catastrophe," the editors of the *Lancet* noted, explaining this odd silence with the report that conference participants had agreed to set Lübeck off limits. "As the causes of that unfortunate affair are still under consideration by the German health authorities," it wrote, "all reference to it was excluded by common consent."[106] Throughout the conference, the official organizers and individual speakers respected the "blackout" and maintained a discreet and tolerant silence.

If any of them harbored misgivings, they hid them well, for at the close of the meeting the Council of the Union "congratulate[d] Prof. Calmette and his collaborators on their splendid work on preventive vaccination against tuberculosis by means of the B.C.G." The Congress, "with the expression of its full confidence," further thanked "the Pasteur Institute of Paris for the generosity with which it places B.C.G. cultures at the disposal of all countries" and "expresse[d] the wish that this work should be carried on, in the hope the outcome may be an efficient weapon in the campaign against tuberculosis."[107] Their position was hardly equivocal, and BCG consequently emerged from the discussion unscathed.

The international reaction apparently reassured the Americans who attended the conference. Opie, director of the laboratory at the Henry

Phipps Institute, was one official American delegate. Trained in bacteriology and pathology at Johns Hopkins and Yale, Opie assumed the post at Phipps in 1923. There, like many of his colleagues, he participated in epidemiological studies of tuberculosis, but he also undertook BCG studies; and he oversaw early and tentative vaccination trials that Phipps conducted in Philadelphia. Thus, Opie was a well-informed and interested observer at the international debate. The report that he presented upon his return to Philadelphia skirted discussion of Lübeck. Instead, he acknowledged that "B.C.G. protects susceptible animals in a limited degree" and that "[m]ost of those who have given B.C.G. to infants found that the death rate from all causes in vaccinated children was much less than in unvaccinated." He further assured that "[t]he observations of those who discussed the subject indicate that B.C.G. employed according to the methods recommended by Calmette is harmless."[108]

If, in deference to the blackout, Opie excised any misgivings from his formal summary of the conference proceedings, he seemed also to exclude them from his personal comment and appraisal. He noted simply that though it was "certainly impossible to state positively that no laboratory device will succeed in returning to the B.C.G. the virulence it has lost, . . . no experimental or clinical evidence indicates recovery of its virulence and capacity to give rise to progressive tuberculous lesions."[109] Nor did Lübeck diminish the Phipps's tentative interest in BCG vaccination.[110] "[T]he percentage of tuberculosis has been less among the [children we have] vaccinated than among the unvaccinated," Opie wrote to Calmette in December 1930.[111] A year later, in an interview with the *Ledger of the Philadelphia College Medical Society*, he publicly endorsed BCG. "At the Phipps Institute," Opie indicated, "we think it desirable that children exposed to danger of contact with tuberculosis be given BCG."[112]

McCoy also offered a candid reassessment of the "tragedy." McCoy had been sent to Europe, in his official capacity, to assess BCG. He traveled widely and evaluated various public, private, and commercial interests in the vaccine. If McCoy had any fears about Lübeck, he too downplayed them. In the summary that he presented to the surgeon general in September 1931, he commented peripherally that in Italy, "'BCG' vaccine was not countenanced for clinical use," and he noted that in Germany "[s]ince the Lübeck experience it has been required that special permission be obtained for the use of 'BCG' on human beings," but he otherwise made no comment on either the Lübeck disaster or the safety of BCG. McCoy focused instead on the issue of commercial licensing. He relayed the information that, although in England "the preparation is not licensed," extensive experimental trials were underway, and a few clinical studies had been undertaken. In Czechoslovakia, Holland, and Germany BCG was produced and used under governmental supervision, though "there is no commercial distribution of the vaccine." In the context of this international activity, McCoy found it "a rather remarkable fact that there never has been made a request for license for this preparation in the United States."[113]

Edward Devine, secretary of the New York Charity Organization Society and director of the Bellevue-Yorkville Health Demonstration, also traveled through Europe during the summer of 1930 to track reactions to Lübeck. As a representative of the NTA, Devine polled the reactions of officials in major European cities. Responses split evenly. In London, Edinburgh, and Belfast, the medical officers advised, "Don't touch it," but in Geneva the acting head of the Health Section of the League of Nations continued to endorse BCG, dismissing the Lübeck incident as a "blunder."[114] In Paris, Amsterdam, Oslo, and Prague, use of BCG was supported, but in Austria "public opinion [was] antagonistic." Devine ultimately turned to Lübeck itself to "hear if possible directly from the Health Department of that city their own version of their sad experience." There, the administrative secretary of the Health Department reassured him that the bacillus on which the vaccine was based had not itself become modified. Instead, "what happened undoubtedly was that in some way the vaccines used had become contaminated with human tuberculosis."[115] Devine too came away convinced that the incident at Lübeck was a careless accident.

The popular response to Lübeck reinforced this interpretation. In a piece written in March 1931 for the *Ladies' Home Journal,* Paul de Kruif assured readers that Lübeck was an isolated tragedy that "was no fault of Calmette or of BCG."[116] Rather than cautioning young mothers against vaccination, de Kruif proposed that "German nationalist newspapers" had sensationalized the incident,[117] and he took the opportunity to promote interest in Calmette's vaccine.

A great popularizer of biomedical achievements, de Kruif confidently believed that the proper application of scientific principles would conquer disease and a host of other social problems.[118] He extended his faith in scientific medicine to BCG and roused public opinion with testimonials to Calmette's good character. De Kruif alternately described Calmette as a brilliant scientist and a "hero" who had achieved his success through simple living, patience, and long hours of hard work rather than any special privilege. De Kruif's account, punctuated with the provocative subtitles "Undaunted," "Saving the Babies," and "Fewer Deaths," thoroughly explained the steps by which Calmette had developed and tested BCG.

It enumerated the many vaccination trials conducted in Europe and North America. De Kruif presented both sides of the story and aired the grievances of Petroff, Watson, and other critics, but he dismissed the opposition as "niggling and unjust" and dwelt heavily on data that "overwhelmingly indicated that BCG was effective." On the off chance that this testimony to Calmette's personal and professional virtues failed to sway his audience, de Kruif appealed to national pride. "Europe is aflame about it," he wrote. "Even in backward Rumania the death rate among 50,000 tuberculosis-exposed but BCG-vaccinated wee ones has tumbled down to 1.3. Yet in our whole land only a few hundred babies have yet had the chance to dodge death by this strange simple trick of BCG feeding."[119] And lest his readers dismiss BCG as irrelevant to American needs, de Kruif reminded them that tuberculosis continued to pose a very real problem. "In America, right now," he cautioned, "380,000 youngsters are known to be tuberculous. . . . $800,000,000 a year is spent to fight tuberculosis. . . . Death from consumption still costs a billion and a half a year."[120] Hence de Kruif hoped that his readers would join him in support of BCG and bring pressure to bear on those who kept it from Americans.

By the 1930s, then, BCG had marshaled some measure of public interest. But even with this increased optimism and support, a residual ambivalence remained. Devine betrayed some of this. "I had a different slant on BCG Thursday evening in dining with my old friends, Prof. and Mme. Fuster," he wrote back to friends in New York. Fuster, Devine explained, was "an intimate" and longtime friend of Calmette; his wife was a social worker in Paris "knowing a great deal about actual living conditions of the poor. Both of them are ardent advocates of insisting on BCG for [infants born to tuberculous] mothers. They think that the danger of infection is immediate, serious, induced almost certainly and almost certainly fatal (considering housing, income, habits, undernourishment, etc., etc.). The danger if any is remote, slight, problematical. They think we take a great responsibility in *not* using it."[121] The decision to use BCG in Paris, Devine recognized, was intimately tied to assessments of poverty; so were the discussions of BCG that took place in New York but in a quite different way. Just as Professor and Mme. Fuster saw it as their duty to save the poor by vaccinating them against tuberculosis, so Devine and others came to wonder whether the use of BCG would not deflect attention away from, and thereby weaken, their efforts to root out the conditions that made people both poor and susceptible to TB. Devine, a social worker with an active and longstanding interest in welfare policy, had a vested interest in casting the debate over vaccination in these terms, but as attention shifted to clinical and epidemiological trials that would determine the efficacy of BCG, others similarly recognized the importance of the question he posed.

Just as an earlier generation of physicians had feared that tuberculin would deflect attention away from the social roots of TB, so some of the early critics of BCG suggested that the vaccine would blind those responsible for TB control to the larger goal of building a multifaceted resistance to the disease. The problem in this respect was not that BCG was demonstrably less effective than the traditional measures of TB control. Rather, the difficulty was precisely that BCG might well appear to provide a useful way of controlling the disease that would then make these other measures expendable. Petroff, for instance, warned that propaganda in favor of BCG "bids fair to engender a false and dangerous security, which would neglect standard and adequate hygienic measures."[122]

While BCG technically and physiologically heightened resistance, the vaccine was thus no solution to the TB problem because it would undermine the essentials of the campaign to build resistance in the broad sense, which included both physiological and sociological dimensions. Such reservations made considerable fiscal and epidemiological sense—once one accepts that TB is a disease of both seed and soil—and they clearly appealed to those researchers who seized on treatment methods that united the goals of destroying microbes, forming healthy tissues, and promoting the habits of life and social conditions that built resistance.

As first impressions gave way to second thoughts, and as private judgment gave way to public pronouncement, the same reservations continued to inform physicians' assessments of BCG's efficacy. Perhaps the best example of this second wave of reaction to BCG is seen in the work of Knopf, a leading authority on TB and one of the first American physicians assigned responsibility to report on BCG in an official public capacity. Knopf spoke for those who continued to recognize that tubercular germs would plant themselves only in an unhealthy soil, and his goal was to till that soil in a manner that made it inhospitable to tubercular infection. Though aware of the hereditary influences that contributed to susceptibility, Knopf continued to focus his attention on environmental conditions. He connected TB to the evils of poverty, child labor, underfeeding, overcrowding, and large families (for which he proposed birth control and even abortion as an antidote).[123] Recognizing the link between social conditions and disease, Knopf consistently advocated both economic and social reform as a means of combating tuberculosis.

Committed as he was to the eradication of tuberculosis among children, Knopf could not ignore BCG, and he paid just tribute to Calmette's vaccine. Still, though essentially well-disposed, Knopf entered the typical American caveat: "Of course, this vaccination should not cause one to dispense with hygienic measures capable of preventing or lessening massive infection."[124]

Knopf articulated his concerns about the threat that BCG posed to existing campaigns against TB still more clearly in a report that he presented to the United States government. The official government delegate to the meeting of the International Union against Tuberculosis held at The Hague in September 1932, Knopf had been asked to provide the surgeon general, the State Department, the War Department, and War Veteran's Bureau with an account of his experiences. He submitted this account in 1933 as part of a larger work in which he discussed war veterans and children side by side. All three sections of his report drew attention to the social as well as the physiological dimensions of tuberculosis, and the chapter he devoted to BCG was sandwiched between discussions of "Psychological and Social Aspects of the After-Care of the Tuberculous," "Outdoor Sleeping Devices for the Tuberculous in City and Country," and "Prevention of Tuberculosis in Children by Breathing Exercises, Outdoor Life, etc."

Lübeck had done nothing to tarnish Knopf's confidence in the efficacy and safety of BCG, but though he remained enthusiastic, Knopf nonetheless refused to divorce the problem of creating physiological resistance from the larger campaign against the disease. In what came to be a familiar American style, he argued that vaccination with BCG was not enough. He warned:

> [W]hatever may be discovered in the future by the workers in tuberculosis laboratories now functioning throughout the civilized world, along the lines of immunity or cure, we must not forget the well known essentials in the prevention of tuberculosis; . . . we must develop the physiques of [our] children to add to the immunity conferred upon them through BCG inoculation in earlier years. We must create a physiological strength to lastingly overcome the inherited physiological poverty. Besides as much outdoor life as possible, the prevention of child labor, the creation of open air schools, I consider judicious breathing exercises the very best means of developing chest capacity, strong lungs, strong voices and resistance to disease in general.[125]

Thus, Knopf would not abandon other measures of tuberculosis control in favor of BCG. BCG, like tuberculin, acted on the host rather than the bacillus, but its action was purely physiological and its use incompatible with the broader, ideological goals of the American campaign against tuberculosis. To Knopf, tuberculosis was a manifestation of deeper social problems, and he viewed the crusade against the disease as part of a larger campaign to breed good citizens. BCG vaccination might confer immunity, but it could not build the resistance that marked those citizens.

In the earliest American debates over BCG, incompatible intellectual and scientific traditions collided. Recognition of the need for a national research agenda and the intricacies of institutional and regulatory processes inhibited efforts to test or adopt the vaccine. But, in addition, American physicians resisted BCG because of the inconsistency between vaccination and the premises that had sustained their anti-TB crusade through the late-nineteenth and early-twentieth century and that, by the 1930s, seemed as vital and appropriate as ever. Like tuberculin, only more radically, BCG challenged the bases of a campaign dedicated to building a combined physiological and sociological resistance. For many American physicians, to accept BCG required that they abandon both their understanding of TB as a physiological-sociological disease and their larger goal of transforming behavior to create good citizens. Ultimately, as we shall see in the next chapter, this proved too high a price to pay.

CHAPTER 5

For Cows, Boys, and Indians: North American Trials of BCG, 1924–1946

"Two factors enter into a discussion when a method of antituberculosis vaccination is based on the use of living micro-organisms," Strasheimer Alburtus Petroff reminded his colleagues. These were: "(1) is the method dangerous, (2) is it effective."[1] As fears about the safety of BCG receded, a new set of worries about efficacy emerged. Like researchers throughout the world, Americans measured efficacy in both physiological and statistical terms. They evaluated the mechanism by which BCG worked and undertook theoretical and experimental analyses of the relationship between allergy to tuberculin and immunity. They scrutinized Albert Calmette's quantitative data and challenged the numerical basis for claims that vaccination reduced mortality and morbidity. In addition, however, American researchers measured BCG vaccination against the standard of other preventatives for tuberculosis, and they asked whether, in light of the conditions that spawned TB, BCG "was enough." This last effort, which led to the formulation of a definition of relative efficacy in which social context became critical, defined the American response to BCG. It served, moreover, once again to unite the biological and social campaigns against disease and to turn attention to the tuberculous "soil."

The early epidemiological trials that Americans conducted demonstrate how deeply physicians shared the assumption that to combat TB one had to eradicate both the biological causes of the disease and the malnutrition, poor housing, lack of self-control, and general poverty that rendered Americans susceptible. Between 1924 and 1960, when Americans and Canadians conducted trials of BCG on cattle, children, and Native Americans—or cows, boys, and Indians[2]—Canadian investigators attempted merely to replicate Calmette's results and reduce tuberculous mortality. Their American colleagues, however, asked additional questions about the relative efficacy of BCG. These physicians and the institutions they represented continued to believe that malnutrition, poor housing, and general poverty predisposed to TB and that belief shaped both the design and the interpretation of their research. They asked not just whether BCG safely reduced mortality but also whether vaccination was superior to measures that both reduced tuberculosis and improved the standard of living. Their interest in these questions of relative efficacy truly distinguished the American response to BCG.

DEFINING EFFICACY

The comparative judgment on which the question of BCG's relative efficacy turned built on several distinct but related observations. One of the earliest objections raised was that Calmette's preventative vaccine was not in itself sufficient to get to the root of the TB problem. At the simplest level this charge of insufficiency addressed the vaccine's technical limitations.

As Americans appraised BCG's efficacy, their concerns ran the gamut from the general and theoretical to the downright picky, but one—the relationship between vaccination and allergy to tuberculin—stood out as critical and exposed far more serious and fundamental questions about the relationship of infection, allergy, and immunity. The difficulties began with the observation that when BCG was administered orally, infants neither routinely nor consistently became allergic to tuberculin. Both in the United States and abroad, 75 percent of unvaccinated children who lived in a tuberculous environment normally reacted positively to tuberculin by the end of their first year of life. Only 26.6 percent of the vaccinees Calmette had drawn from tuberculous homes and 7.6 percent of those he had drawn from nontuberculous environments became tuberculin positive. Reaction rates taken at the end of two years were little better, and after four years only half of Calmette's vaccinees regularly tested positive.

Calmette did not equate immunity with allergy to tuberculin. He had adopted a parasitic model of tuberculosis, and in his opinion immunity occurred when a few live, avirulent bacilli continued to exist within the body. American physicians disagreed. They almost unanimously accepted Robert Koch's assertion that a positive reaction to tuberculin formed a necessary precondition of immunity to TB. Thus their preoccupation with tuberculin conversion reflected fundamental scientific disagreements, but it also had significant, practical implications. Accustomed to associating immunity with allergy to tuberculin, American physicians knew no other way of gauging whether vaccination had taken. Hence, whether or not BCG could actually produce immunity without allergy, the editors of *Journal of the American Medical Association* argued that it left physicians without a benchmark of its efficacy.[3]

Clinicians and experimentalists returned again and again to the matter of tuberculin conversion and sought alternative measures of the immune state. Some, like Eugene Opie and William Hallock Park, tried to circumvent the problem. Opie, no more successfully, attempted to gauge BCG's efficacy by examining tubercle formation. Park concentrated on devising a vaccination method that would render recipients tuberculin positive, for in his experience whether BCG was administered orally, interally, or subcutaneously made a difference in the response to tuberculin.[4] In the wake of these efforts, Opie summarized the sentiments of many of his colleagues when he observed, "Immunity to tuberculosis has a number of inconvenient features."[5] Petroff, who again played a key role in the debate, tipped the entire problem on its head and fundamentally reframed the relationship between infection and immunity. Rather than asking how in the absence of a positive reaction to tuberculin one could gauge the efficacy of BCG or how one could modify the method of vaccination to produce a positive reaction, Petroff questioned the very meaning of the positive reaction to tuberculin. If BCG, which was meant to produce immunity to tuberculosis, routinely failed to render vaccinated individuals tuberculin positive, Petroff argued, then a positive tuberculin reaction ought logically to be interpreted as a sign of infection. He consequently proposed that when vaccinated children belatedly became tuberculin positive, this reaction indicated that BCG had failed.[6] This time, Petroff did not disagree with Calmette's premises. He accepted the assertion that immunity was not synonymous with allergy to tuberculin, but he now argued that an allergy to tuberculin must signify infection.

Even if BCG did safely confer immunity, it had technical limitations. It appeared to have a short duration, and it could be given only to newborns or to the very few others who had never been exposed to tuberculosis. In other words, both the action of the vaccine and the population that it might affect were understood to be limited. Hence, Calmette's "preventive" was "not enough," and it would be necessary to supplement BCG with other measures. Given its limitations, the question of whether BCG provided any better protection than standard preventative measures that were already in place—and that, even with the advent of BCG, presumably would still supplement vaccination—became crucial.

The *Times* earliest reports had set the stage. In an editorial entitled "His

Preventive Not Enough," the *Times* used language strikingly reminiscent of earlier assessments of tuberculin to compare the results of vaccination with traditional measures of TB control. "These are the results that for years have been accomplished in many instances by careful attention to diet, habits and environment, especially as were conducted in sanatoria," the *Times* correspondent suggested, and they were "accomplished there not because of any mysterious benefits from air or climate in those places but because rules can be followed better in them than in most homes."[7] When he dismissed the need for BCG in 1928 Petroff also raised the issue of relative need. "In the United States and Canada where the campaign against tuberculosis is made very effective by the use of various sociological and health measures," he argued, "mortality and infection in childhood have decreased to a very low level, and we cannot see why such a prophylactic as advocated by the French investigators should be introduced at present."[8]

Statistical concerns reinforced these apprehensions. By the late 1920s, substantial empirical evidence could be marshaled to support the argument that BCG reduced tuberculous mortality and morbidity. The sheer number of the studies and their overwhelmingly positive conclusions forced even BCG's staunchest critics to admit that vaccination offered at least some measure of protection.[9] However, the amassed evidence did not convince Americans, who felt that the French data often appeared much more extensive than they actually were.

As William Charles White, Petroff, and other critics closely assessed Calmette's work, they focused initially on the quality of the data. Though by January 1, 1927, Calmette's research team had vaccinated 43,283 children, they had used a much smaller population for their statistical assessments. Sufficient comparative data existed for only 1,050 vaccinees.[10] Moreover, Calmette's American critics noted that although the French researchers had distributed questionnaires to a large number of tuberculosis dispensaries in order to elicit broad information from a wide variety of sources, only a small percentage had responded. Yet Calmette based his evaluation of general tuberculous mortality, at least in part, on the response to these questionnaires.

Attacks on Calmette's statistics gradually focused in on his use of controls. "Dr. Calmette's vaccine ingested by children has had wide use in Europe," White observed, "but when one examines the statistical data already published one is impressed by the lack of control data upon which to base conclusions as to its value."[11] In an apparent effort to make its data more comprehensive and representative, the French team had drawn comparisons between its test group and the general population. Their attempt to estimate mortality from "general death rates and from reports of studies for other purposes and from other periods"[12] seemed equally flawed. Moreover, no data had been collected for the period 1924–1927, during which extensive antituberculosis programs had been implemented and during which death rates from TB had presumably declined. "It is a matter for regret," White's editorial in the *Journal of the American Medical Association* concluded, "that in an experiment so far reaching and so extensive, care was not taken to secure control figures that might have made the published results more convincing."[13]

The still more serious charge was of selective data collection. Petroff alleged that Calmette had "selected figures for comparison which were in his favor" and had chosen his vaccinees according to criteria that made them incomparable with the nontest population. He accused Calmette, as well, of treating his populations differently. He had separated the vaccinees but not the controls from the infective environment.[14] Opie also took issue with the different treatment accorded subjects and controls, which he believed skewed the research results. He further chastised Calmette for failing to analyze the ways in which this differential treatment might have affected his results. Opie then fused objections to Calmette's presentation of data and his experimental design in the charge that Calmette's team had calculated mortality in the test and control populations differently. When they calculated the death rate for their test population, Opie noted, the French researchers excluded any tuberculous deaths that occurred during the first ten days; however, they included these early deaths in their statistics for the controls.[15]

The observation "that vaccination [with BCG] not only lowers the mortality rate from tuberculosis but also lowers that from all causes of death"[16] seemed to confirm charges of Calmette's selectivity. Other investigators, working on other public health problems, had previously encountered and explained away a similar phenomenon.[17] Now, however, the general good health of Calmette's subjects fueled the allegations that his two populations were incomparable and had not been chosen according to the same criteria of health and hygiene. Some, like the editors of the *Journal of the American Medical Association,* suggested that "[t]he care and education which precede and follow vaccination, must render as preferred the group of children and families studied."[18] Others, like Petroff, turned attention to the original home environment and argued that "one must consider that there is also a social difference in the two groups of mothers."[19]

The ease and speed with which American researchers attributed Calmette's results to social differences among the control and test populations betrayed their deep-seated conviction that such differences shaped the epidemiology of TB. Where Calmette assumed that general good health was a by-product of the eradication of TB, the editors of the *Journal* and other Americans assumed that general good health was the precondition for resistance to TB. This assumption, alongside the conviction that existing tuberculosis control measures worked, became a fundamental basis of American efforts to measure the efficacy of BCG. Again and again, American researchers insisted on judging Calmette's preventative against the measures, programs, and approaches already in place. In short, beyond understanding the immunological processes and beyond questioning the statistical evidence, American physicians brought to their study of BCG a notion of relative efficacy. "We have now reached the cross-road and must decide as to what course we must pursue in our campaign against tuberculosis," Petroff warned. Presenting the alternatives, he defined the American dilemma. "Shall we tuberculize the whole world by adopting Calmette's method of vaccination with living microörganisms?" he asked. "Or shall we continue those preventive methods, adopted some years ago in this country and Canada, and so successfully employed in reducing the mortality from tuberculosis and preventing infection in infants?"[20] Even as killed vaccines, therapies like sanocrysin, and new avenues of research offered alternatives, and even as the MRC promoted lab-based research, American physicians clung tenaciously to traditional measures of disease control.[21]

THE CANADIAN TRIALS

A comparison of American and Canadian vaccination trials illustrates the ways in which an unshakable faith in the value of existing measures and a continued commitment to a multifaceted conception of resistance shaped American attempts to evaluate BCG. At its first meeting, the Canadian ACTR affirmed the need for vaccine research. Soon thereafter, it supported its verbal commitment by allocating funds to both experimental and epidemiologic investigations. It gave priority to analyses of prophylactic inoculation and bacterial transformation and especially to "repetition of the vaccination experiments made by Calmette and Guérin and the duration of immunity."[22] The ACTR had no staff to undertake these investigations but instead subdivided the research problems among the best qualified Canadian medical and veterinary scientists. Thereafter, the ACTR coordinated and managed the individual studies. It met yearly to review the progress of research and to revise common goals.[23]

Under the auspices of the ACTR, Canadian medical and veterinary scientists engaged in an integrated, well-planned effort to determine whether Calmette's claims could be verified and duplicated. Ultimately, the tests of BCG that they conducted on cattle, on children in Quebec, and on Native Americans in Saskatchewan sought to determine whether vaccination really combated TB as dramatically and effectively as Calmette had reported it did. The trials on cattle, with which they began, offered a mixed assessment. When the ACTR first met, E. A. Watson and A. C. Rankin had already obtained the BCG culture from Lille and begun tests of the vaccine. Because the ACTR keenly appreciated the dangers of tuberculous cattle, it actively encouraged Rankin and Watson's efforts.[24] At the second meeting of the ACTR, each took the floor. Rankin's preliminary report supported the use of BCG. By October 1925, he had vaccinated ninety-eight calves, whom he had subsequently exposed to tuberculous animals and fed on contaminated milk. Two months later, he measured the tuberculin reaction of the vaccinees and of controls whom he had similarly exposed to infection and reported that "the [ten] uninoculated calves—with one exception—were found to have reacted more vigorously than the inoculated."[25] Rankin, unlike his American colleagues, accepted Calmette's interpretation of the relationship between allergy and immunity and interpreted this difference in reactivity to mean that the inoculated animals were less vulnerable to TB. He supported his conclusion with the evidence that none of his vaccinees presented any signs or symptoms of active tuberculosis. Watson tempered Rankin's enthusiasm. At the time, he felt reasonably confident that Calmette's results could be replicated, but he remained unsure of BCG's safety and hence provided only a tentative endorsement of BCG.[26]

Despite Watson's reservations, the ACTR recommended further vaccination trials. The impetus came partly from growing awareness of the human costs of tuberculosis among industrial workers and especially among children. It came as well from Dr. J. A. Baudouin, professor at the School of Applied Social Hygiene at the University of Montreal. Baudouin and his staff had formal ties with both Calmette and the Pasteur Institute. Their personal allegiance to Calmette along with their professional preference for French medicine predisposed them favorably toward BCG. At the second meeting of the ACTR, Baudouin made an explicit case for human vaccination trials.[27] The ACTR respected his interest and authorized the University of Montreal to proceed.

Over the next two years, Baudouin cooperated with the Pasteur Institute in an attempt to replicate Calmette's findings. To ensure comparability, he requested that Calmette appoint a member of his staff to oversee the Montreal trials; A. Petit soon assumed the role of liaison. When he moved from Paris to Montreal, Petit imported Calmette's protocol and a strain of BCG. Thereafter, he regulated production of the vaccine while Baudouin supervised clinical trials.[28] Perhaps because he entered into BCG research with the goal of affirming rather than testing the validity of Calmette's results, Baudouin introduced no innovations. Unlike Park, who had experimented with different methods of vaccination, Baudouin followed Calmette's protocol exactly and administered BCG orally to newborns. Baudouin's allegiance to Calmette's product and technique did not completely sway his judgment. A former Rockefeller Foundation fellow who had studied at Johns Hopkins, Baudouin had a keen interest in epidemiology, statistics, and social hygiene. He consequently recognized flaws in Calmette's study design, which he attempted to rectify by selecting equal numbers of subjects and controls. Moreover, he matched these carefully for age, socioeconomic, and "contact" conditions.

Baudouin's preliminary results confirmed Calmette's claim that BCG safely and effectively reduced tuberculous mortality. By 1928, the staff at the University of Montreal had vaccinated almost 700 infants with a method that Baudouin felt sure replicated Calmette's. After presenting a preliminary but positive report to a League of Nations conference on BCG vaccination,[29] Baudouin extended the trial so that by 1934 his study population included 5,126 infants. In a review of this work Baudouin reported unprecedented reductions in mortality. "[I]t is found that the mortality rate in the vaccinated group of 1–12 months was only one-quarter of that of the unvaccinated group," he wrote "and in the second group of 1–7 years approximately one third."[30] Striking as the general reduction was, the death rate among vaccinated children who were exposed regularly to tubercular infections and the age-adjusted rates even more clearly confirmed BCG's efficacy. Almost 600 of Baudouin's vaccinees lived in regular, close contact with an adult who had been diagnosed as tuberculous; yet, despite this proximity, the overall tuberculous death rate for these children was four-and-a-half times less than that of a comparable group of unvaccinated children. When Baudouin adjusted these data for age, he found that, for children under one year, "the [tuberculosis death] rate was only 8 per thousand in comparison with 49 per thousand in the unvaccinated group—six times as great."[31] On the basis of these findings, Baudouin concluded that BCG provided a particularly effective means of reducing mortality in children under one year of age who lived in close contact with tuberculosis.

Baudouin succeeded in replicating Calmette's results so well, in fact, that he reproduced some of the same trouble spots that had excited Calmette's American critics. For example, like Calmette, Baudouin found that BCG vaccination reduced not just tuberculous mortality and morbidity but also morbidity and mortality from other causes, or, as he put it, the "health record of the vaccinated group is more favorable than that of the unvaccinated group."[32] Rather than lowering his estimate of BCG's efficacy, Baudouin took the general improvement in health as further confirmation that he had successfully replicated Calmette's results. When he discovered that with every year "the results are even more favorable in the vaccinated group than were recorded in the previous years," the realization that this increase ought to be attributed, at least in part, to the "larger size of the groups under observation" did not dampen his enthusiasm. Baudouin unabashedly concluded that "the findings tend to show more and more conclusively with each succeeding year of observation, that BCG vaccination against tuberculosis must be included as part of a complete campaign for the control of this disease."[33] By 1941, he had vaccinated 44,734 infants. Among all subjects, whose ages ranged from infancy to fifteen years, BCG reduced mortality by an average of 61 percent; among infants under one year, the vaccine reduced mortality by 66 percent. In no circumstance had the oral administration of BCG proven dangerous.[34]

Nor did vague insinuations that a close association with Calmette "compromised" the validity of his research trouble Baudouin. As his trials proved increasingly successful, Baudouin grew increasingly modest and took measures to improve his credibility. In 1933, he asked Armand Frappier, a Rockefeller fellow who had studied with both Calmette and Petroff, to join his research team. Frappier had intimate knowledge of arguments both in favor of and against BCG, which he critically applied to vaccine production and epidemiological analysis.

To guarantee the integrity of his statistical work and to stave off the sort of attack that had been launched against Calmette, Baudouin also invited J. W. Hopkins, a statistician for the Division of Biology and Agriculture of the National Research Laboratories in Ottawa, to provide an independent evaluation. Hopkins's extensive appraisal, completed in 1941, supported Baudouin's conclusion that BCG safely reduced tuberculous mortality. To ensure that he provided an accurate assessment of efficacy, Hopkins limited his analysis to data concerning vaccinees who lived with tuberculous adults. "The morbidity figures," he wrote, "exhibit striking differences in favor of the vaccinated children," and, "under the conditions of this investigation, the oral administration of BCG vaccine at birth substantially reduced the incidence of tuberculosis during the third, fourth and fifth years of life."[35]

Subsequent trials that Frappier and Baudouin conducted further confirmed that BCG vaccination reduced tuberculosis mortality substantially, and they won international praise.[36] Frappier's BCG laboratory, now housed at the Institute of Microbiology and Hygiene of Montreal, expanded production and began to distribute vaccine throughout Canada. The success of the Montreal trials convinced the Quebec provincial Department of Health to advocate broader vaccination programs. In Montreal and in other cities throughout Quebec, hospital staff began to regularly vaccinate newborn "contacts." By 1949, the Quebec Department of Health had also implemented an extensive school vaccination campaign.[37]

Concern about tuberculosis among children drew attention to the parallel problem of disease among the native population. The Federal Department of Health's 1923 survey of preschool and school-age children suggested that tuberculosis was an enormous threat to Canada's native population. The findings of a study conducted by the Fort Qu'Appelle Sanatorium, in Fort Qu'Appelle, Saskatchewan, confirmed the fears; at Fort Qu'Appelle, and other sanatoria on the Canadian prairies, Native American admissions had increased markedly.[38]

Both the ACTR and the Canadian Tuberculosis Association (CTA) responded to these early cries of alarm by commissioning further studies. To better assess the problem, the ACTR appointed R. G. Ferguson, medical director of the Fort Qu'Appelle Sanatorium, to conduct a study of "tuberculinization" of Native Americans in the surrounding area.[39] On the assumption that allergy to tuberculin provided an indication of exposure to infection, Ferguson initiated wide-scale tuberculin testing. He looked as well for evidence of tubercles and other signs of active disease. The CTA encouraged the federal Department of Indian Affairs to undertake a similar survey of Pacific Coast Indians.[40]

Both Ferguson and the Department of Indian Affairs found further cause for concern. Most of the 315 schoolchildren that Ferguson tested had signs of active disease or recently healed infections.[41] Response rates to tuberculin among native and white children differed so significantly that Ferguson called for immediate intervention. The preliminary report of the Pacific Coast survey, delivered to the 1926 meeting of the CTA, was more cautious. The department had only just begun its work and would not offer more than "impressions," but these confirmed Ferguson's findings. Tuberculosis was more prevalent among Pacific Coast Indians than in the average white population, and a disproportionate number of cases existed in the under-fourteen population. Because fewer cases appeared among those over forty years of age, the department also proposed that Native Americans experienced a more virulent form of tubercular disease.

Unlike his colleagues in the Department of Indian Affairs, Ferguson was unwilling to ascribe his findings to a different, "Indian" form of TB.[42] Instead, he argued that natives were particularly susceptible to TB because they had only recently been exposed to infection. Evidence of lower mortality among the Métis, or mixed-blood, population and the observation that as successive generations became tuberculinized the death rate fell supported this argument.[43]

Hence, Ferguson's call to arms, despite its urgency, did not initially ring with desperation. He held out hope that, with time, mortality among the native population could be brought in line with that of the general Canadian population. Moreover, he found the socioeconomic conditions under which the tribes lived marginal but not appalling. "The nourishment and general condition of these children was good," Ferguson observed, "and compared favorably with any group of white children previously examined in Saskatchewan." Thus, "while the incidence was much larger than would be found among white children," Ferguson believed that "[t]aken altogether, the evidence of tuberculosis is of such a character as to show a marked advance in resistance against disease."[44]

Over the next several years, as depression and drought exacerbated the economic difficulties of Western Canada, Ferguson's optimism rang increasingly hollow. By 1933, the health of Canadian native peoples had deteriorated generally, and tuberculosis mortality increased to the point that it was ten times greater than in the white population.[45] An average of 68.7 percent of the children who lived on the reservation in the area of Fort Qu'Appelle had been infected before they reached the age of ten; in some areas, as many as 91 percent were infected.[46] Yet while mortality and morbidity increased, the high costs of isolating and caring for consumptives within sanatoria ensured that fewer and fewer Native Americans received the help they needed.

As traditional measures of tuberculosis control failed the Fort Qu'Appelle Indians, Ferguson considered BCG. In 1932, he proposed to the ACTR that he and A. B. Simes, the medical director of the Qu'Appelle Indian Health Unit, mount a vaccination trial.[47] The proposal passed easily, for it satisfied both the practical needs of those who feared for the health of Native Americans and the more theoretical interests of those who sought further confirmation of BCG's merits.[48] At its meeting of April 7, 1931, the ACTR had unanimously agreed on the safety of BCG and issued the statement that "use of BCG as a vaccine, particularly when applied parenterally, confers a degree of resistance."[49] However, despite this affirmation, some members of the ACTR considered the "problem of vaccinial immunity" unresolved and called for further study. The Fort Qu'Appelle Indians, riddled as they were with tuberculosis, offered what seemed to be an ideal test population.

Ferguson began work in 1933 with an initial population of all infants born on reserves under the jurisdiction of the Qu'Appelle Indian Health Unit. At first, Ferguson vaccinated his subjects orally, using BCG produced in Montreal by Frappier. In 1934, however, he vaccinated a small, secondary group intracutaneously and, like Park, found this method preferable. Consequently, after 1935, he continued to use the BCG produced in Montreal but vaccinated all his subjects intracutaneously.[50] Ferguson also modified Calmette's study design to guard against some of the harsher methodological criticisms. His view of susceptibility was both contagionist and evolutionary, and he believed that lack of prior exposure was a key determinant.[51] In deference to these environmental circumstances, Ferguson paired "[f]amilies of comparable status in respect of housing, sanitation and certain other economic and social factors likely to affect the health of children."[52] One child of each pair received BCG vaccine; the other became the control. Ferguson took additional care to ensure that he, unlike Calmette, could not be accused of choosing test and control populations differently or treating them selectively. The general death rate during the first year of life was comparable in his two groups, and both subjects and controls remained in a highly infectious environment.

By 1938, Ferguson's preliminary results indicated that BCG vaccination reduced mortality among Native American children who lived in a highly infectious environment by 75 percent.[53] These results justified an appeal for an expanded trial in which BCG would be used both on Native American infants and on the tuberculin-negative nurses who worked closely with TB patients. Partly out of caution and partly because his attention shifted temporarily to the study of nurses, Ferguson did not report again until 1946, when he once again attested to the efficacy and safety of BCG. Protection was not "absolute," he conceded, but it was "considerable."[54] Three years later, Ferguson offered further endorsement of BCG. During the twelve-year period during which the trial was in place, 306 infants had been vaccinated and 303 served as controls. Six cases of tuberculosis and two tuberculosis deaths had occurred among the vaccinees; twenty-nine cases and nine deaths occurred in the controls. Adjusted for population, these figures suggested a fivefold difference in both mortality and morbidity.[55] Ferguson and Simes thus concluded that "BCG conferred valuable protection in a highly infectious environment."[56]

By the mid-1940s, the various BCG trials conducted under the auspices of the ACTR mostly confirmed Calmette's claims. Vaccination, an experimental technique used before 1946 only in Saskatchewan and Quebec, was employed thereafter in every province. BCG vaccination did not constitute a large portion of the Canadian crusade against TB when viewed from a financial perspective, but recognition of its usefulness in preventing disease among particularly susceptible populations was growing.[57]

THE AMERICAN TRIALS

Quite the opposite proved true south of the border. Institutionally, no equivalent of the ACTR developed to sponsor and coordinate American BCG trials. Individual private laboratories, such as the Phipps Institute of the University of Pennsylvania, the Tice Laboratory of the University of Chicago, and the New York City Department of Health, undertook the major American studies, and the NTA acted as a clearinghouse. But the differences were not simply institutional. Between 1930 and 1946, American trials contributed steadily to doubts about vaccination campaigns as those who conducted them and those who evaluated them continually questioned the relative efficacy of BCG.

Tests on Cattle and Children

Like the Canadians and French before them, American researchers began to test BCG on cattle. The majority of their trials, performed under the auspices of agricultural colleges like that at Cornell, soon indicated that BCG worked and convinced even such harsh opponents as Petroff that BCG conferred some protection. However, unlike Rankin and Watson, who at this point supported BCG—or at least withheld judgment—Petroff introduced the criticism that would guide further American trials. Americans could not restrict their discussions of efficacy to analyses of BCG's ability to reduce tuberculous mortality, he insisted; they needed to determine as well whether the vaccine worked more effectively than existing measures of control. In Petroff's assessment it did not. As we saw earlier, Petroff built his case by making the charge of selectivity and by testifying to the value of isolation schemes. Loyal to the hygienic measures that Americans and Canadians had adopted, he deemed these effective and opposed any proposal to supplant them. When those less convinced than he suggested that BCG would effectively reduce bovine TB in areas where testing and isolation had failed, Petroff stood firm. He attributed the persistence of bovine tuberculosis not to the inadequacies of existing TB control measures but to the sloppiness of those farmers and public authorities who failed to enforce them rigorously. Hence, Petroff suggested that vaccination, rather than reducing disease, might actually lead to a resurgence of infection. In this context he argued that vaccination might "engender a false and dangerous security which would neglect standard and adequate hygienic measures."[58]

Strongly as Petroff might argue that testing, isolation, and the slaughter of infected cattle had reduced rates of bovine tuberculosis, he could not make the same case for measures to limit human disease. Attempts to destroy the tubercle bacillus and to produce preventatives and cures had repeatedly failed, and infection rates remained high. However, if Petroff's reluctance to abandon educational and sanatorium based efforts in favor of a vaccine that had been demonstrated to be both safe and effective seems peculiar, the ensuing discussion of human vaccination trials indicated that he was no isolated crank. In further assessments of the vaccine, Americans repeatedly argued that BCG was less effective and appropriate than existing hygienic means of control.

The first human trials conducted in the United States exposed these concerns about relative efficacy. In 1927, after he had assured himself that BCG was safe, Park initiated a human vaccination trial. He chose for his study infants from tuberculous households in the New York City area whom local hospitals and clinics referred to him. Park vaccinated half the children with BCG, left the other half as controls, then followed both groups for new cases and mortality. In 1929, he reported his initial findings. Because he had vaccinated 183 babies of whom only 87 were by then over one year, Park qualified his results; still, he concluded that in this small population BCG vaccination had indeed proven simple, safe, and effective. Park found a significant decline in tuberculous mortality within the test population. The nontuberculous death rate was comparable in both groups, but TB caused 8.6 percent of deaths among the controls and only 1.2 percent among the vaccinees.

Baudouin, on the basis of similar results and a virtually identical trial, had concluded that BCG was highly effective,[59] but Park seemed reluctant to accept his own numbers. He acknowledged that "BCG vaccination is easy, harmless, and provides some immunity of unknown duration," but, like Petroff, he equivocated on the question of precisely how much protection BCG actually afforded. A major problem in assessing the immunizing value of BCG, he argued, resulted from difficulties in obtaining suitable cases and controls. "There are few fit cases for BCG vaccination in New York City," he maintained, first, because "social conditions are much better here" than in other countries and, second, because "the general health intelligence of the masses being higher in this country, the family understands better how to protect the babies."[60] Factoring these social determinants of resistance into his equation, Park now proposed that one could not isolate the component of protection that BCG produced. He suggested that the observed decline in tuberculous mortality might not be attributable to vaccination. Tuberculosis, he warned, had "bacterial, constitutional and social causes," and his trial had not adequately controlled for the social causes, especially what he called the "health intelligence" of the subjects.[61] This argument about the health intelligence of subjects attracted a significant American following and drew the notice of researchers, like Opie, who included it in their own analyses.[62]

Park had once again resorted to the old argument of "incomparable" vaccinated and control populations. The apparent decline in tuberculosis mortality that followed BCG vaccination, he proposed, was "misleading, because the BCG and control groups are not equally exposed to tuberculosis."[63] This suggestion led Park into a logical trap to which he was apparently oblivious. Because so many of the doubts about Calmette's work arose from his allegedly inappropriate selection of subjects and controls, Park, to avoid similar criticisms, boasted that he had carefully constructed his control statistics from "the mortality rate of babies coming from tuberculosis families . . . and given the same hygienic care as the vaccinated ones except the vaccination itself."[64] Though he should therefore have been unwilling to ascribe differences in mortality or morbidity to differences in population, he was not. "[T]he control families," he suggested, "are on average less intelligent and less cooperative than the vaccinated ones. Due to the lower intelligence, the social conditions of the family are lowered also."[65] He consequently believed that the families in the control population would less frequently adopt behaviors that protected against infection. Hence, he postulated that the controls were more frequently exposed to sputum than the vaccinees and were therefore at greater risk. Park had now worked the problem of relative efficacy into his study design, and as he continued his trial, he openly examined the question of whether BCG or "social factors" offered the true explanation for the declining tuberculosis death rate.

By 1933, Park had extended his trial to include over 1,000 subjects. His earlier efforts convinced him of the superiority of parenteral vaccination over either oral or interal, and he consequently switched methods. Of 413 babies vaccinated parenterally, only 0.5 percent died of tuberculosis, while 2.8 percent of his 608 controls died from TB. BCG seemed particularly effective among infants exposed to a constant source of infection. Among those known to have been in contact with positive sputum, 0.9 percent of the vaccinated group died from tuberculosis compared with 4.2 percent of the nonvaccinated.[66]

Yet Park still would not endorse the vaccine. "In order to evaluate the effect of the BCG vaccine on the mortality rate," he wrote, "scoring of the other influencing factors is necessary."[67] He argued again that the efficacy of BCG could not be fully established until researchers had matched the control and test populations for "all the more important factors which can have an influence on the development of tuberculosis or the escape from it."[68] Among these factors he included a category that he designated as "social and constitutional." In this category he included family earnings, family size, number of rooms in the family dwelling, birth weight, general health of the baby, ventilation and light in the apartment, cooperation of the family, and intelligence of the parents in regard to care of the baby. Before any definitive conclusions about the efficacy of BCG could be drawn, Park suggested, each test subject should be assigned a "Social Score". A composite of the above factors, that score would range from a low of 0 to a high of 100. BCG's ability to prevent tuberculosis in the low-scoring, or "handicapped," group would be a true measure of its efficacy.

Tests on Native Americans

Despite Park's reservations, interest in BCG grew. In 1933, the New York State Medical Association sponsored an open debate at which Dr. Konrad Birkhaug presided. Trained in Norway, Birkhaug had moved to New York, where he became a physician at the New York State Board of Health. Having learned of BCG in Europe, Birkhaug had continued to study the vaccine after he immigrated to the United States. However, he had found the American research climate chilly. "It has appeared of late to many European investigators," Birkhaug complained, "that conservatism in American medicine was carried a little too far in not giving BCG a trial in this country." Park's results seemed to him to break the ice. "It is a hopeful sign," he wrote, "to have the clinical results of vaccination with BCG in New York. . . . These studies afford a valuable corrective to the attitude assumed by Drs. Petroff, Medlar, Sasano and Watson in this country that BCG is a dangerous virus capable of producing progressive tuberculosis."[69] Birkhaug optimistically interpreted Park's work as having clearly demonstrated that BCG produced a higher degree of immunity to tuberculosis more consistently than did natural exposure. He also claimed that the vaccine seemed the most promising means of controlling tuberculosis presently available. The time had consequently come, he insisted, for Americans to measure its effects in the populations most prone to the disease.

In the United States, as in Canada, children were one of the vulnerable populations that Birkhaug identified; Native Americans were another. By the early 1930s, Americans had become critically aware of the extent to which tuberculosis was decimating Native American communities.[70]

The calls for "Indian assimilation,"[71] first made at the turn of the century, had taken their toll as Native Americans, both off the reservations and on, adopted an impoverished and crude facsimile of the "white" lifestyle, which compromised their health. Through the first decades of the century, Progressive reformers had regularly exposed the problem,[72] and in 1923 the NTA joined in the effort by presenting a report on "tuberculosis among the North American Indians" to Congress.[73] The Office of Indian Affairs responded quickly to the NTA's demands for an investigation by surveying the "Indian" tuberculosis problem, and the report that it issued in 1932 underscored the particular susceptibility of Native Americans. Among the many tribes tested, virtually every adult reacted positively to tuberculin. The reaction was double that found in rural white populations; it was one-third again as great as that found among rural blacks.[74]

Birkhaug's appeal reinforced these concerns and paved the way for BCG trials on Native Americans. In 1935, Opie responded by recommending an extension of Park's trial.[75] One year later, Phipps, in conjunction with the Bureau of Indian Affairs (BIA), began a long-term trial of BCG vaccination on Native Americans. Phipps had already tested BCG on a minor scale. At about the time of Lübeck, Opie and his staff had vaccinated a small number of children in Philadelphia who came from tuberculous homes. Committed to reducing tuberculosis among blacks, whom it deemed particularly susceptible to TB, Phipps had also approached the Rockefeller Foundation with a proposal to "vaccinate the colored population of one or more southern States." Calmette himself endorsed the project enthusiastically, but it seems never to have gotten off the ground.[76] Instead, Phipps cooperated with the Rockefeller Foundation in a study of "protective inoculation against tuberculosis in Jamaica."[77] Now, Phipps combined its various interests and talents in a study of tuberculosis among Native Americans.

Esmond Long and Joseph Aronson, both on staff at Phipps, became consultants to this new venture. Long, who later assumed the directorship of Phipps, had trained as a pathologist. While a graduate student at the University of Chicago, he developed tuberculosis. Thereafter, he moved to Saranac Lake, where he studied under Allen Krause and E. R. Baldwin. In 1923, Long moved to Philadelphia and began work at Phipps. He devoted most of his time to studies of the tuberculin reaction, which he conducted with Florence Seibert, and to investigations of nutrition, metabolism, and the chemistry of tuberculosis.[78] Long, however, also bore the mark of his years with Krause, and as he later explained, he and the clinical staff at Phipps understood TB as "a problem of the environment, the way people had to live, . . . [as] overwhelmingly a social and economic problem."[79] This interest drew him to epidemiological studies of tuberculosis among Native Americans. With the BIA, Long had conducted a tuberculosis survey of the Papago Indian area of southern Arizona, which demonstrated how widespread tuberculous infection was.[80] He was also interested in racial differences in tuberculous mortality. Concern for the "underlying basis for the high susceptibility of young females of the Negro and Indian races" led him to examine hereditary and environmental bases of nutritional differences in these populations.[81] It led, as well, to an assessment of the need for BCG.

In the United States, as in Canada, tuberculosis among the native population posed both an epidemiological and a clinical problem. Mortality was high; yet traditional sanatorium-based methods of treatment seemed impracticable and ineffective. As a result, BCG vaccination presented an important alternative, which Aronson, trained in bacteriology, epidemiology, and clinical medicine, well recognized. Aronson, like Ferguson, appreciated that vaccination had practical advantages. He also realized that the conditions on reservations provided an ideal opportunity to "determine the effectiveness of BCG vaccine in the control of tuberculosis in a population having high morbidity and high mortality."[82] Furthermore, because few attempts had been made to curtail TB and because Native Americans had not been educated about the causes of the disease, such a trial would also gauge whether BCG was effective in the absence of isolation and the social improvements Park deemed so important.

In early 1936, Aronson, J. G. Townsend, R. Saylor, and I. Parr—of the Office of Indian Affairs—moved into the interior. They selected a test population from Native Americans who lived in southeastern Alaska and on the Pima Agency (Arizona), the Wind River Agency (Wyoming), the Turtle Mountain Agency (North Dakota), and the Rosebud Agency (South Dakota). These tribes represented a variety of racial and cultural types with different social, economic, and dietary habits.[83] All the subjects fell between the ages of one and nineteen; all were tuberculin-negative. Between February 1936 and February 1938, Aronson, Saylor, and Parr vaccinated 1,565 Indian children with BCG; they simultaneously administered a placebo of sterile saline solution to 1,459 controls. They followed both groups for three years and performed tuberculin tests and chest X-rays at yearly intervals.

In a preliminary assessment of the trial, conducted at the end of three years, Aronson concluded that "[t]he results obtained thus far indicate that both mortality and morbidity from tuberculosis are significantly lower among those vaccinated with BCG vaccine than among the unvaccinated control group."[84] But he went no further. Instead, he cautiously advised that "[n]o definite conclusion should be drawn at this time as to the protective value of the vaccine."[85] The vaccination program had been in effect for only a short time, Aronson explained, and he wanted to reserve final judgment until the trial had been in progress longer.

With time, Aronson became more convinced of BCG's merits. By 1946, the results of Aronson's extended trial showed that vaccination reduced deaths from TB significantly and that six times as many controls as vaccinees developed tubercular disease. Moreover, while the incidence of new cases remained constant with age among the controls, it declined significantly among the vaccinees. On the basis of this evidence, Aronson concluded that "BCG vaccination is associated with marked protection against the development of tuberculosis as measured by mortality and morbidity."[86] Because he had carefully matched the test and control populations for age, sex, socioeconomic status, and as many other variables as possible, Aronson additionally argued that the vaccine, and the vaccine alone, had produced the results.

Aronson's impressive work appealed to his colleagues at Phipps, but it failed to convert the unconverted. Like Park and Calmette before him, Aronson had found that general mortality declined in the vaccinated population. His observation that the general death rate of the controls was almost double that of the vaccinees seemed to belie the claim that there was no inherent or socially induced difference in the vitality of the two groups.[87] Now, however, his critics seized on the fact that tubercular infections had declined naturally throughout North America. Between 1935 and 1945, tuberculosis mortality in the death-registration states dropped from 50/100,000 to 37/100,000. This drop affected both white and nonwhite populations.[88] The reduction in disease rates, apparent everywhere and even among nonvaccinated Native Americans, led critics to argue that Aronson could not possibly gauge the impact of BCG. He could not attribute the entire difference in mortality and morbidity to vaccination, they maintained, for at best he had isolated the component of declining mortality and morbidity that BCG might have caused.[89]

Even Aronson hedged on this issue. Though he had carefully matched his controls at the start of the trial, he had not monitored changes that might have occurred with time in their social and economic status. He later admitted that "the logical approach to the development and evaluation of a specific immunizing agent against tuberculosis requires not only an understanding of immunity but an appreciation of the many factors that make such an evaluation difficult. These factors include variations in the biology of the tubercle bacillus, the susceptibility of the host, the pathogenesis of the disease, the degree of exposure, social and economic factors."[90] To better test the validity of his conclusions, Aronson felt compelled to monitor the social and economic changes on the reservations. Over the next nine years, he collected additional data that would enable him to determine whether vaccination or improved living conditions produced the reductions in disease that he observed.

Aronson's willingness to admit the influence of social and economic factors testified to the power and pervasiveness of the belief that tuberculosis could not be understood in simply bacterial or physiological terms. In what was now standard American style, Aronson proposed that "[t]uberculosis, unlike most infectious diseases, has not shown definite cyclic epidemics. Increases in the occurrence of the disease have usually been associated with the ravages of war, or post-war conditions, with famine, or with marked economic depression."[91] The conditions of economic and social distress that predisposed to TB in the general population also affected Native Americans. When he provided background information about his test population in 1942, Aronson recognized that "[t]he incidence of tuberculous infection is associated with living conditions." Among the Sioux Indians on the Rosebud Agency, marked differences in infection and reactivity to tuberculin existed among those who attended mission schools and those who attended county public schools. Similarly, in Alaska, "where housing conditions are good, only 2 per cent of preschool children were tuberculin positive . . . in striking contrast to 24 per cent reactors among the same age group . . . where many families live together in large clan houses." Aronson attributed these differences and the high rates of the disease on the reservations to poverty and crowding. "The children attending the county schools came from more or less widely separated ranches where living conditions were more or less comparable to [those of] the white population," he wrote, "while those attending the government and mission schools came from the crowded, poorly housed families living under conditions which would compare with [those of] an urban slum."[92]

Aronson, like others before him, attributed susceptibility to social conditions that engendered disease. He repeatedly dismissed hereditarian explanations, maintaining that "the Indian as a race, is not peculiarly susceptible to tuberculosis." Locating his own work within the context of other studies, he argued that "the high rate of tuberculous infection and disease among Indians may be attributed, at least in part, to social and bionomic factors. That similar factors play a role among the white population has been definitely shown by Edwards in his case-finding survey in New York City. Of a total of 133,062 persons X-rayed, the incidence of

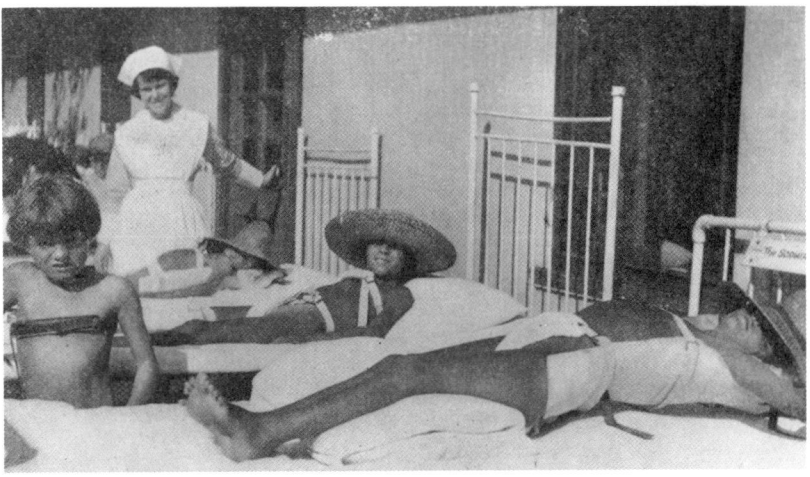

Native American Children
Source: R. I. Harris, "Heliotherapy in Surgical Tuberculosis," American Journal of Public Health *16 (1926): 689.*

active tuberculosis varied from .4% among high school students to 5.3 percent among transients and homeless persons."[93] Thus, Aronson did not differ with his critics on the question of the social determinants of TB. He agreed that the general decline in tuberculosis reflected social progress, including improvements in housing, diet, and education.

However, Aronson was not convinced that improvements had taken place on the reservations, nor was he convinced that they were the primary cause of declines in TB. The status of the tribes had altered over time, and both his own observations and data provided by the superintendent of each agency suggested that the Indian Service field nurses had effected the most dramatic changes. They had modified habits of child care, provided information about the sources of infection, and issued instructions about the value of hygiene. But though Aronson willingly credited the nurses with having helped to reduce the spread of disease, he would not correlate declining infection with any other change in the social and economic status of the tribes. No evidence of a significant improvement in housing or diet existed, he argued. "Housing continues to be inadequate and overcrowding has probably increased with a growing population. Cash incomes are larger, but there is no exact information concerning expenditures. Dietary habits have remained unchanged or show a continuing change from traditional native foods to those used by the neighboring white population."[94] Consequently, Aronson attributed declining rates of infection primarily to vaccination with BCG. He confidently and enthusiastically endorsed the vaccine, and he recommended its widespread use.

The Park Study Revisited

While Aronson grew increasingly convinced of BCG's merits, other investigators became more and more skeptical. In 1946, the same year in which Aronson published the preliminary findings of his trial, an update of Park's New York City trial appeared. Park by this time had died, but his collaborators, M. Levine and M. Sackett, had continued his work. In the report they now issued, Levine and Sackett reached conclusions that were diametrically opposed to Aronson's.

Between 1933 and 1946, Levine and Sackett closely studied over 1,000 children. Guided both by Park's earlier concerns and by experiences in almost fifty other vaccination trials, they had divided their subjects evenly into vaccinees and controls, and they had taken particular care to minimize economic and social differences in the two test populations. Unlike Baudouin—who, once he had established that vaccinees and nonvaccinated controls lived under identical conditions, readily accepted the efficacy of BCG—Levine and Sackett repeatedly emphasized the importance of comparable controls.[95]

The initial results of Levine and Sackett's study confirmed Park's early observation that vaccination safely and effectively conferred immunity to tuberculosis; however, like Park, they qualified their conclusions in ways that reintroduced the question of relative efficacy. Their qualifications revealed, moreover, the ways in which old and deep-seated prejudice created definite assumptions about the structure and goals of American antituberculosis campaigns. Despite the positive results of their trials, Levine and Sackett warned that "[a]s a public health measure, the routine vaccination with BCG of children from tuberculous homes is less advantageous than removal of the tuberculous subject from the home."[96] The data from their study did not alone support this conclusion. Statistically, the effects of isolation and of vaccination did not differ significantly. In the text of their paper, Levine and Sackett also reaffirmed that exposure to microbes did not correlate simply with infection; many people were exposed to tubercle bacilli but did not become ill.

However, isolation of the infected subject had advantages that vaccination did not. Once public authorities had removed tuberculous subjects from the home, they could attend to the "intelligence and cooperation of parents," the "economic conditions,"[97] and the other social determinants of infection that Levine and Sackett, like Park before them, identified as important. Thus, their conclusion once again raised the cry for public health and social programs that would both eradicate both the "seed" and the general social and constitutional determinants of the disease, and it posed the challenge for the next generation.

After 1924, Americans carved out a range of objections to BCG. They began by challenging the safety of the vaccine. Later, they questioned its efficacy. As they stripped away these objections layer by layer and discarded them, they resorted to the claim that, in the United States, mass vaccination with BCG would not be an appropriate public health measure. After 1945, as the PHS assumed increasing responsibility for tuberculosis control, the symbolic question of whether an effective campaign against tuberculosis should focus narrowly on the bacterial causes of infection or should also attack the poverty that bred the disease continued to inform the American debate over BCG.

"Not a Substitute for Approved Hygienic Measures": BCG and the Postwar Campaign against Tuberculosis

The Second World War marked a turning point in the American campaign against TB. As we saw in earlier chapters, no centralized governmental agency for the study or control of TB existed before the war. The experiences of illness, American understandings of susceptibility and risk, the shifting authority of medical science, and concerns about the jurisdiction of the state all played a role in delimiting state activity. However, in the era that followed the war, Americans mobilized the institutions and authority of the state to control tubercular disease. New understandings of the relationships among science, individual behaviors, and the jurisdiction of the state formed part of this process, as did an altered assessment of risk.

"Historically, tuberculosis has been a predominantly urban disease in the United States," Milton Roemer of the West Virginia Health Department argued in 1949. "Associated with poverty, congested housing, poor nutrition, and over-exertion, tuberculosis has taken its greatest tolls in the slums of the big city."[1] During the 1930s, the Social Security Act and the work of Surgeon General Thomas Parran brought public health into the limelight, and federal efforts to regulate and combat tuberculosis also expanded. New case-finding surveys initiated in rural populations surprised public health authorities, however, by revealing widespread tuberculosis. "If tuberculosis is the classical 'social disease,'" Roemer subsequently observed, "the socio-environmental factors contributing to its occurrence are today found most strikingly in rural parts of the United States."[2] As control of TB became part of a national program of public health, the relationship of TB to (rural) poverty and the problem of controlling a disease that was at once physiological and sociological became increasingly thorny, and so did the debates over BCG.

MOBILIZING THE INSTITUTIONS OF THE STATE

World War II served as a catalyst for the development of tuberculosis-control activities within the PHS. Before the war, no centralized governmental agency for the study or control of the disease existed, and public responsibility was diffuse. The mounting of the war effort drew to Washington many of the personnel who had worked informally to establish a federal program of tuberculosis control, among them Herman Ertresvaag Hilleboe. Hilleboe, who received degrees in medicine and public health from the University of Minnesota, was a practicing physician, epidemiologist for the Minnesota State Department of Health, and chief of the Medical Unit of the State Division of Social Welfare. In 1939, Parran invited him to establish a case-finding program within the PHS. Hilleboe accepted the offer, and on July 1, 1939, received a commission as senior assistant surgeon. Over the next year, he expanded case-finding efforts, coordinated the activities of various state tuberculosis-control programs, and almost single-handedly formed a federal tuberculosis-control program.[3]

The power of individual personalities like Hilleboe did not alone spur the federal government to action; war experiences brought home the need for a concerted campaign against disease. Abroad, in battle-torn Europe, tuberculosis mortality rose again. Americans might link this rise to social and economic experiences that they did not share—to hunger, cold, inadequate clothing and housing, and the prevalence of other diseases—but they could not entirely dismiss TB as a foreign problem. American mortality continued to decline, but the pace of decline slowed after 1940, and after 1942 the new case rate rose sharply in both civilian and military populations.[4] Immigrants also posed a renewed threat, as medical inspection of Japanese evacuees from the West Coast indicated that many had active or latent TB.[5] The draft for World War II, like that for World War I, disclosed how many Americans were tuberculous and unfit for military service. A significant percentage of recruits later received treatment for or were discharged with tuberculosis. "These individuals represent a staggering potential cost to the taxpayer in terms of disability pensions alone," analysts warned.[6]

Tuberculosis once again posed a national threat, which politicians, physicians, and the general public recognized, but little administrative machinery existed to combat it. By 1938 Canadians had successfully built the control of tuberculosis into the full-fledged Medical Research Council. Before the war, members of Congress and their constituents continued to lobby intermittently and unsuccessfully for integrated, federal programs of TB control. During the 1910s and 1920s, their cry for a tuberculosis-control division had provoked sharp jurisdictional disagreements about welfare services. By the late 1930s, with the Social Security Act in place, many of the earlier jurisdictional disputes had apparently been resolved as most Americans came to acknowledge the federal government's responsibility to provide some kinds of relief and as the machinery needed to administer policy developed. Still, though these legislative and administrative changes prompted additional pleas for active federal involvement in TB control, opposition remained. Bill S. 2547 (1939) proposed the creation of a division of tuberculosis control and drew support not just from members of Congress but also from physicians and private citizens, who in letters and petitions made it quite clear that they deemed existing machinery and legislation inadequate.[7] "The control of tuberculosis is an important public health problem in the United States" that demands immediate attention, discussants of the bill advised, and they pushed hard for federal intervention.[8] Nonetheless, this bill ultimately failed.

Moreover, the leaders of the opposition included none other than Parran, who in his official capacity as surgeon general staunchly opposed the creation of a division of TB control. Parran, who engineered the public campaign against venereal disease, advised against a similar attack on TB. "I do not see any need," he insisted in July 1939, "for a special 'commission' to deal particularly with the tuberculosis problem with respect to either its public health aspects or rehabilitation and vocational training and guidance of arrested cases."[9] Parran based his opposition on two distinct arguments that replicated some of those given in the earlier debate. His first objection addressed the issue of administrative control. "I am strongly of the opinion that any further dispersion of administrative responsibility in the conduct of the public health activities of the federal government," he wrote, "would be harmful to the work and only add to the confusion which now exists in many states as a result of the necessity of dealing with different agencies on a federal level."[10] Though Parran feared that the creation of a tuberculosis-control division would produce administrative chaos, he might as easily have hoped that a centralized division would coordinate tuberculosis control and eliminate bureaucratic overlap.

Parran's second objection was based in his respect for federalism. Whatever he might say or do about other diseases, Parran could not divorce the control of tuberculosis from more general social programs, administration of which fell rightly, he thought, to the states. In a letter to then Congressman Warren Magnuson, he explained that Titles V and VI of the Social Security Act had already made ample provision for the social services needed by the tuberculous, that the federal government had no right to tread upon the states' turf, and that it could achieve its goals quite simply by making direct grants-in-aid to the states.[11] Thus, Parran maintained that a division of TB control would be, at best, redundant.

Popular support for Bill S. 2547 and the country's entry into the war soon forced Parran to reconsider his opposition. In response to mounting national concern about disease and to fears about the increasingly heavy toll that TB exacted in Europe, Bill H.R. 3968 (1941) was introduced in the House; it authorized annual appropriations for grants to states that would extend and improve tuberculosis-control programs. Parran, who two years earlier had affirmed the states' responsibility for TB control, supported the legislation. "There is no doubt that this bill is directed to a National Problem which requires both additional research, study and experimentation," he wrote. In contradistinction to his earlier position, he now labeled H.R. 3968 a stopgap in that it provided funds to the states for treatment and prevention but did not attack the root of the problem.

> TB is among the major causes of death in the United States, and it strikes with special force among young adults who constitute this Nation's great force of industrial workers. The only effective treatment presently known entails a prolonged and expensive regimen of care which overtaxes the resources of most individuals and is beyond the reach of the average or less than average family income. This situation creates a vicious circle of recurrence in the lower income brackets, and often has the effect of depleting an individual family's resources, and at the same time, removing opportunities for their recovery.[12]

Because of these links to poverty and industry, Parran understood that the tuberculosis problem was "already generally recognized and accepted as a public responsibility," but he lamented that the "equipment to meet it is entirely inadequate."[13] In what appeared to be a reversal of his earlier position, he now supported the creation of an Office of Tuberculosis Control within the State Services Bureau of the PHS, and he placed Hilleboe at its head.[14] Still haunted by debates over federalism and states' rights, he justified his actions by separating the medical from the social aspects of disease and by working primarily through the State Services Bureau to link venereal-disease control to TB control and to broaden casefinding efforts.

The Office of Tuberculosis Control was a wartime unit designed primarily to "prevent the expected war-time rise in tuberculosis incidence and fatality in the United States."[15] Under Hilleboe's direction, it turned primarily to case finding and follow-up services. It conducted x-ray examinations of workers in the war industries and their families, followed newly diagnosed cases, and attempted to develop a workable system of reporting the cases it discovered to state and municipal agencies. The limited services that the office could provide soon seemed insufficient, and Parran, who had become surgeon general in 1936 in order to realize his "American Dream" that "health for all people is an attainable goal,"[16] soon lobbied for the expansion of tuberculosis-control services. When reorganization of the PHS began in 1943, he gave priority to tuberculosis.

The Public Health Service Act of July 1, 1944, expanded the scope of that federal agency generally, and it made specific provision for the creation of a separate Tuberculosis Control Division. Congress awarded the division a budget of $10,000,000 for the fiscal year ending June 30, 1945, and the Public Health Service Act ensured allocation thereafter of "sums sufficient" to enable the division to fulfill its duties. These duties included the development of "more effective measures for the prevention, treatment, and control of tuberculosis," research, and the provision of money and human resources to assist the activities of states and their "political subdivisions."[17]

Much like Parran's crusade against venereal disease, the campaign against tuberculosis that the division launched in its early years focused on the detection and treatment of cases.[18] In his speeches, Parran linked the two diseases. He acknowledged that TB, like venereal disease, could not be "prevented without the cure of infected persons,"[19] and by 1945 the division identified "tuberculosis case finding" and "isolation and treatment of persons with active infectious tuberculosis" as priorities.[20] However, in sharp contrast to the development of the campaign against venereal disease, neither Parran nor his staff made much effort to reduce tuberculosis to a purely biological problem. Though he fully believed that TB "would go" if every health department worked to discover and treat new cases, when he placed the disease in context Parran conceded that "full employment with a high level of national income, healthful housing, and improved nutrition are essential to the program."[21]

Those who ran the division agreed. Unlike the Canadian ACTR, which drew its members primarily from pathology, bacteriology, and biochemistry labs within the government or universities,[22] the PHS chose staff with experience in epidemiology and child hygiene. Hilleboe had previously directed the Tuberculosis and Crippled Children's Programs of Minnesota. Carroll Palmer, who guided the division through the 1940s and 1950s, similarly moved from child hygiene to tuberculosis.[23] As they made their transition, these researchers continued to examine the links between medical and social problems. Though they deemed existing measures inadequate and called for "research in methods of treatment, which includes search for a drug or biologic that will prove efficacious in the control of tuberculosis," they ranked these quests for cures only among the "auxiliary methods of control."[24] More immediate and important, in the view of the division's chief, were "after care and rehabilitation of the patient" and "protection of the families of the tuberculous against economic distress."[25] In 1942, Hilleboe and Palmer began a cooperative investigation of "the effects of war and industrialization on tuberculosis," for which they received funding from the NTA.[26] The division supported their interest in the connections between tuberculous disease and an impoverished social environment by sponsoring not just medical research but also investigations into poor nutrition, poor hygiene, and the economic poverty and dependency associated with TB.[27] It appointed a full time "medical-social" consultant and employed a corps of social workers.[28]

THE FIRST BCG CONFERENCE

The newly formed Tuberculosis Control Division also turned its attention to BCG. In this area too, it betrayed its concerns about the links between tuberculosis and poverty. By 1946, American clinical and experimental trials generally confirmed the safety and efficacy of vaccination, and after the publication of the Park and Aronson trials, support for BCG increased. So, however, did the opposition. The Tuberculosis Control Division consequently sponsored a conference to evaluate the divergent opinions. On September 7, 1946, representatives of the PHS and of major American and foreign research laboratories met in Washington to debate the "BCG question."

Immediately, the lack of American consensus emerged. Hilleboe, chief of the new division, opened discussion with a summary of the principles that underlay Albert Calmette's original work and with a detailed review of trials conducted both at home and abroad. "Although extensive vaccinations have been carried out in Europe and South America, and careful studies undertaken in the United States," he concluded, "BCG vaccination has not been widely accepted in this country."[29] Joseph Aronson and Johannes Holm, a representative of the State Serum Institute in Copenhagen, immediately attempted to shake Americans from their apparent indifference. Aronson presented the results of his Native American trials, which, he reported, had reduced mortality sevenfold. Holm, with evidence from trials conducted in Denmark, endorsed BCG still more enthusiastically. The joint testimony of these two experienced and reputable physicians underscored the need for serious reconsideration of the effectiveness of BCG vaccine in the control of tuberculosis.

The PHS responded exceedingly cautiously to Aronson and Holm. The participants at the BCG conference recognized the need for additional vaccination trials but only in particularly vulnerable groups, which it identified as "various tribes of American Indians; inmates and employees of mental institutions; employees of general hospitals and sanatoria in which the danger of infection is excessive because control measures are lacking; medical students in schools in which the services include exposure to tuberculous patients; and persons economically and socially underprivileged, among whom tuberculosis mortality is very high."[30] Moreover, they once again made the plea for national research. Before drawing final conclusions on the efficacy of BCG, the participants recommended, the PHS ought to sponsor cooperative investigations "with recognized research groups throughout the nation, especially in population groups highly exposed to tuberculous infection," and "set up a controlled study in a community with population of 100,000 or more."[31]

In essence, the concerns raised at the 1946 conference differed little from those that had guided American studies over the course of the previous twenty years. Participants questioned the safety of BCG; they questioned its efficacy; and they reached the consensus that vaccination reduced morbidity and mortality. Like others who had reached similar conclusions before them, however, the delegates warned again and again against the hasty adoption of BCG, then shifted to the question of whether vaccination provided an appropriate alternative to other measures of control.

The voice of J. Arthur Myers prevailed in this discussion. Myers, director of tuberculosis activities at the Minneapolis Division of Health, chief of tuberculosis services at the Minneapolis General Hospital, and professor of medicine, preventive medicine, and public health at the University of Minnesota, had worked formerly with Hilleboe. His early pioneering studies of the tuberculin reaction had mapped the extent of infection in the United States. They built moreover on Strasheimer Alburtus Petroff's earlier suggestion that sensitivity to tuberculin might sometimes be a sign of susceptibility of the disease. First infection, of either children or adults, Myers argued, was usually benign, but it carried a "double health liability." Those who suffered it often fell prey to "re-infection tuberculosis," a far more problematical disease, with a "strong tendency to progress and cause much destruction of tissues and result in illness and death."[32] Hence, though a majority of the children who reacted positively to tuberculin never developed tubercular disease, there were "many, who in later life, because of dissipation, overwork, worry, malnutrition and poor housing conditions," could not keep the germs dormant.[33]

Myers consequently placed a premium on measures that would prevent first infections and deemed this "much sounder policy than any method aimed at immunization, which at best is questionable and which allows subsequent contamination."[34] The evidence of declining rates of tuberculous mortality and the steadily decreasing number of tuberculin reactors reassured him that such a sound policy existed in the United States. The evidence prompted him, as well, to oppose particularly the widespread use of BCG vaccine in areas with a low percentage of tuberculin reactors. In Myers's view, "the tuberculin test is the only fine screen available in the diagnosis of the first infection type of tuberculosis in children,"[35] and BCG vaccination reduced its utility.

The conference participants heeded Myers's advice by attempting, while investigation proceeded, to restrict production of BCG. That task seemed relatively easy. Drug companies, it should be remembered, had originally shown little interest in Calmette's vaccine. As we saw earlier, problems associated with the production of tuberculin—the stronghold that Saranac Lake retained over the "market," the PHS investigation of the Von Ruck brothers, and the technical difficulties of manufacturing a strong and reliable product—had combined with fears of BCG's virulence to scare off even the most ambitious and mercenary of labs. Even after the studies that followed Lübeck essentially cleared BCG, commercial manufacturers steered clear, for they found it "not very suitable for commercial exploitation since it must be used within a few days after production."[36] Prior to 1947, therefore, control of American production of BCG rested in two academic laboratories: the Phipps Institute of the University of Pennsylvania and the Tice Laboratories of the University of Illinois (Chicago), which made small quantities solely for research purposes. Still, the first BCG conference took the precaution of advising strongly against the issue of any license for commercial manufacture of BCG and against the distribution of vaccine to general practitioners for use in private practice. The participants suggested, as well, that Phipps and Tice be brought under the PHS umbrella and made part of a national BCG laboratory, which would be established to produce the vaccine used in any American trials.

These efforts to control production, distribution, and use of BCG soon hit a roadblock. In 1946, Konrad Birkhaug, the Norwegian physician who had so enthusiastically endorsed William Hallock Park's trials, used his influence to establish a BCG laboratory within the New York State Department of Health. Changes in New York State legislation, which included elimination of the "means test" and effective establishment of the "principle of free diagnosis and treatment of tuberculosis by public agencies," seemed to encourage research on BCG.[37] Under the direction of Hilleboe, who had left the PHS to assume the position of New York State commissioner of health, New York became the first state to produce BCG.

As the eradication of tuberculosis came within scientific and legislative reach, New York took the lead by both producing BCG and using it to "protect groups seriously exposed to infection."[38] The state cautiously authorized use of BCG only in "limited groups," and it charged Hilleboe, in his official capacity as commissioner of health, to control distribution strictly. However, these "limited groups" included diverse populations, among them nurses, medical students, hospital personnel, those known to have household exposure, and "population groups with high tuberculosis morbidity and mortality rates."[39] Moreover, after the first vaccinations in 1947, aspirations for the program quickly grew. Information about BCG soon became part of official state publicity. A BCG booth appeared at the annual state TB exhibition, and the state incorporated bulletins about BCG into a statewide traveling TB demonstration. Information stimulated popular demand. Hence, Albany, Buffalo, Farmingdale, Ithaca, Kingston, New York City, Rochester, Syracuse, and Oneonta soon became sites of new vaccination programs. The state additionally made plans to begin vaccination in the mental institutions that fell under the jurisdiction of the Department of Mental Hygiene.[40]

New York's initiative spurred the PHS to action. The opening of the New York State BCG lab had coincided with the installation of Leonard Scheele as the new surgeon general and of Robert Anderson as the new director of the Tuberculosis Control Division. Under their leadership the PHS moved more quickly on BCG. In early 1947, the division began a long-term vaccination trial among school children in Muscogee County, Georgia. Soon thereafter it began another trial in Puerto Rico.[41] Simultaneously, the National Institutes of Health (NIH) began to conduct laboratory-based investigations of both BCG and killed antituberculosis vaccines.

RURAL TRIALS OF BCG: MUSCOGEE COUNTY AND PUERTO RICO

By the late 1940s, TB was no longer principally an urban problem. Women, children, and immigrants had slowly graduated from the category of risk, and tuberculosis was recast as a disease of "rural life" and of "the older age groups."[42] Morbidity disproportionate to opportunities for infection surprised the epidemiologists who studied TB in rural populations, and they soon shifted attention from "bacterial contacts" to racial characteristics and then to social conditions.[43] "The remarkable decline in the tuberculosis death rate since about 1900," Roemer explained, "has been due in the main to urban developments. Improvements in housing and nutrition, rises in real wages, isolation and treatment of cases in sanatoria have doubtless all played their part."[44] Rural poverty, he then suggested, "has its effects on the problem of tuberculosis, as does the squalor of city slums."[45] Some rural Americans also lived in shockingly overcrowded dwellings, had undernourished children, and attained below-average educational levels—including education about personal hygiene and living habits. Yet nonindustrialized areas enjoyed few of the benefits of urban reform; their residents remained victims of low income, low population density, and all the resultant inadequacies in health care services.[46]

Nowhere did the problems Roemer described appear more acute than in Puerto Rico and Muscogee County. In 1948, the tuberculous death rate in Puerto Rico hovered at 179/100,000. This rate was a significant reduction from the peak of 332/100,000 recorded in 1933, but it nonetheless greatly exceeded rates found anywhere in the continental United States.[47] In the South, tuberculosis mortality had declined little in the period between 1940 and 1946, and in absolute terms the death rate remained high.[48] Muscogee County, which encompassed the city of Columbus and a surrounding rural population of over 20,000, had earlier served as the site of a PHS venereal disease demonstration, and it seemed to pose a distinctive problem. When the PHS used Muscogee in 1946 to conduct a special census on experiences with tuberculosis, early results indicated that mortality was very high. Many residents of Muscogee County and Puerto Rico also lived in tremendous poverty. Thus, like the Native Americans before them, they provided researchers with an opportunity both to address an immediate health problem and to gauge the efficacy of BCG vaccine against the backdrop of social circumstance.

The design and interpretation of the trials conducted in Puerto Rico and Muscogee once again exposed the concerns about relative efficacy that underlay American assessments of BCG. Both trials took the form of long-term follow-up studies that together would evaluate trends in tuberculosis mortality, determine the efficacy of vaccination, and assess the effects of the vaccine within a broader epidemiological context. As it implemented its trials, the PHS took care to safeguard itself against the many criticisms that had been leveled against other vaccination studies. It attempted to "gain as complete a knowledge as possible of the community so that all factors which influence the spread of tuberculosis could be evaluated."[49] It endeavored to define a large enough population; to choose adequate controls; to conduct preliminary, communitywide x-rays and tuberculin tests that would measure the extent of tuberculous infection; to offer BCG to a select group of school children; and to collect detailed information about the socioeconomic conditions of vaccinees and controls.

Those who conducted the trials also undertook a careful evaluation of the tuberculin reaction. BCG's critics still seemed uncertain about the relationship between infection, allergy to tuberculin, and immunity. During the 1930s, as the combination of tuberculin testing and radiography became an increasingly popular diagnostic tool, inconsistencies in the findings of these two screening methods emerged. Particularly in the South, those who tested positive to tuberculin often had a negative chest x-ray. At first, researchers attributed these discrepancies to differences between older tuberculins and newly introduced products. However, it soon became clear that something much greater was at stake, and the question of whether the reaction to tuberculin signified infection, immunity, or something completely different generated a heated debate.

At a tuberculin conference that the PHS sponsored in Hagerstown, Maryland, in the fall of 1938, Esmond Long had drawn a critical distinction between "infection incidence" and "case finding." Long, like many of his predecessors, distinguished between infection and disease and maintained that those who tested positive to tuberculin were infected but need not necessarily become cases.[50] The Hagerstown conference warned that the tuberculin reaction was unreliable and ought to be interpreted very cautiously.[51] But if tuberculin allergy provided no indication of cases, one participant suggested, were not "extensive and costly [case-finding] programs" essentially on the "wrong track" and a waste of the taxpayer's money?[52]

Over the next decade, American physicians continued to debate the meaning of tuberculin allergy and its implications for public health initiatives. The PHS soon became a party to this debate. In July 1944, Hilleboe wrote to Myers inquiring about his work. "I have been getting quite a few comments on your article," he wrote. "Apparently some of the boys were concerned about the scientific basis upon which you base the statement that a positive tuberculin means live organisms in the body. If you would care to give me the pathological studies upon which this statement is made I would be delighted to have an opportunity to defend you."[53]

These questions became critical as the PHS staff embarked on its trials. BCG, it should be remembered, had been developed for use only among nonreactors to tuberculin. Despite uncertainty about the significance of the tuberculin reaction, by the early 1940s most American physicians agreed that allergy resulted from prior infection, which, in the absence of clinical disease, left the host resistant to reinfection. Tuberculin-positive nurses who worked in close contact with TB patients, and others in similar circumstances, routinely seemed protected.[54] Hence, a majority of American physicians presumed nonreactors to tuberculin to be free of tuberculous infection, vulnerable to infection, and the primary source of new cases.

Evaluations of the early trials conducted in Muscogee and Puerto Rico challenged both this standard interpretation and the very premise that underlay BCG vaccination. Starting in the spring of 1946, the PHS and the local health department encouraged all Muscogee residents over five years of age to be screened with x-rays and tuberculin. By 1950, 64,136 residents—46.4 percent of the census population—had complied. During the first year of the trial, 15,000 school children were screened, and a total of 26,542—60 percent of the five- to nineteen-year-olds in the census population—ultimately participated. Thus, though voluntary, the Muscogee trial became one of the largest and most comprehensive studies of BCG ever conducted.

Preliminary assessments of infection rates in Muscogee raised the first red flag. These rates indicated that at age twenty, 35 percent of whites and 60 percent of blacks were tuberculin sensitive. Such high levels of tuberculin allergy were not on their own surprising, nor was the observation that reactivity increased with age. However, the equally large percentage of young reactors did strike the investigators as "almost incredible" and quite suspect: 54 percent of white children and 63 percent of the black children were tuberculin positive.[55] Despite their misgivings about these rates, directors of the trial felt that they had no alternative but to immediately exclude the "positive" subjects from the study. Protocol dictated that BCG could be administered only to tuberculin-negative children. Hence, only nonreactors, under twenty years of age who also had negative chest x-rays became eligible for vaccination.

To assess the effect BCG had on tuberculin conversion, the PHS staff administered a second tuberculin test six months after vaccination. They presumed at this time that "allergy in the vaccinated group represented only the effect of BCG"; hence, they revaccinated children who tested negative. Three years later, they again recalled the subjects, tested them with tuberculin, and revaccinated those who remained tuberculin negative. Both the six-month and three-year recall produced unanticipated results. Those who conducted the trial fully expected that "nearly the optimum degree of allergy" would be shown in a tuberculin test conducted six months after vaccination; yet, though 90 percent of the white children showed some reaction at this stage, only 41 percent reacted in a "significant" way.[56] After three years, only 75 percent reacted in any way to tuberculin, and, of these, only 23 percent had a response that could be considered "positive."[57] At each of the test periods, vaccinated children responded in much the way that they had done earlier; those who showed little or no allergy at six months also reacted only slightly at three years.[58] This low reactivity was inconsistent with other BCG trials, in which vaccination seemed routinely to produce "a high degree of allergy, which means a typical tuberculin reaction to a small dose of tuberculin."[59] Hence, either the "take" of BCG or the tuberculin test was problematical.

Even more perplexing than the low level of allergy in the vaccinated group was the large percentage of nonvaccinated controls who later reacted positively to tuberculin. George Comstock, epidemiologist and tuberculosis-control officer of the Muscogee County Health Department, had designed the trial carefully and assigned nonreactors randomly to test and control populations on the basis of alternate birth years. Hence, he could not resort to the earlier explanation of population difference. Nor could he claim any unusual conditions of tuberculous exposure. Still, though they had failed to react to 100 TU (tuberculin units) three years earlier, 66 percent of the controls now reacted in some degree to a 5 TU dose.

These early findings might have reflected shortcomings in the vaccination method, flaws in the tuberculin test, or peculiarities in the test population, but members of the PHS staff, especially Lawrence Shaw, the chief statistician of the Immunization Section of the Field Research Branch of the Tuberculosis Control Division, quickly directed their critique to BCG. The observations made in Muscogee County, he suggested, demonstrated that one could not attribute tuberculin conversion to vaccination, nor could one credit BCG with the protection this conversion might afford. In a point at once substantive and methodological, Shaw warned:

> From the viewpoint of obtaining sound scientific knowledge on the production of tuberculin allergy by BCG vaccination, the present study brings out the tremendous importance of having equivalent observations on a comparable control group of unvaccinated persons. In the absence of the controls, it is almost certain that most of the reactions in the vaccinated would have been attributed to BCG. An entirely different conclusion is quite admissible: that there was very little residual effect of BCG after 3 years, for BCG cannot be considered as essential in producing the major part of the allergy observed.[60]

Shaw conceded that "the fundamental relationship between allergy to tuberculin and immunity to tuberculosis is still a highly controversial matter,"[61] and the part BCG played in this process also remained unclear. Still, he concluded that BCG had limited value.

Early reports from Puerto Rico intensified the confusion. The PHS had designed its trial as an "island-wide mass program for children," which it hoped might relieve an immediate public health problem, and between September 1949 and May 1950 it initiated BCG vaccination programs at over 1,400 schools. Local staff performed both tuberculin tests and vaccinations. The PHS publicized the program widely through newspapers, radio, and door-to-door visits, and during the summer of 1950 it attempted to broaden its initiative by inviting nonenrolled, school-age children to also receive BCG at a nearby school. Later, it expanded the study to include preschoolers. Compliance in the school population reached almost 45 percent, but fewer preschoolers and nonstudents participated.[62] In all, the campaign reached nearly 200,000 children. As had been the case in Muscogee, only tuberculin-negative children were considered eligible for vaccination. In an effort to ensure that its results would be accurate, unbiased, and beyond reproach, the PHS also adopted the system of allocation employed in Muscogee; it assigned subjects and vaccinees randomly, on the basis of birth year, to maintain comparability between test and control populations.

In Puerto Rico as in Georgia, evaluation of the relationship between allergy and immunity became critical. Those who designed the Puerto Rico trial extended their investigations to a new group of subjects so that they might better measure the efficacy of BCG. They used as controls both unvaccinated tuberculin-negative children and children who, though they had not been vaccinated with BCG, reacted positively to tuberculin. This innovation allowed them to compare more directly the efficacy of BCG and that of more traditional measures of tuberculosis control. The use of comparable populations of BCG-vaccinated subjects and controls who were either tuberculin-positive (reactors) or tuberculin-negative (controls) would enable the PHS to assess morbidity more closely; it would provide, as well, a measure of the number of those new cases that BCG vaccination would prevent.

The innovation, however, produced findings that once again challenged the meaning of tubercular infection and the premises of BCG vaccination. Preliminary morbidity and mortality data provided contradictory assessments. The morbidity data, acknowledged to be "deficient in the completeness of the reporting and the accuracy of diagnosis," suggested that there had been two cases of tuberculosis among the controls, six among the vaccinees, and seventy-five among the reactors. The mortality data provided a rather different picture; there had been four deaths among the controls, one among the vaccinees, and twenty-four among the reactors. The preliminary findings of the study suggested that the "vaccinated are faring better than the controls." However, instead of emphasizing the extent to which vaccination reduced mortality, Shaw and Palmer, who presented the preliminary data, stressed that "there has been a considerable concentration of tuberculosis mortality in the tuberculin reactors." Thus, in Puerto Rico, nonreactors to tuberculin did not constitute the population at greatest risk of developing TB. Rather, the data suggested that 75 percent of new cases occurred among the nonvaccinated reactors to tuberculin.[63]

The possibility that tuberculin reactors represented the population at greatest risk now became critical to assessments of BCG, for if the majority of cases occurred in those already tuberculin positive, vaccination could have little effect. In a review essay on the "status of BCG," Shaw and Palmer began to make this case. Briefly summarizing the Muscogee trial, Aronson's trial, the Puerto Rico trial, and one other trial underway in Ohio mental hospitals, Palmer and Shaw assessed the data as "contradictory" and as providing conflicting assessments of the value of BCG. In Muscogee, in Puerto Rico, and on the reservations, BCG appeared to be "of value," but in Ohio "essentially no difference between the vaccinated and controls" existed.[64] Hence, Palmer and Shaw argued, on the one hand, "[i]t is possible that, in the Indian and Puerto Rico mortality data, there may be early signs that BCG, under certain circumstances, could be useful in tuberculosis control." But they proposed, on the other hand, that "these studies do not indicate that tuberculosis in this country would be more effectively controlled by adding mass vaccination programs."[65] Palmer and Shaw found that, despite their differences, all the studies agreed "on the point [that] a very large proportion of the tuberculosis which appears in each population during the first few years after the vaccination program occurred in the group who were not vaccinated because they had already been infected."[66] The "tuberculosis problem" in the United States, they consequently concluded, was the tuberculin reactor.

Almost twenty years earlier, Wade Hampton Frost, renowned professor of epidemiology at Johns Hopkins University and a staff member of the PHS, had made much the same proposal. After carefully reviewing age selection data, Frost concluded that mortality was lowest among the class of adults that had least exposure to the tubercle bacillus during its youth and that "the present high rates in old age are the residual of higher rates earlier in life."[67] Tuberculosis differed from other infectious diseases, Frost maintained, in that "age and prior exposure bring no such immunity against tuberculosis as they establish against many of the acute infections";[68] hence, rather than conferring protection, prior exposure became one determinant of vulnerability.

The staff of the Tuberculosis Control Division knew Frost's arguments well. In June 1946, its chief tipped his hat to Frost when he opposed widespread use of BCG in the United States on the grounds that "epidemiological studies, particularly analyses by such scholars of public health as Wade Hampton Frost, raised pertinent questions as to the permanent value of vaccination against tuberculosis."[69] Palmer had worked alongside Frost at Hopkins and Hagerstown, where he had grown to admire the senior epidemiologist. Now he and Shaw continued the work that his mentor had begun and paid an epidemiological tribute to Frost by redefining the American tuberculosis problem. In Muscogee and in Puerto Rico, Palmer and Shaw suggested, the greatest risk of disease existed among those previously exposed to tuberculous infection or, in other words, among reactors to tuberculin. "Muscogee County in Georgia may not be entirely representative of the whole country," they concluded, "but, since the effect of the vaccination program there is imperceptible, it seems that there is little reason to expect very different results in other communities."[70] Deferring once again to Frost, they endorsed his earlier assertion that "for the eventual eradication of tuberculosis it is not necessary that transmission be *immediately and completely* prevented" but rather that "infection spreading cases . . . [be kept] to a minimum."[71]

If Palmer and Shaw couched their assessments of BCG in cold, epidemiological terms, once again other concerns lay quite close to the surface. When it conducted its census in Muscogee County, the PHS collected both data on experiences with disease and information on housing conditions that would serve as "an index of socioeconomic forces."[72] "For a long time, it has been felt that socioeconomic factors have great influence on the development of tuberculosis, the fate of infected persons, and the readiness with which patients accept treatment," Comstock explained. "Lack of knowledge about the normal group as well as the restriction of many socioeconomic studies to selected population groups, has prevented an adequate determination of the role of these factors both in the development of the disease and in the behavior of tuberculosis patients."[73] A health inquiry that the U.S. House Committee on Interstate and Foreign Commerce launched in October 1953 revisited these arguments. The inquiry began with the observation that "despite medical advances, TB remains the most important communicable disease problem in the United States" and that "tuberculosis is a very costly and crippling disease for men and women in their most productive years."[74] It consequently confronted the PHS on the scope and success of its antituberculosis campaign. In particular, the inquiry challenged policy regarding use of BCG. Its chairman read extensively from statements made by eminent American and European physicians who enthusiastically supported the vaccine. He noted the widespread use of BCG in Europe, and he asked the PHS to justify its persistent opposition to vaccination. As representatives of the Tuberculosis Control Division testified, they once again brought the discussion of BCG back to the relief of poverty.

The statement of Anderson, now chief of the Tuberculosis Control Division, contained well-worn arguments about the social origins of TB. Anderson did not dispute BCG's worth. He even called it a good vaccine, but he argued that it was not the best means of controlling TB. TB differed from the self-limited diseases, against which vaccines were regularly employed, Anderson carefully explained. He based this assessment, in part, on immunological considerations and, in part, on the observation that tuberculosis was not simply a bacterial disease. In language that resembled the earlier discussions of seed and soil, Anderson identified the tubercle bacillus as one cause of TB—the specific cause—but drew attention to the "precipitating and predisposing causes." Among these he included "prolonged physical and emotional strain, malnutrition, fatigue, overcrowding, low economic status, poor personal hygiene, and silicosis."[75]

Increases in tuberculosis in war-torn Europe, Anderson suggested, revealed the close association between tuberculosis and social and economic disruption. He suggested, as well, that European nations had turned in despair to BCG:

> Subsequent to the Second World War, under conditions of great social and economic disturbances, with poor nutrition, poor housing and lack of rest, many people in war-devastated areas succumbed to tuberculosis. Many of the affected areas had little in the way of hospital facilities, nurses or laboratories to cope with this increase in the TB problem. BCG became the tool of control of tuberculosis since it could be used among people throughout the world in the absence of adequate treatment facilities and personnel.[76]

Reviving concerns raised in debates over Park's and Aronson's trials, Anderson testified that European assessments of BCG's efficacy were "confused because of the fact that in those countries social conditions, standards of living and nutrition have also changed subsequent to the war."[77] European trials had not controlled appropriately for social and economic changes, which could on their own produce a decline in tuberculous mortality and morbidity; hence, they offered no real indication of the vaccine's efficacy.

Anderson then turned the problem inside out. He argued that because

Americans had been able to maintain high standards of living and enforce hygienic measures of tuberculosis control, they had kept mortality and morbidity in check. As a result, they had no need for BCG. Vaccination, in his view, was a last resort that was neither necessary nor appropriate in the United States. Anderson's confidence in American health, American wealth, and American campaigns against tuberculosis did not completely sway his inquisitors. His testimony rested on a transparent party line, or mythology; the committee members well knew that American achievements in tuberculosis were nowhere near as grand as Anderson claimed.

Each time the PHS rose to congratulate itself on its achievements, it also confessed its shortcomings. In 1949, Surgeon General Scheele proclaimed that, after a long period in which the fight against TB had slowed, "rapid progress is now being made in halting the spread of this disease."[78] Three years later, he again lamented that, "[a]mong the communicable diseases, tuberculosis remains a major health problem." The new case rate, Scheele recognized, had declined only slightly in the calendar year 1951, during which 119,000 new cases of TB were reported. Moreover, "[f]or every tuberculosis death, there were four new cases reported in 1951— the highest such ratio yet recorded."[79] Thus while Scheele took pride in the "marked decline in tuberculosis deaths," he nonetheless warned that "methods, facilities and knowledge must be extended and strengthened if full control of the disease is to be achieved."[80]

The chairman of the health inquiry consequently questioned Anderson closely about the epidemiology of TB. "Are the reported cases of tuberculosis in this country on the increase or decrease?" he bluntly demanded. Anderson confessed that rates of disease had remained constant, but he excused the epidemiological steady state by attributing it to improved case-finding programs and new standards of reporting.[81] When asked whether BCG might not be a useful supplement to existing measures of control, Anderson emphatically denied it. "Indiscriminate use of BCG here," he argued, "[could] divert attention from the control activities which are serving the Nation well and which, under the circumstances prevailing in the United States, could lead to the virtual eradication of tuberculosis. It is our feeling that we must be very careful not to imperil the gains we are making with proved control methods."[82] Like so many others before him, Anderson weighed BCG against existing measures of control and found it wanting.

Palmer's and Shaw's assessments and the health inquiry put a damper on American studies of BCG. In 1953, New York State abruptly ended its investigations of BCG. Offering no further explanation than that "changes in the program of the Division have been made for eminently practical reasons," the director of the Division of Laboratories and Research suddenly announced that "[t]he BCG laboratories have been closed."[83] Field studies in New York and elsewhere similarly came to an end.

THE CHALLENGE OF ANTIBIOTICS

The introduction of new antibiotics offered opportunities to both cure and prevent disease and, at a critical moment, provided real alternatives to BCG. Between 1943, when the American bacteriologist Salman Waksman discovered streptomycin, and the introduction in 1952 of isoniazid (also known as INH), a series of chemotherapeutic breakthroughs posed the first significant alternative to BCG and inspired new hopes for the prevention and cure of TB. Unlike penicillin and other early antibiotics, which those who attempted to use soon recognized to "have no effect on TB,"[84] streptomycin had obvious bactericidal and bacteriostatic properties.[85]

However, it soon became apparent that the new wonder drugs could not deliver all they promised. From the time of its introduction, the actual efficacy of streptomycin was unclear. Shirley Ferebee, a biostatistician employed by the Tuberculosis Control Division, immediately expressed doubts about the structure of the streptomycin trials, which she openly criticized as not sufficiently rigorous.[86] On Ferebee's recommendation, the PHS commissioned new studies, which revealed streptomycin to be both too strong and not strong enough. When administered in doses sufficient to cure infection, streptomycin quickly produced a strain of drug-resistant tubercle bacilli.

In 1948, the Tuberculosis Study Section of the NIH established a steering committee to examine streptomycin, and the statement it issued introduced further reservations. The statement identified two distinct sets of concerns. One centered on the uncertain findings of therapeutic trials of streptomycin. "It is the judgment of the members of the Steering Committee that the value of streptomycin in the treatment of pulmonary tuberculosis is unproved at present," the statement cautioned, "and that further research is necessary to establish its place in the treatment of this disease." The committee did not restrict itself to questions about efficacy however. As with BCG, it made the safety of streptomycin a second issue. "Although certain dramatic effects have been observed . . . ," the committee warned, "[t]he serious toxic effects may outweigh any beneficial therapeutic effect."[87] Thus, by 1949, the recognition that "the unfortunate thing about streptomycin is that it is sometimes toxic" had become common, and physicians restricted use of the drug to those "forms of tuberculosis which are ordinarily fatal."[88] Use of para-aminosalicylic acid (PAS), a bacteriostatic agent developed in England in 1949, resolved some of the problems.[89] PAS prolonged the activity of streptomycin and, when administered in combination with it, allowed for use of smaller doses of streptomycin, which had fewer side effects and longer duration.

Still, other objections to the antibiotic regimen remained. The problem of how to "judge activity" or identify suitable cases for treatment was one. "It is generally agreed that we have excellent methods for establishing the *presence* of tuberculosis," Walsh McDermott wrote to Long in early 1947, "yet . . . [a] large part of our time is occupied in attempting to decide whether or not a particular individual with obvious tuberculosis is or is not capable of continuing at work. We will soon have to decide in addition whether that individual should or should not receive antibacterial therapy."[90] Though McDermott, esteemed director of medical research at the ATS, editor of the *American Review of Tuberculosis,* researcher and professor in medicine and public health at Cornell University Medical College, enthusiastically supported antibiotics, he recognized that the tasks of determining who needed treatment, who was eligible for treatment, and who had been cured posed innumerable difficulties.[91]

Isoniazid, a derivative of isonicotinic acid, promised more than either streptomycin or PAS. It had bactericidal properties, and it seemed both to work specifically on mycobacteria and to be particularly effective against actively dividing cells. It could be used in combination with PAS and streptomycin to treat tuberculosis, but it seemed almost as effective on its own. Most important, isoniazid differed from other antibiotics in that it could be used as a preventive rather than as a cure. When prescribed for those who were exposed to tuberculosis in their families or households or for those who had recently become tuberculin positive, isoniazid promised to contain the early infection and convert it into a protective state.[92]

However, isoniazid presented its own difficulties. In 1954 the Tuberculosis Control Division confidently reported that isoniazid alone could cure as effectively as any combination of drugs,[93] but by 1955 evidence of resistant bacteria and of toxicity had emerged.[94] Isoniazid was effective only when taken in long-term, massive doses, but use of the drug in this way seemed to correlate with liver damage and even liver cancer. Moreover, the complicated, lengthy isoniazid regimens prevented many patients from complying fully with the treatment. "Isoniazid prophylaxis," Long later reflected, was "at best a cumbersome procedure,"[95] and the large number of patients who failed to finish the prescribed course complicated assessments of its efficacy.[96] Chemotherapy, one physician warned, was transforming TB from a "killer" to a "crippler," for as patients abandoned treatment, resistant organisms became a larger and larger problem, and relapses occurred with greater frequency.[97]

BACK TO BCG

The limitations of chemotherapy returned attention to BCG. Aronson marshaled new evidence in the vaccine's support,[98] and Sol Roy Rosenthal at Tice, similarly rallied to BCG's defense.[99] As the debate grew increasingly heated, the ATS, the medical arm of the NTA, recognized the need for another BCG conference. The PHS and Tice cosponsored the meeting, which was held on October 17, 1955; the agenda included discussion of vaccines and immunology in tuberculosis, epidemiological factors pertinent to prevention, and alternative preventive agents. Palmer presented the most recent data from Puerto Rico and Muscogee County. Equal time was allotted to Rosenthal. Well organized and well attended, the meeting did little to ease the tension. Aronson and Rosenthal, backed by the philanthropist Mary Lasker, placed pressure on the PHS to endorse BCG. Taking his cues from Palmer and Shaw, the surgeon general resisted.[100]

In the aftermath of the conference, several distinct lines of opposition to BCG emerged. One of these was represented in a conflict between Rosenthal and the PHS. Rosenthal remained a steadfast and impassioned advocate of BCG. His numerous studies routinely indicated that vaccination worked,[101] but, like the Von Rucks a generation earlier, Rosenthal engaged in a constant battle with the PHS, at the heart of which lay questions about vested interests. After the abrupt closure of the New York State BCG lab, his institute became the major American producer of BCG, and as a result the PHS immediately viewed Rosenthal's trials with suspicion. "Dr. Rosenthal, the principal producer of BCG vaccine in this country, desires that BCG be more widely used," Anderson explained to the surgeon general in 1955. Because Rosenthal had a financial interest in BCG, the reliability and validity of his research trials seemed questionable. In the eyes of the PHS, he had a "vested interest."[102] As in the earlier Von Ruck incident, the authority of those who produced a therapy was pitted against the authority of those whose duty it was to safeguard the public.

Other forms of opposition also surfaced. Palmer, Shaw, and Comstock had continued to follow the incidence of tuberculosis among reactors to tuberculin, and as they reviewed results from Muscogee and Puerto Rico, they continued to redefine the tuberculosis problem. As they did so, they offered a bipartite critique of BCG. First, unmoved by evidence that the new-case rate remained steady, Comstock, Palmer, and Shaw argued that rates of reactivity to tuberculin had fallen so low as to render the risk of new infection slight.[103] Tuberculosis, they consequently suggested, had lost its status as a major health problem, with one exception. The results of the BCG trials conducted in Muscogee and Puerto Rico suggested that among those who were already infected and who therefore reacted positively to tuberculin, the disease continued to take its toll. In 1956, Myers lent weight to this conclusion by formally redefining the relationship between infection and disease. Positive reactors to tuberculin, Myers now suggested, represented "cases." These individuals harbored signs of disease that physicians had overlooked in the past. He claimed, however, that new radiographic techniques "demonstrated that lesions are always to be found in tuberculin reactors, but the minuteness of the lesions often made it difficult to locate them at autopsy and to locate them in most cases on x-ray film."[104]

Second, evidence from Muscogee and Puerto Rico suggested that little tuberculosis had occurred "among those eligible for vaccination, whether or not they were vaccinated."[105] Instead, tuberculosis posed the greatest danger to infected individuals, who through poor hygiene and bad habits reinfected themselves. Only those who did not take proper precautions, whose behavior predisposed toward disease, ran the risk of continued infection. BCG—a passive, immunological measure designed solely for use in nonreactors to tuberculin—could do little to prevent the resurgence of disease in this population. Once again, Palmer and Shaw congratulated Americans on the measures they had already implemented and downplayed the usefulness of BCG. Estimates of the vaccine's efficacy, they came to argue, had been greatly inflated because researchers had not restricted their analysis to the occurrence of tuberculosis in tuberculin-negative controls. They suggested that the data indicated that BCG would reduce TB within that segment of the population by a mere 25 percent.[106]

Hence, Palmer and Shaw advised American officials not to waste their efforts on BCG but to concentrate instead on the prevention of "re-infections and breakdowns." Even in Puerto Rico, where the risk of infection vastly exceeded that of the rest of the United States, such measures—which encompassed educational programs, routine screening, and isolation of the diseased—had worked. They had minimized the risk of infection from the social and physical environment. Thus, the PHS concluded that vaccination had no value in the population at greatest risk of becoming ill with tuberculosis, and it offered only minimal protection to nonreactors to tuberculin. In this context, it was unclear "that the advantages of using BCG would outweigh the disadvantages of losing the tuberculin test as a diagnostic and case-finding tool."[107]

Aronson disagreed. Experiences with the disease seemed to him to belie the assessments of risk among reactors to tuberculin. "Myers believes that a positive tuberculin reaction must be evaluated as a pre-requisite to the development of progressive and fatal tuberculosis," he quipped in 1957, but, he asked, if every tuberculin reactor represented a disaster waiting to happen, why did physicians find so few cases of TB among reactors, and why did every reactor not become a case? The logic of the argument seemed to him to be based on both erroneous hypotheses and faulty data.[108]

Opie, Long, and many others were similarly "astonished to find that Myers's opinion concerning the relation of negative and positive tuberculin reactions to subsequent clinical disease still has a vogue."[109] Palmer and Shaw had emphasized the clinical dangers and epidemiological importance of "reinfection tuberculosis." In this population, the x-ray, not the tuberculin test, was the critical diagnostic tool. Even Myers acknowledged that "the tuberculin test gives no aid in the diagnosis of the reinfection type of tuberculosis," where the "roentgenogram is the most valuable aid in detection."[110] Moreover, as Myers's opponents had once suggested, neither x-rays nor tuberculin tests actually did anything to prevent infections. BCG did. Hence, the argument that vaccination widened the population that needed screening seemed irrational to those who believed that the routine vaccination of children would effectively eliminate the need for screening.

The peculiar responses to tuberculin found in Muscogee County seemed to further undermine arguments about the value of tuberculin testing and the susceptibility of tuberculin reactors. In 1953, even Palmer had admitted that "the time has come, it is apparent, for wider consideration of the proposition that tuberculin sensitivity in human beings is very often not due to tuberculous infection."[111] Puzzled by the Muscogee study and by other studies like it, he amassed a large body of epidemiological and statistical evidence indicating that sensitivity to tuberculin depended much more on place of residence than on contact with tuberculosis. He argued:

> [This evidence] leads directly to the conclusion that most of the sensitivity brought out only by strong doses of tuberculin is not caused by tuberculous infection, at least not by the same organism or by the same mode of infection responsible for tuberculous disease in human beings. This conclusion, supported by the findings of several previous studies challenges the traditional assumption that all tuberculin sensitivity is necessarily of tuberculous origin and postulates the existence of at least two main sources of tuberculin sensitivity in human beings.[112]

Because Palmer had found greatest sensitivity among residents of the southeastern states, his work threw into doubt the Muscogee and Puerto Rico findings. In both areas, it remained unclear whether the subjects who tested positive to tuberculin had a primary infection or whether they reacted to something else. These questions applied particularly to Puerto Rico, where no chest x-rays had been performed. If something other than exposure to tubercle bacilli could provoke a positive reaction to tuberculin, then Palmer's and Shaw's claims for the diagnostic value of tuberculin fell flat, and their conclusions about reinfection tuberculosis became highly dubious.

Closer analysis of the trials drew attention to additional problems. With the exception of those trials of BCG that Palmer and Shaw had assessed, every vaccination study conducted in the United States suggested that BCG was effective, Aronson objected in 1957.[113] Confronted with a wealth of evidence that contradicted their conclusions, Palmer and Shaw dismissed the other studies on largely methodological grounds. Yet in the eyes of some critics they did not judge their own work by applying the same high standards that they applied to others. For all its concern about method, the PHS had been remarkably lax about ensuring that its two trials were ultimately comparable. The Puerto Rico staff, unlike their counterparts in Muscogee County, did not x-ray the child participants. The age of the subjects in Muscogee ranged from five to twenty years and in Puerto Rico from one to eighteen years. More important, the two trials employed different vaccines and methods of vaccination. Ingestion of BCG was by now out of vogue, but no standard technique had replaced Calmette's original method, and different producers and proponents of the vaccine adopted different techniques. Hence, in Muscogee, participants received BCG (produced by Tice) by the "multiple puncture" method that its producers preferred; in Puerto Rico, subjects received intracutaneous injections of vaccine manufactured at the New York State BCG lab. These differences complicated efforts to compare the outcomes of the trials.[114] Inconsistent methods of case finding had also been adopted. Most important, as Palmer and Shaw admitted, "[t]he definition of what would be accepted for present purposes as a case of tuberculosis differed somewhat in the two trials." In Puerto Rico, "any person reported as having tuberculosis or as dying of the disease was accepted as a case," and "[i]n line with policy of not disturbing the existing diagnostic procedures in any way, no attempt was made to verify the accuracy of the diagnosis."[115] In Muscogee County, far more rigid standards applied.

Like Park and others who had feared that the different mortality statistics found among vaccinees and controls reflected fundamental differences in those populations, Palmer frequently stressed the importance of maintaining "comparability." He took the selection of controls extremely seriously, and in the mid-1940s challenged the results of a classic Swedish BCG study on grounds of selectivity. Data obtained from the vaccination of conscripts formed the basis of the Swedish trials. The Swedish authorities had offered BCG vaccine to all conscripts, and they had taken those who accepted the vaccine as their subjects while leaving those who rejected it as controls. Palmer objected that those who complied and those who did not represented fundamentally different populations.[116] The boys who took BCG, he reputedly said, were boys of a different moral fiber, who obediently followed orders. Palmer had consequently ensured that when American trials of BCG were planned in 1946, it was clearly understood that "it was unacceptable to vaccinate all who were willing to be vaccinated and use those who refused as controls."[117]

Yet Palmer had not ensured this condition in Puerto Rico. There, the vaccination campaign had been made a "political issue," and Palmer, Comstock, and Shaw acknowledged that, "as a result of adverse publicity directed against vaccination, large numbers of parents (and some of the children themselves) refused to have anything to do with the program or accepted only the tuberculin test."[118] In Palmer's own terms, those who refused vaccination were the sort who resisted orders and, hence, could well be of different moral fiber or socioeconomic standing than those who accepted. Thus, he might have invoked fundamental differences in the populations to account for the results obtained, but he did not, and he made no effort to correct for such factors.

"A FALSE SENSE OF SECURITY": THE 1957 REVIEW OF BCG

By 1957, the debate over BCG had become particularly contentious, as news that the British Medical Research Council would endorse BCG stoked the already-heated dispute and lent support to BCG's American advocates. Like the PHS, the British council had originally opposed use of BCG, primarily on grounds that the vaccine was unsafe and that French trials did not provide ample evidence of efficacy.[119] By the mid-1950s, however, British trials had relieved many of the earlier misgivings. In 1956, the British Medical Research Council issued a first progress report in which it advised that BCG would reduce mortality by at least 55 percent with few apparent complications.[120] As the trial continued, all the prior objections were erased, and Great Britian joined the many nations that administered BCG. The United States was consequently left alone in its opposition, and BCG's advocates used this isolation to sharpen their knives.

The PHS launched another investigation. On June 14, 1957, an Ad Hoc Advisory Committee on BCG met in Washington to "review and prepare recommendations on Public Health Service BCG policy and program."[121] The members of the committee included such authorities as Long, McDermott, and James Perkins, the managing director of the NTA. Faced with the same challenge that three other committees of investigation had faced, the 1957 Ad Hoc Advisory Committee reviewed the earlier efforts. The committee examined the conclusions of its 1946 predecessor one by one, and over and over again it found itself in agreement. In 1946, the BCG conference had recommended that the vaccine not be made commercially available or be distributed to private doctors; the 1957 committee concurred. In 1946, the conference had called for further research on the relationship between allergy and immunity, on the proper method of vaccination, on the need for revaccination, and on the efficacy of vaccination in "groups highly exposed to tuberculous infection"; each step, the 1957 committee agreed, had been appropriately taken.[122] The earlier conference had ultimately concluded that BCG "affords only incomplete rather than absolute protection."[123]

> [In addition,] the most effective methods of controlling tuberculosis in the general population are (a) further improvement of living conditions and the general health, (b) reduction of tuberculous infection, which can be accomplished by modern public health methods and the unremitting search among presumably healthy individuals for patients with infectious tuberculosis, (c) prompt and adequate medical and surgical treatment of patients with active disease, (d) segregation and custodial care of those not amenable to accepted forms of therapy and (e) adequate rehabilitation.[124]

It stressed that BCG vaccination "must not be regarded as a substitute for approved hygienic measures or for public health practices designed to prevent or minimize tuberculous infection and disease."[125] In the mid-1950s, eminent American physicians agreed that the earlier "statement was adequate for current use. Consequently no changes were made and the policies continue as before."[126] The 1957 committee concurred.

It justified its position with self-congratulatory affirmations of the singularity of the United States. "In those places of the world where tuberculosis is a national emergency and where prosecution of the usual control methods is impossible," it advised, "it is understandable that BCG has been given extensive application. In this country, where we are not faced with the same deficiencies, the medical profession for the most part has not advocated the widespread use of the vaccine."[127] Once again, the committee reaffirmed its faith in existing measures of control, and it openly expressed its fears that "indiscriminate use" of BCG would undermine those measures. BCG, it believed, should not be seen as an alternative to or substitute for "approved hygienic measures." Ultimately, the committee concluded, "vaccination may lead to a false sense of security which could result in failure to observe precautions that would otherwise be taken."[128]

WHENCE THE OPPOSITION? ANTIBIOTICS AND A NEW THERAPEUTIC OF SOCIAL REFORM

In 1959, a group of experts from around the world met at the Arden House, in Harriman, New York, to yet again evaluate American policy governing use of BCG. That same year, the British Medical Research Council assigned vaccination a more prominent place than it had previously had in its campaign against tuberculosis and advocated greater use of BCG, which its trials found both safe and 80 percent effective.[129] Just a few years later, representatives of the Canadian Public Health Association and the Department of National Health and Welfare would call similarly for more extensive use of BCG, which had "been on trial for 40 years," and had proven to be safe and 80 percent effective and to confer protection that lasted for ten years.[130] But at the Arden House, representatives from the PHS replayed and refined old themes as they once again declared that tuberculosis "is in part a sociological as well as a biological problem."[131] Saluting declining mortality and morbidity, they reaffirmed the worth of existing tuberculosis-control measures, advocated the use of antibiotics, and opposed the adoption of BCG.[132]

During the 1940s and 1950s antituberculosis drugs had not passed beyond the experimental stage, and their safety and efficacy had not, as yet, been fully determined. Clinical trials conducted to assess the worth of these drugs proved controversial, and they pointed from the start to many hazards associated with chemotherapy. The need for combination doses and long terms of treatment discouraged patients from complying with complicated therapeutic regimens. Moreover, early studies suggested that the side-effects of isoniazid ranged from toxicity to liver damage and cancer. The resurgence of TB during the late 1980s and early 1990s, with the emergence of new drug-resistant strains, testifies to the validity of these early concerns.

Nonetheless, the PHS promoted preventive drugs—streptomycin, isoniazid, and PAS among them—and educational and rehabilitative services. Precise data on expenditures are incomplete, but the figures that exist in published reports of the PHS and in records of the Tuberculosis Control Division indicate that through the 1950s the Tuberculosis Program typically spent more on "prophylaxis evaluation," "therapy evaulation," and "educational and technical information" than on vaccination. The figures for 1959 were, respectively, $650,000, $250,000, $55,000, and $35,000. They also expended considerable sums in "technical assistance to state and local health agencies" in order to support medical, nursing, social, statistical, educational, laboratory, administrative, and home-care services.[133]

Given the problems inherent in chemotherapy and chemoprophylaxis, why did the PHS not subject these agents and BCG to the same degree of scrutiny? And why did it opt for experimental drugs over BCG? The comparative expenses of chemoprophylaxis and vaccination are arguably part of the answer. Mass vaccination programs generally incur high costs, and BCG would be no exception. However, in the first stages, use of antibiotics was also expensive. Streptomycin initially cost twenty dollars per gram, which rendered the three-gram-per-day dose prohibitively expensive.[134] By the mid-1950s, the cost of the antimicrobial drugs had dropped considerably, but the per-diem rate still exceeded five dollars.[135] In order for isoniazid to be effective, patients had to take it for a period of at least one year, which brought the cost of medication to nearly $2,000. Necessary supplements to treatment, which included screening, rehabilitation, and the services of medical and advisory staff, made the full costs considerably higher. Moreover, though the declining number of tubercular infections meant that chemoprophylaxis could be concentrated on a small population, the PHS recognized that as the number of people with tuberculosis declined, they became more difficult and costly to locate.[136] Combined, the costs of providing routine tuberculin screening, antimicrobial drugs, and rehabilitation remained so high that as late as 1966 the PHS again lamented that "[t]uberculosis has been and still is the costliest of the communicable diseases in the United States—both in terms of human lives and dollars."[137] By one estimate, each case of tuberculosis cost at least $15,000.[138]

Another line of inquiry points to the relation between BCG, antimicrobial drugs, and the broader aims of the American campaign to "build resistance" to TB. The initial appraisals of BCG and antibiotics suggest that American physicians continued to value a multifaceted resistance to tuberculosis; as they engaged in debates over BCG and antimicrobial drugs, this goal once again loomed large. Neither BCG nor antibiotics, early assessors warned, provided a panacea. Neither offered an alternative to established methods of control. The steering committee of the NIH warned in its initial statement on streptomycin that "rapid improvement induced by this drug, may be temporary and therefore less helpful to the patient than slower improvement, similar in degree, resulting from the development of immunity uninfluenced by chemotherapy."[139] Antimicrobial drugs, the committee thus feared, might interfere with and undermine the benefits of traditional hygienic and dietetic methods of controlling tuberculosis. Even advocates of antibiotic treatment, McDermott among them, feared that these products would interfere with the natural development of host resistance. "If we pursue this course of action," he wrote, "we will need also to search for methods of enhancing the resistance of the host to tuberculous infection after the latter has been partially or temporarily inhibited by antibacterial therapy."[140] McDermott warned his colleagues not to lose sight of host resistance, and he recommended that those interested in this end keep in mind such factors as "the influence of posture on healing" and "the nutritional aspect of the problem."[141]

Such concerns became common and surfaced throughout the 1950s. In March 1955, the PHS and the New York State Department of Health cooperated in sponsoring a conference on "current concepts of the drug treatment of non-hospitalized tuberculosis patients." The department appreciated that "modern treatment of tuberculosis with drugs and resectional surgery has made great changes in the management of this disease and in the outlook" and wished to make the findings known to its county, city and district health officers. A memo from Commissioner Hilleboe and Robert Plunkett, director of the Division of Tuberculosis Control, dutifully informed these officers of the various drugs available for treatment and of their strengths and limitations. Though optimistic, the department warned of the uncertainties that continued to surround antimicrobial therapy. "The action of the drugs is known to be only bacteriostatic or suppressive but not eradicative," Hilleboe advised; "drug treatment is therefore seldom definitive of itself. This means that drug treatment is an addition to the other methods of treating tuberculosis and not a substitute for them, particularly bed rest. Because of the peculiar nature of the disease, what basically determines its outcome in a given patient is the bodily resistance to the disease—natural or acquired or both."[142] As Hilleboe clearly indicated, American campaigns against tuberculosis continued to rely on diet, hygiene, "rest and other things," which rendered the soil resistant to the seed. He and Plunkett, like investigators of an earlier generation, remained loyal not just to the goal of building resistance but also to the methods by which that goal had been accomplished.

While Hilleboe, Plunkett, and McDermott stressed the physiological dimensions of resistance, neither they nor their colleagues forgot that resistance also had a sociological component. An important difference between BCG and antibiotics was that despite early fears use of isoniazid and streptomycin could be reconciled with the larger goals of a campaign to build a combined physiological-sociological resistance in ways that BCG could not be.

Here, a comparison with earlier debates over tuberculin is suggestive. Though they ultimately became responsible for closing down sanatoria, in their early stages drugs both could be and regularly were used within these institutions. There was no reason to expect that new chemotherapeutic and chemoprophylactic agents would reduce the need for tuberculosis hospital beds, Anderson, chief of the Division of Tuberculosis Control, noted in 1952; if anything, he commented, these drugs should increase the need for hospital places.[143] As an earlier generation had guarded against the use of tuberculin in private practice, so a new one advised against the use of drugs outside of hospitals. In 1955, Hilleboe warned that the advantages of "drug treatment outside the hospital" were primarily financial but that any savings of public monies effected thereby were false economies, for the assumption that "drug treatment outside the hospitals is an entirely satisfactory substitute for an adequate period of hospitalization under competent medical guidance" was "utterly fallacious."[144] One year later, Dr. James Waring, the president of the Colorado Foundation for Research in Tuberculosis, made the case that the successful treatment of active disease could be achieved only when an experienced sanatorium physician administered chemotherapy. Home care or outpatient treatment, he argued, were only "permissible and practical provided an experienced physician keeps in close touch with a cooperative patient."[145] Economic concerns marked the arguments of this new generation. Declining mortality, they clearly realized, placed tuberculosis hospitals in jeopardy of extinction.

In the years before 1960, American physicians rarely administered antituberculosis drug regimens outside of hospitals.[146] The justification they often gave for this practice was that, when used within sanatoria and tuberculosis hospitals, antituberculosis drugs became an "adjunct to the basic bed-rest."[147] Streptomycin, though it did not itself act to improve host resistance, could thereby be made consistent with other efforts to build resistance—diet and rest chief among them. Thus, if antibiotics focused on the seed, they did not compromise efforts to nourish the soil.

Isoniazid appeared to have an additional advantage in that it not only was consistent with the rehabilitative goals of the campaign to build resistance, which continued to focus on diet and rest, but seemed actually to reinforce these goals. Though its mode of action was not yet understood, isoniazid appeared to act on both bacillus and host. More important, those who worked with isoniazid soon recognized that it affected the metabolism of the host. "Isoniazid is a metabolic inhibitor of a normal metabolic pathway," investigators later explained, and "the drug stimulates appetite leading the patient to greater food consumption, increased weight gain and presumably better nutrition which in itself may be having a therapeutic benefit."[148] Hence, the use of antibiotics in general and of isoniazid in particular meshed with the physiological goals of the campaign to build resistance to TB. They could be used within hospitals and sanatoria as part of or as adjuncts to programs based on diet and bed rest, which invigorated the host.

But just as late-nineteenth- and early-twentieth-century sanatoria had sought to build more than a physiological resistance, so the larger goal of creating social well-being informed the twentieth-century campaign against TB. Here again, the comparison with tuberculin and earlier methods of building resistance is illuminating. BCG, like tuberculin, built resistance by acting on the host rather than on the bacillus, but just as Allen Krause, Luther Emmett Holt, and others in an earlier generation had believed that physiological resistance was not enough, so this new one believed that resistance was far more than physical. Throughout the 1950s representatives of the PHS repeatedly defined tuberculosis as "in part a sociological as well as a biological problem."[149] In continually reinforcing this link between tuberculosis and socioeconomic conditions, those who represented the PHS proved themselves to be the intellectual grandchildren of that earlier generation. They sought not only to reconcile new tuberculosis control measures with older, established procedures but also to use them in ways that would build a combined physiological and sociological resistance.

Their concern for the social as well as the physiological rehabilitation of patients is apparent in the discussions of the treatment of nonhospitalized patients that took place during the 1950s. "A highly important disadvantage of treatment outside of hospitals," Hilleboe wrote in the 1955 memo, "is the impossibility of providing the essential extramedical services for patients which the modern tuberculosis hospital does provide, namely education, diversional and occupational therapy, counselling, testing, vocational guidance, training, job placement and social services."[150] Cure of tuberculosis, he made clear, depended on infinitely more than physiological improvement. It depended as well on such factors as "suitable home environment," "adequate nutrition," and "proper health education for both patient and family."[151]

Like those who, a generation earlier, had advocated sanatorium regimens, Hilleboe recognized the modern tuberculosis hospital as the proper home for these extramedical measures, in part because they would be provided nowhere else. In the absence of a social-welfare system, the hospital assumed many roles. "The provision of medical and surgical treatment is only one of the basic functions of the modern tuberculosis hospital," he wrote. "Another is the segregation of sources of infection to reduce the spread of tubercle bacilli, and still another is the education of patients concerning the necessary adjustment of their lives to their impaired physical condition, as well as the methods of preventing the spread of infection to others, especially members of their households."[152] Social rehabilitation remained an important function of the tuberculosis hospital. Within its walls, patients learned discipline and the essential tenet of citizenship—that one should act to protect the interests of both self and others. These "fundamental measures of tuberculosis control cannot be accomplished for patients treated outside of hospitals, particularly those who have not had a previous period of hospitalization," Hilleboe and Plunkett feared.[153]

BCG, unlike isoniazid, could not be used in sanatoria or hospitals; it did not complement and supplement the hygienic, dietary, and educational programs. It did not promote the discipline or habits of life that led to a combined biological and social resistance. Rather, it obviated the need for institutionalization, "further improvement of living conditions and the general health,"[154] and the healthful and hygienic practices that the PHS and ATS repeatedly insisted were needed to render the soil resistant to tubercle bacilli. BCG promised on its own to achieve this end. Isoniazid alternatively provided a means of linking regimens for physiological reform with exhortations to proper living. Prescribed prophylactically, isoniazid was easily combined with educational programs. Employed in hospitals or, as later on, under the close supervision of visiting nurses, isoniazid, Americans hoped, would combat disease at both physical and social levels. However, neither hospitals nor American social services could long support these interventions. Worthy as the goals of American tuberculosis control programs were, the campaign to build a combined physiological and sociological resistance was unrealistic, could not alone create the material conditions needed to combat TB, and could not succeed without parallel economic and social reforms.

Restoring History to Understand the Resurgence of Tuberculosis

Tuberculosis is once again a fearsome disease. National magazines and newspapers repeatedly warn of epidemics and drug-resistant strains and predict the wildfire spread of dangerous microorganisms for which there is no available cure. As it ponders the mysteries of "Paradise Lost" and the "Disease That Rose from Its Grave," the American popular press focuses repeatedly on poverty, liberty, and responsibility.[1] Illegal immigrants, the homeless, and those "reluctant patients" who fail to take their pills are at the heart of the epidemic. At a city-run TB clinic, the *New York Times* reported, physicians "adjusted doses for patients suffering side effects and cajoled reluctant patients to take their pills—offering free lunches, tokens and car rides to other appointments."[2] Detention poses a less friendly alternative but is used, despite the infringement of rights, to control those who pose a public health threat because "they have repeatedly failed to take their medicines."[3]

These are old and familiar problems, which Clio, the muse of history, puts into perspective. From the time they began to use chemotherapy and chemoprophylaxis in the 1950s, American physicians recognized the risks. Drug-resistant strains began to appear soon after streptomycin was introduced. Patients' failure to comply with cumbersome INH programs exacerbated the problem. As one physician complained, "Because the medication must be taken daily, 5 times a week for one year, it will not be easy to carry out the program."[4] Administration of drug treatments outside of hospitals further compromised success. "Cooperation on the part of the patient and conformance with the medical recommendations," Herman Ertresvaag Hilleboe and Robert Plunkett observed, were hard to ensure. "There is evidence," they noted, "that patients do not take oral drugs which have been dispensed to them at the time of their periodic visit to an outpatient or field clinic. . . . The failure to keep clinic appointments is still another problem."[5] By 1967, some American researchers estimated and feared that many patients failed to take their pills over 75 percent of the time.[6]

Equally familiar is the limited role assigned to BCG. Despite changes in disease patterns and social experience, Americans continue to ignore vaccination as an option for tuberculosis control. In September 1992, as Canadian papers warned of an "American-Style Outbreak," provincial health ministers reinstituted BCG vaccination programs for vulnerable populations.[7] In October 1992, in the last of a five-part series on tuberculosis, the *New York Times* reported that, "Stymied by Resurgence of TB, Doctors Reconsider a Decades-Old Vaccine."[8] In September 1993, when a Reuters News Agency release reported a "discovery" that was seen as an "important step" toward the development of a vaccine, it made no mention of BCG, and it erroneously stated that "a vaccine has been in existence since the 1930s, but does not protect against the transmission of pulmonary tuberculosis."[9]

The purpose of this book is not to suggest that Americans should adopt BCG nor to blame today's epidemic on past policy. Rather, at a time when TB again poses a major public health hazard, and Canadian health care has become one model for American reform, it asks us to explore important differences in national policy. In particular, it raises questions about the links between health policies and the material provisions made to care for the poor who developed TB. The difference between American and Canadian experiences, one might argue, owes less to scientific or medical decisions not to vaccinate than to a disjuncture between the aspirations and rhetoric of American TB control programs and the state's ability materially to transform social and economic conditions or alter attitudes toward poverty. In essence, laudable as the goals of American physicians were, they could not alone provide the social improvements and high level of awareness needed to eradicate TB.

This work has shown that a range of intellectual, institutional, and ideological forces shaped the formation of American policy. Scientific and immunological debates raged throughout the thirty-year period during which BCG was studied. The absence of an American equivalent of the Pasteur Institute and the defensive posturing of researchers who tried to establish a national scientific style helped to determine BCG's fate. So did epidemiological changes. Tuberculous mortality declined during the first half of the twentieth century. By 1955, mortality among even the most vulnerable populations, American Indians and Eskimos, had dropped. By 1960, TB no longer ranked as a major killer of young adults; it appeared, instead, as a less dramatic plague of the elderly.

When viewed from a parochially American perspective, any one of these intellectual, institutional, or epidemiological factors might justify the American response to BCG. But, once again, a comparative perspective enriches and complicates the analysis. The Canadian case is particularly suggestive. In Canada, as in the United States, tuberculous mortality fell throughout the first half of the twentieth century. Canadian mortality, in fact, fell more sharply than American mortality.[10] Similarly, trends in the incidence of new cases followed a parallel course in the two nations with, once again, the Canadian rate charting a slightly lower path than the American.[11] Comparable patterns existed among the native populations of Canada and the United States, the groups at greatest risk; after 1953, tuberculous mortality among Canadian Indians remained well below 100/100,000.[12]

Yet Americans and Canadians interpreted these epidemiological shifts differently. In the United States, Carroll Palmer, Lawrence Shaw, J. Arthur Myers, and George Comstock argued that the number of tuberculin re-actors had declined sufficiently to obviate the need for BCG. They pro-posed that improvements in the standard of living and traditional measures of tuberculosis control had so reduced mortality that further intervention appeared unnecessary, and they feared that a vaccine that rendered its subjects tuberculin positive would actually undermine existing efforts. Canadian authorities, surveying a similar epidemiological vista, reached quite different conclusions. Pointing to "the leveling off of morbidity and mortality, the occurrence of several sharp epidemics in different provinces, and the problems of drug resistance," they argued that "[d]espite great advances in tuberculosis control . . . tuberculosis still constitutes the ma-jor infectious disease problem in Canada."[13] Though case rates had de-clined, an official spokesman maintained, each new case had ample opportunity to infect many others. Hence, on the basis of the accumu-lated evidence, he deemed American opposition to BCG unfounded, dis-missed as "exaggerated" fears that widespread BCG vaccination would lead to the loss of the tuberculin test as a diagnostic and epidemiological tool, and pronounced mass vaccination with BCG both necessary and justified.[14]

In this instance, then, the divide that separated the United States from Britain, Canada, and much of the rest of the world was not epidemio-logical. The campaign against tuberculosis was, at least in part, a cam-paign against poverty, and, to Americans, BCG seemed to challenge the fundamental principles of that larger effort. Here, the biological and sociopolitical goals of the campaign against tuberculosis dovetailed neatly, so that even if isoniazid had not become available, powerful ideological reasons for opposing BCG would still have persisted. The American debate over use of BCG borrowed terms from the broader debate over social welfare then taking place. Just as the Progressives who worked to combat tuberculosis tied TB to poverty and betrayed their deep-seated beliefs about the origins of social decay, so did those who battled TB in the era of the New Deal. Progressives, who attributed poverty to ignorance and inadequate or squandered opportunity, hailed education as an instrument of social reform. They employed it similarly in their battle against tuberculosis, for in both instances they believed education would help to create an independent and healthy citizenry. By the time of the New Deal, assumptions both about the nature of poverty and about the appropriate solutions to that problem had shifted. The poor, framers of the Social Security Act realized, required not just opportunity but also assistance—financial or otherwise—that would redress imbalances. But even at the height of the New Deal, a gap existed between rhetoric and action. As many recent scholars have shown, Americans remained deeply uncomfortable with notions of dependency, institutionalized poor relief, and state intrusion into private life. Thus New Deal programs strove to provide measures that were enabling rather than protective or, in the words of James Patterson, to create "doors" not "floors."[15]

Distrust of protectionism filtered into American discussions of TB control, as debates in the United States over Papworth Village settlements betrayed. Papworth Village was an English settlement for the care of chronic tuberculosis patients. Though it combined elements of rehabilitation and care, Papworth differed from the American sanatorium in that it did not represent one stop on the road to recovery. Because its founder, the physician Sir Pendrill Varrier-Jones, did not believe that tuberculosis was curable, Papworth, like the sanatorium in Thomas Mann's *Magic Mountain,* kept its patients. It provided inpatient care, sometimes followed by outpatient services in a nearby village, where it also employed patients at standard union rates of pay. Instead of training patients for full reentry into the outside world, Papworth made its patients dependents of a permanent, subsidized colony.[16]

In 1954, William Dahlgren, of the Pottenger Sanatorium in Monrovia, California, proposed that a settlement like Papworth be established in the United States. Dahlgren's letter provoked a tense discussion in which the underlying goals of the American crusade against tuberculosis surfaced. One argument raised against building a settlement like Papworth in the

United States was that antibiotics would soon make the "chronic victim" a relic of the past. Another argument was based on personal freedom. "It is difficult to explain all the reasons why this type of colony has never taken hold in the United States," Robert Anderson wrote in one of the many letters exchanged. "Among them are the apparent disposition of the American culture not to propose or accept regimentation. . . . It is doubtless a matter of subtle but decisive differences between the cultural complex of the two nations."[17] Fears of protecting the poor and of creating a dependent subclass seemed central to that cultural difference. "The Papworth Village type of colony has never taken hold in this country," Paul Pamplona, senior surgeon of the Tuberculosis Control Division, explained in September 1954, for "[o]ur effort, rather, has been to educate tuberculosis patients in proper techniques to prevent the spread of the disease and to return them to normal life through programs of rehabilitation. . . . According to the physical, emotional, and medical limitations of each patient they are given an opportunity for training and are oriented in a new life compatible [to] their abilities."[18]

As Dahlgren enlisted senators, representatives, and public health officials from California in support of his cause, these affirmations of American difference recurred again and again. Americans approached the problem of the chronic tuberculosis patient differently than did the British, as Edward Bloomquist, medical director and chief of the Tuberculosis Program within the Division of Special Health Services, wrote. In the United States, he suggested, "emphasis [is] given to preventing chronic tuberculosis from developing, rather than caring for the chronic cases after they become established."[19] Fears of protectionism also emerged in the rhetoric that surrounded BCG, as, for instance, when Strasheimer Alburtus Petroff, William Hallock Park, Anderson, and others feared that BCG would provide a "false sense of security" that would lead to laxity and disorder.

Over the course of a century, American rhetoric made, indeed seized on, the association between tuberculosis and poverty. The presumed relationship between class and the disease melded with peculiarly American assumptions about poverty to constrain the administrative and legislative responses to tuberculosis control. Because Americans viewed TB as a disease that required both social and medical responses, at the turn of this century they concentrated responsibility for its control in sanatoria and voluntary agencies. Later, when the federal government assumed primary responsibility for the American crusade against tuberculosis, the link with poverty was not lost. The genealogy of federal control over TB is suggestive. In Canada, federal jurisdiction over tuberculosis began with the ACTR. Child of the NRCC, a scientific, research-oriented body, the ACTR shared the goals of its parent. However, in the United States, federal authority in the area of tuberculosis derived from the Social Security Act. Born of social reform, the Tuberculosis Control Division of the PHS formed part of a larger campaign to relieve poverty and to improve the welfare of ordinary citizens.

Hence, rather than simply focusing on microbes, the Tuberculosis Control Division sought as well to eliminate the social factors that predisposed toward the disease. It made this commitment clear in 1944, when, it set as its goals medical research into the poor nutrition, poor hygiene, poverty, and dependency associated with TB. It made this commitment clear in its choice of staff. It made this commitment clear when, in 1950, the Tuberculosis Control Division became part of the Division of Chronic Diseases,[20] thereby ensuring that victims of tuberculosis would receive medical treatment and "also physical, mental and social rehabilitation."[21] It made this commitment equally clear in epidemiological assessments conducted during the 1950s, which examined the influences of marital and economic status on susceptibility to TB.[22]

Well into this century, a range of American physicians, whose interests led them into the lab and into the community, continued to take the social dimensions of TB seriously. Like earlier generations of physicians, they inextricably tied the campaign against TB to social reform. They allowed the understanding that both physiological and sociological factors fertilized the tubercular soil to draw their attention toward research on resistance—on tuberculin, heliotherapy, and nutrition. They further allowed that understanding to color their therapeutic judgments by consistently preferring a form of treatment that would permit them to teach their patients broad behavioral lessons. The realization of this goal depended on economic prosperity and robust social-welfare programs that would mold a self-sufficient, enlightened population. Until the 1970s, TB hospitals and physicians worked in concert with the state and the people to deliver these services and provide not just vaccination but an "antitoxin of self-respect." During the 1950s and 1960s, as physicians, public health officials, and social workers debated the relative merits of various treatment programs, they acknowledged the need to make a range of services widely and publicly available. At a meeting of the NTA-PHS joint staff held in June 1957, for example, Floyd Feldmann of the NTA "brought up the emotional aspect of treatment clinics," which he feared "may be construed as a form of socialized medicine." James Perkins, managing director of the NTA, quickly dismissed Feldmann's concerns. "[G]overnment hospitals and clinics for TB are socialized medicine, if one wants to call it that," he argued.

"[B]ut since we are dealing with a communicable disease the control of which is the responsibility of the health department, it has been accepted by organized medicine. Physicians might be resentful but the principle is not new. It would be a new practice in many communities."[23]

However, since the mid-1970s, those limited social services that did exist have been eroded. Health care and preventive medicines have grown increasingly expensive and inaccessible to those in greatest need.[24] BCG still marshals little support, and its medical alternatives have proven limited. But, equally important, the medical effort to create a combined physiological/sociological resistance has survived at a rhetorical level that is divorced from material intervention.

Thus, tuberculosis remains a disease of the socially disadvantaged. On August 12, 1994, an official with the International Union against Tuberculosis and Lung Disease commented, "You never hear about TB in North America because of who gets it these days: immigrants, natives, poor people and AIDS patients for the most part."[25] As the United States once again confronts disease, poverty, and the need for social reform, the lessons of history are worth reviewing.

Notes

ABBREVIATIONS USED IN THE NOTES

Journals

AJMS	*American Journal of the Medical Sciences*
AJPH	*American Journal of Public Health*
Am. Rev. TB	*American Review of Tuberculosis*
Anns. Inst. Past.	*Annales de l'Institut Pasteur*
BHM	*Bulletin of the History of Medicine*
BMJ	*British Medical Journal*
BMSJ	*Boston Medical and Surgical Journal*
CLC	*Cincinnati Lancet and Clinic*
CMAJ	*Canadian Medical Association Journal*
DMW	*Deutsche Medizinische Wochenschrift*
IJHS	*International Journal of Health Services*
JAMA	*Journal of the American Medical Association*
JHM	*Journal of the History of Medicine*
NOMSJ	*New Orleans Medical and Surgical Journal*
SJMS	*Southern Journal of Medical Science*
Trans. NASPT	*Transactions of the National Association for the Study and Prevention of Tuberculosis*
Trans. NTA	*Transactions of the National Tuberculosis Association*

Manuscript Collections Cited

Baldwin Papers	Papers of E.R. Baldwin, National Library of Medicine, Washington, D.C.
Becker Papers	Papers of Florence Deakins Becker, Library of Congress, Washington, D.C.
Long Papers	Papers of Esmond R. Long, National Library of Medicine, Washington, D.C.
National Archives (NA) Records of the NIH	RG 52A–208: Immediate Office of the Director, Mail and Files, Washington, D.C. RG 443: Old Investigations, Washington, D.C.

Records of the PHS   RG 90–0425: General Classified Records, Group ix, General Files (1936–1944), Washington, D.C.
RG 90–0425–32, RG 90–0470, and RG 90–0470–132: General Files (1924–1935), Washington, D.C.
RG 90–62A–177: Records of the Tuberculois Program: Institutions, and Records of the Tuberculosis Control Division: Meetings, Conferences, and Congresses, Suitland, Md.
RG 90–62A–2748: Records of the Department of Health, Education and Welfare/Office of International Health, Subject Files, Suitland, Md.
RG 90–64A–645: Records of the Tuberculosis Program, Suitland, Md.
RG 90–73E–0058: Records of the Centers for Disease Control Tuberculosis Program, Suitland, Md.

Opie Papers   Papers of Eugene L. Opie, American Philosophical Society, Philadelphia

Pritchard Papers   Papers of Elizabeth Gaitlin Pritchard, National Library of Medicine, Washington, D.C.

Walsh Papers   Papers of Joseph Walsh, College of Physicians of Philadelphia

INTRODUCTION

1. Reports are legion. For a representative few, see "New Strain of TB," *Toronto Globe and Mail* (August 15, 1992), A5; Robert Baltimore, "Distribution of AIDS Resembles That of TB," *New York Times* (December 17, 1987); Michael Specter, "Panel Proposes Stronger Steps to Curb TB," *New York Times* (November 30, 1992), A1, B1; "Neglected for Years, TB Is Back with Strains That Are Deadlier," *New York Times* (October 11, 1992), A1. See also "Deadly, Untreatable TB Strain Plaguing US Puts Canadian Health Officials on Red Alert," *Montreal Gazette* (October 4, 1992), A1, A6; "A Deadly Return," *Newsweek* (March 16, 1992), 53.

2. The phrase "costliest of communicable disease" was used frequently during this period. See "Public Health Service Recommendations on the Use of BCG Vaccination in the United States," *Morbidity and Mortality Weekly Report* (October 15, 1966), 350. The primary cause of nineteenth-century deaths, TB ranked among the top ten causes of death well into the twentieth century. Until 1900, TB claimed over 200 of every 100,000 American deaths per year. Thereafter, it continued to surpass other infections, such as polio, in both fatality and prevalence. As late as 1965, pneumonia and influenza were the only other infectious diseases ranked among the leading causes of American deaths. Cressy L. Wilbur, *Tuberculosis in the United States* (Washington, D.C.: GPO, 1908); United States Bureau of the Census (USBC), *Historical Statistics of the United States, from Colonial Times to 1970* (Washington, D.C.: GPO, 1975), vol. 1, 77. See also U.S. House, Select Committee on Population, *Domestic Consequences of United States Population Change, 95th Cong., 2d sess.,* 1978.

3. USBC, *Historical Statistics*, vol. 1, 58–77.

4. Ralph Chester Williams, *The United States Public Health Service, 1798–1950* (Washington, D.C.: Commissioned Officers Association of the United States Public Health Service, 1951), 774; United States Department of Health, Education and Welfare (USDHEW), *Tuberculosis in the United States: Status of the Disease in the Early Sixties,* Public Health Service (PHS) Publication 1036 (Washington, D.C.: GPO, 1963), 23–24.

5. Eleanor Roosevelt's experiences with TB are well hidden. I first stumbled upon them through a reference in Jerry Gladman, "The Fight against Tuberculosis—The White Plague," *Toronto Sun* (March 8, 1992), 43, which led to a frustrating search for further information. Though her autobiography recounts a bout of "pleurisy" in 1919 that her physician warned her might be tuberculous, Roosevelt makes no mention of her illness, nor do standard biographies. However, in *Eleanor, The Years Alone,* her biographer Joseph Lash quotes a letter from Dr. James Halsted to James Roosevelt commenting on Mrs. Roosevelt's death. In it, Halsted observes, "Unfortunately she had an old tuberculosis lesion dating back to 1919, the scars of which were shown in the x-rays of her chest. . . . The tuberculosis which was activated by steroid treatment spread rapidly and widely throughout her body and was resistant to all kinds of anti-tuberculosis treatment. This was the cause of her death.'" Letter from James Halsted to James Roosevelt, March 25, 1966; quoted in Joseph P. Lash, *Eleanor, The Years Alone* (New York: Norton, 1972), 331.

6. See Allan M. Brandt, "Polio, Politics, Publicity and Duplicity: Ethical Aspects in the Development of the Salk Vaccine," *International Journal of Health Services (IJHS)* 8 (1978): 257–269.

7. "Present Policy of the American Trudeau Society on BCG Vaccination," *American Review of Tuberculosis (Am. Rev. TB)* 57 (1948): 544.

8. USDHEW, *The Arden House Conference on Tuberculosis* (Washington, D.C.: GPO, 1960).

9. The best discussions of the ways in which bacteriology transformed public health are provided in Barbara G. Rosenkrantz, *Public Health and the State: Changing Views in Massachusetts 1842–1936* (Cambridge, Mass.: Harvard University Press, 1972); Judith Walzer Leavitt, *The Healthiest City: Milwaukee and the Politics of Health Reform* (Princeton, N.J.: Princeton University Press, 1982); Naomi Rogers, *Dirt and Disease: Polio before FDR* (New Brunswick, N.J.: Rutgers University Press, 1992). For other discussions, see George Rosen, "The Bacteriologic, Immunologic and Chemotherapeutic Period, 1875–1950," *Bulletin of the New York Academy of Medicine* 40 (1964): 483–494; George Rosen, *A History of Public Health* (New York: M.D. Publications, 1958); George Rosen, *Preventive Medicine in the United States, 1900–1975* (New York: Prodist, 1977); R. H. Shryock, *The Development of Modern Medicine: An Interpretation of the Social and Scientific Factors Involved* (1939; reprint, Madison: University of Wisconsin Press, 1979); C.E.A. Winslow, *The Evolution and Significance of the Modern Public Health Campaign* (New Haven: Yale University Press, 1943).

10. Jesse L. Steinfeld, "Introduction and Conference Goals," in USDHEW, *Status of Immunization in Tuberculosis in 1971: Report of a Conference on Progress to Date,* National Institutes of Health (NIH) 72-68 (Washington, D.C.: GPO, 1972), 127.

11. Robert Koch, "Die Aetiologie der Tuberculose," *Berliner Klinische Wochenschrift* 19 (1882): 221–230. Translation: Joseph Eichberg, "The Etiology of Tuberculosis, Being a Translation of the Original Article of Dr. Robert Koch as Presented at the Meeting of the Berlin Medical Society," *Cincinnati Lancet and Clinic (CLC)* 49–50 (1883): 439, hereafter referred to as Koch, "Aetiologie," Eichberg trans.

12. Rosen, "Bacteriologic."

13. Allen K. Krause, "Solving Tuberculosis, a Many Sided Problem" (address to the Open Meeting of the Ninth Session of the Mississippi Valley Conference on Tuberculosis, Columbus, Ohio, September 12, 1921), printed as "The Tuberculosis Problem" in Allen K. Krause, *Rest and Other Things* (Baltimore: Williams & Wilkins, 1923), 98.

14. Examples of a vast body of scholarship include Thomas McKeown, "A Historical Appraisal of the Medical Task," in Gordon McLachlan and T. McKeown, eds.,

Medical History and Medical Care: A Symposium of Perspectives Arranged by the Nuffield Provincial Hospitals Trust and the Josiah Macy Jr. Foundation (London: Oxford University Press, 1971); P. Wright and A. Treacher, eds., *The Problems of Medical Knowledge: Examining the Social Construction of Medicine* (Edinburgh: Edinburgh University Press, 1982); G. Risse and R. Numbers, *Medicine without Doctors, Home Health Care in American History* (New York: Science History Publications, 1977); S. Reverby and D. Rosner, "Beyond the Great Doctors," in S. Reverby and D. Rosner, eds., *Health Care in America, Essays in Social History* (Philadelphia: Temple University Press, 1979); Roy Porter, "The Patient's View: Doing Medical History from Below," *Theory and Society* 14 (1985): 167–174. A superb analysis of the strengths and weaknesses of the new social history of medicine is provided in John Harley Warner, "Science in Medicine," *Osiris*, 2d ser., 1 (1985): 37–58.

15. See, for example, Joseph Eyers, "Prosperity as a Cause of Death," *IJHS* 7 (1977): 125–149. Eyers writes: "The remaining 95% of the variation [in the overall death rate that cannot be accounted for by suicide] was for a long time reconceptualized under ideas which made the social origins of disease seem irrelevant. While the mid-nineteenth century reformers, from Chadwick and Farr onward, had seen the ultimate origins of urban disease in poor housing, deficient nutrition and unsanitary living conditions, the rise of the germ theory of disease in the late nineteenth century removed the focus from the conditions favoring infection of individuals to the germs themselves, and the impetus of reform shifted from general social equalization to specific and narrow public health measures," 127. In support of his statement, Eyers cites Rosen, *A History of Public Health*.

16. Both sentiments are expressed in a joint statement that the PHS and the American Trudeau Society issued in 1948; they are expressed as well in the proceedings of the Arden House Conference, sponsored by the PHS in 1959. USDHEW, "Present Policy of the American Trudeau Society on BCG Vaccination," *Arden House*, 4.

17. For discussions of the theoretical and historiographic problems that studies of the middle classes pose, see Stuart M. Blumin, *The Emergence of the Middle Class: Social Experience in the American City, 1760–1900* (New York: Cambridge University Press, 1989); Anthony Giddens, *The Class Structure of the Advanced Societies* (New York: Harper & Row, 1975).

18. I use *ideology* here, as Shklar does, to mean nothing "very complicated. It refers simply to political preferences, some very simple and direct, others more comprehensive." Judith Shklar, *Legalism: Law, Morals and Political Trials* (Cambridge, Mass.: Harvard University Press, 1986), 4. More specifically, I use the term in the manner prescribed by Geertz, who identifies ideologies as "cultural symbols" for programmatic preferences. For Geertz, ideologies act as "maps of problematic social reality and matrices for the creation of collective conscience." Clifford Geertz, *The Interpretation of Culture* (New York: Basic Books, 1973), 220. My analysis is also informed by anthropological studies of illness and disease, such as those of Taussig. He argues that "the signs and symptoms of disease, as much as the technology of healing, are not 'things-in-themselves,' are not only biological and physical, but are also signs of social relations disguised as natural things." Michael Taussig, "Reification and the Consciousness of the Patient," *Social Science and Medicine* 14 (1980); 3.

19. Robert Wiebe, *The Search for Order* (New York: Hill and Wang, 1967).

20. Though historians have appreciated these ideological foundations of disease control programs, they have most often portrayed them as corrupting influences. See, for example, Allan Brandt, *No Magic Bullet: A Social History of Venereal Disease in the United States* (Oxford: Oxford University Press, 1986). An alternative presentation can be found in Sylvia Noble Tesh, *Hidden Arguments: Political Ideology and Disease Prevention Policy* (New Brunswick, N.J.: Rutgers University Press, 1988).

21. Barbara Bates, *Bargaining for Life: A Social History of Tuberculosis, 1876–1938* (Philadelphia: University of Pennsylvania Press, 1992); Sheila Rothman, *Living in the Shadow of Death: Tuberculosis and the Social Experience of Illness in American History* (New York: Basic Books, 1994).

CHAPTER 1: DISEASE AND THE AGRARIAN ORDER

1. Villemin presented his initial evidence that consumption was inoculable and contagious in *Du tubercule au point de vue de son siège, de son évolution et de sa nature* (Paris: J.-B. Ballière et fils, 1861). This work attracted little attention from the *American Journal of the Medical Sciences (AJMS)*, which mentioned Villemin's work in neither the sections it devoted to foreign news nor its "Quarterly Report on the Progress and Improvements of Medical Science." The *AJMS* did contain several discussions of the contagiousness of diphtheria, but the communicability of consumption was addressed only obliquely. If representatives to meetings of the American Medical Association or state medical societies discussed Villemin's hypothesis, those who reported the meetings to the *AJMS* did not deem the discussions newsworthy. Villemin's work also did not appear in discussions in the *Boston Medical and Surgical Journal (BMSJ)*, or the *Philadelphia Medical Times*.

2. Lemuel Shattuck, *Report of the Sanitary Commission of Massachusetts, 1850* (reprint, Cambridge, Mass.: Harvard University Press, 1948), 94.

3. This quote, for example, is from Austin Flint, *A Treatise on the Principles and Practice of Medicine*, 4th ed. (Philadelphia: Henry Lea, 1873), 287.

4. James H. Cassedy, *American Medicine and Statistical Thinking, 1800–1860* (Cambridge, Ma.:Harvard University Press, 1984).

5. C. F. Volney, *A View of the Soil and Climate of the United States*, trans. and ed. Charles Brockden Brown (Philadelphia: J. Conrad, 1804), 223–264, quoted in Cassedy, *American Medicine*, 10.

6. "Dr. Rush's Thoughts upon the Cause and Cure of Pulmonary Consumption," *BMSJ* 3 (1830): 249. See also Benjamin Rush, "An Inquiry into the Comparative State of Medicine, in Philadelphia, between the Years 1760 and 1766, and the Year 1809," in Benjamin Rush, *Medical Inquiries and Observations*, 4th ed. (Philadelphia: M. Carey, 1815).

7. Cassedy, *American Medicine*, 7. See also Samuel Forry, "Statistical Researches Relative to the Etiology of Pulmonary and Rheumatic Diseases, Illustrating the Application of the Laws of Climate to the Science of Medicine," *AJMS* 1 (1841): 13–54; Daniel Drake, *A Systematic Treatise, Historical, Etiological and Practical, on the Principal Diseases of the Interior Valley of North America as They Appear in the Caucasian, African, Indian and Esquimaux Varieties of Its Population* (Cincinnati: W. B. Smith, 1850). Nineteenth century medical texts regularly invoked the wisdom of Forry and Drake on regional differences in the incidence of consumption. See, for example, Leonidas Merion Lawson, *A Practical Treatise on Phthisis Pulmonalis; Embracing Its Pathology, Causes, Symptoms, Treatment* (Cincinnati: Rickey, Mallory, 1861), v.

8. Henry G. Wiley, "Pulmonary Consumption," *BMSJ* 18 (1838): 6.

9. See, for example, "Statistics of Mortality by Consumption," *BMSJ* 26 (1842): 18.

10. Shattuck, *Report*, 94.

11. For contemporary accounts, see Waldo I. Burnett, "A Consideration of Some of the Relations of Climate to Tubercular Disease," *BMSJ* 47 (1853): 149–53, and Bennet Dowler, "Geography of Consumption in the United States," *New Orleans Medical and Surgical Journal (NOMSJ)* 14 (1857): 312–323; compare later accounts, such as Cressy L. Wilbur, *Tuberculosis in the United States* (Washington, D.C.: GPO, 1908); Anthony M. Lowell, *Tuberculosis* (Cambridge, Mass.: Harvard University Press, 1969), 7–8; USBC,

Historical Statistics of the United States (Washington, D.C.: GPO, 1976), vol. 1, 58, 77. See also James H. Cassedy, *Medicine and American Growth, 1800–1860* (Madison: University of Wisconsin Press, 1986), 50–54.

12. Shattuck, *Report*, 103.

13. Samuel Cartwright, "The Treatment of Pulmonary Consumption," *NOMSJ* 14 (1857): 291.

14. See Drake, *Systematic Treatise*; see also Samuel Forry, "Statistical Researches Relative to the Etiology of Pulmonary and Rheumatic Diseases, Illustrating the Application of the Laws of Climate to the Science of Medicine," *AJMS* 1 (1841): 13–54; and see Dowler, "Geography."

15. "M. Louis on Consumption," *BMSJ* 29 (1844): 470. Empirical research conducted during the mid decades of the nineteenth century—such as the studies of Pierre Louis—renewed debate over the role in consumption of "hereditary influence."

16. See, for example, Lyman Barton, "Inoculation with Tuberculous Matter," *BMSJ* 29/30 (1843–1844): 301–302.

17. "Curability of Pulmonary Consumption," *BMSJ* 29 (1843): 343–344. The editorial constitutes a review of Wm. A. M'Dowell, *A Demonstration of the Curability of Pulmonary Consumption, in All Its Stages, Comprising an Inquiry into the Nature, Causes, Symptoms, Treatment and Prevention of Tuberculous Diseases in General* (Louisville, Ky.: Prentice and Weissinger, 1843).

18. "Dr. Rush's Thoughts," 250.

19. Samuel George Morton, *Illustrations of Pulmonary Consumption; Its Anatomical Character, Causes, Symptoms and Treatment. To Which Are Added, Some Remarks on the Climate of the United States, the West Indies, etc.,* 2d ed. (Philadelphia: Biddle, 1837), 216. Compare Samuel George Morton, *Illustrations of Pulmonary Consumption; Its Anatomical Character, Causes, Symptoms and Treatment* (Philadelphia: Key and Biddle, 1834), 120.

20. Lawson, *A Practical Treatise on Phthisis Pulmonalis*, 409.

21. "Dr Flint on the Treatment of Phthisis," *BMSJ* 69 (1863–1864): 87.

22. Samuel Cartwright, "Remarks on Dysentery among Negroes," *NOMSJ* 11 (1854): 162–163; see also Cartwright, "Treatment."

23. Rollin Gregg, "Synopsis of an Unpublished Work on Consumption and Kindred Maladies," *Transactions of the Homoeopathic Society of the State of New York* (1866): 209–227; William A. Hawley, "Report on Clinical Medicine. Case of Phthisis Pulmonalis," *Transactions of the Homoeopathic Society of the State of New York* (1865): 337.

24. I. T. Talbot, "Introduction to the Progress of Homeopathy in Massachusetts," *Transactions of the Homoeopathic Society of the State of New York* (1865): 92–93.

25. Charles Cullis, "Report of the Consumptives Home," *Transactions of the Homoeopathic Society of the State of New York* (1869): 509–510.

26. See, for example, "Record of Clinical Cases, Samuel Gregg of Boston," *Transactions of the Homoeopathic Society of the State of New York* (1866): 78–79; see also Cullis, "Report," 509–511.

27. Hawley, "Report on Clinical Medicine," 337.

28. Ibid., 338.

29. Talbot, "Introduction," 92.

30. This quote, for example, is from "Annual Address, Homoeopathic Society of Northern New York," *Transactions of the Homoeopathic Society of the State of New York* (1870): 726–727. A discussion of the broader context of interchange between allopaths and homeopaths can be found in W. Bruce Fye, "Vasodilator Therapy for Angina Pectoris: The Intersection of Homeopathy and State Medicine," *Journal of the History of Medicine (JHM)* 45 (1990): 317–340.

31. A. R. Morgan, "Consumption in America," *Transactions of the Homoeopathic Soci-*

ety of the State of New York (1869): 667–672; D. H. Beckwith, "Climatology and Its Relation to Respiratory Diseases," *Transactions of the American Institute of Homeopathy* 23 (1870): 226–237.

32. C.M.W., "Homeopathy in Massachusetts," *BMSJ* 14 (1859): 486.

33. For a discussion of the meaning of the term *diathetic*, see Erwin H. Ackerknecht, "Diathesis: The Word and the Concept in Medical History," *Bulletin of the History of Medicine(BHM)* 56 (1982): 317–325. The *Index Medicus* listed consumption under general diseases, diathetic or constitutional—as opposed to exanthematous or xymotic. General textbooks from the 1860s, 1870s, and 1880s most frequently classified it as both a local disease of the lungs and a constitutional cachexia. See, for example, John Eberle, *A Treatise on the Practice of Medicine*, 6th ed. (Philadelphia: Grigg and Elliot, 1845); John Hughes Bennett, *Clinical Lectures on the Principles and Practice of Medicine*, American ed. (New York: S. and W. Wood, 1860); Flint, *Treatise*; John Syer Bristowe, *A Treatise on the Theory and Practice of Medicine*, 2d ed. (London: Smith, Elder and Company, 1878); Robert Bartholow, *A Treatise on the Practice of Medicine*, 2d ed. (New York: D. Appleton, 1889).

34. Todd Savitt and James Harvey Young, eds., *Disease and Distinctiveness in the American South* (Knoxville: University of Tennessee Press, 1988). Warner has also written extensively about southern medical distinctiveness. For a summary, see John Harley Warner, *The Therapeutic Revolution* (Cambridge, Mass.: Harvard University Press, 1987).

35. In lieu of the classification of ages by counties and their subdivisions, the births, marriages, and deaths, the church and school statistics," DeBow wrote, "I have inserted, as of wider interest, county tables in the following particulars—of population, white, free-colored and slave, native and foreign, male and female." J.D.B. DeBow, *A Statistical View of the United States, Embracing Its Territory, Population—with Free Colored and Slaves; Moral and Social Condition, Industry, Property and Revenue, the Detailed Statistics of Cities, Towns and Counties; Being a Compendium of the 7th Census to Which Are Added the Results of Every Previous Census, Beginning with 1790, in Comparative Tables, with Explanatory and Illustrative Notes, Based upon the Schedules and Other Official Sources of Information* (Washington, D.C.: A.O.P. Nicholson, 1854), 1.

36. Bennet Dowler, "Statistical Researches on the Ration of Mortality from Pulmonary Consumption in the Northern and Southern States as Proved by the Mortality Statistics of the Seventh Census (1850)," *NOMSJ* 14 (1857): 312–323, quote on 318.

37. "Health and Longevity in America," *BMSJ* 58 (1858): 265–266.

38. Dowler, "Statistical Researches," 318.

39. Ibid., 320.

40. Ibid., 320; in many ways, Dowler's essay formed part of a more pervasive lament for the misunderstood South. For examples of this genre, see "Reviews: Report of the Sanitary Commission of New Orleans on the Epidemic Yellow Fever of 1853," *NOMSJ* 11 (1855): 524–557, especially 550–551.

41. "Health of New Orleans, from the New Orleans Medical News and Hospital Gazette," *BMSJ* 57 (1858): 516.

42. Dowler, "Statistical Researches," 321.

43. E. M. Pendleton, "Pulmonary Diseases as Affected by Climate, etc." *Southern Journal of Medical Science (SJMS)* 6 (1866): 432–436.

44. "Diseases of Negroes," *BMSJ* 3 (1830–1831): 547–548.

45. "Examples of Longevity in the Colored Race, in 1860, All except One Being in the Southern United States," *NOMSJ* 18 (1861): 150–151; "Mortality of Negroes in America," *SJMS* 1 (1866): 312–313.

46. Cartwright, "Remarks on Dysentery," 162.

47. USBC, *Mortality Statistics of the Seventh Census of the United States* (Washington, D.C., 1855); see also Lawson, *A Practical Treatise on Phthisis Pulmonalis*, 223–226.

48. Cartwright, "Remarks on Dysentery," 155.

49. Samuel Cartwright, "Diseases and Peculiarities of the Negro Race," *DeBow's Review* 11 (1851): 64–69, 331–336, quote on 331–332.

50. Cartwright, "Treatment," 289–297.

51. Ibid., 295.

52. "Mortality of Negroes in America," *SJMS* 1 (1866): 312.

53. Thomas P. Atkinson, "On the Anatomical, Physiological and Pathological Differences between the White and the Black Races," *Transactions of the Medical Society of Virginia* (4th sess., 1873): 111.

54. "Mortality of Negroes," 313.

55. Editors of the *Boston Medical and Surgical Journal*, "Review of Atkinson's 'Differences between the White and Black Races,'" cited in Atkinson, "On the Anatomical," 65.

56. "Mortality of Negroes," 313.

57. "Commentary," *Medical Times and Gazette*, reprinted in ibid., 313.

58. Josiah Nott, "Instincts of Races," *NOMSJ* 19 (1866): 12, 147.

59. Atkinson, "On the Anatomical," 111.

60. Ibid., 113.

61. Nott, "Instincts of Races," 12.

62. "Mortality of Negroes," 313.

63. Stanford E. Chaillé, "Vital Statistics of New Orleans," *NOMSJ* 23 (1870): 61–65, quote on 8–9.

64. Ibid., 43, 45.

65. USBC, *Historical Statistics*, vol. 1, 63 (Table B193-200).

66. The first Canadian census provided population and mortality data for Quebec, Ontario, Nova Scotia, and New Brunswick. This figure was arrived at by adjusting the number of deaths provided per province for population.

67. Cyrus Ramsay, "The Statistics of Some of the Diseases of New York and London, a Paper Presented to the Medical Society of New York, 1863," cited in *AJMS* 46 (1863): 203. Canada urbanized and industrialized less rapidly than the United States. However, Canadian cities similarly harbored the tuberculous, and the difference between patterns of urban and rural mortality loomed large. In 1870, the average tuberculous death rate reported for rural Ontario was 134/100,000 and for Quebec 163/100,000, but in the Maritimes (where mining, paper, and fishing industries were well established), in Toronto, and in Montreal, mortality exceeded 200/100,000. The 1881 census, reflecting the expanded Confederation and including mortality data for Prince Edward Island, British Columbia, Manitoba, and "the territories" of Alberta and Saskatchewan, indicated that, following the trend in the United States, the average tuberculous death rate had dropped to 156/100,000. Still, this average hid tremendous local variations that again reflected patterns of urbanization and industrialization. If mortality was low in the prairies and had fallen in rural Ontario, it had risen in Montreal and Toronto and some Maritime cities to over 300/100,000. Mortality in New Brunsick and Nova Scotia remained close to 200/100,000. It was lowest in the territories—Saskatchewan, Alberta, and the North (42/100,000)—and in Manitoba (42/100,000). Caution must be used in assessing these trends, for the low rate may in fact be an artifact of limited data and hence might skew the average.

This analysis is based on the Canadian censuses of 1870 and 1880; compare George Jasper Wherrett, *The Miracle of the Empty Beds* (Toronto: Univeristy of Toronto Press, 1977), 15, appendices. In Canadian cities, mortality continued to increase until 1900.

For further discussion, see George Jasper Wherrett, *Tuberculosis in Canada: Report for the Royal Commission on Health Services* (Ottawa: Queen's Printer, 1965); G. C. Brink, *Across the Years, Tuberculosis in Ontario* (n.p., n.d.); Katherine McQuaig, "Public Health in Canada" (master's thesis, McGill University, 1981).

68. A concise example of Jefferson's views can be found in Query 19 in Thomas Jefferson, *Notes on the State of Virginia* (New York: Harper and Row, 1964), 156–159.

69. "Country Life," *DeBow's Review* 29 (1860): 615.

70. Cartwright, "Treatment," 295.

71. Henry Ingersoll Bowditch, *Consumption in New England* (Boston: Ticknor and Fields, 1862), v.

72. Ibid. Bowditch's work received wide and favorable reception. The *AJMS* and other medical journals reprinted synopses of his work, and standard medical texts referred frequently to his argument. Flint was one physician who, following Bowditch, examined the influence of climate on the development of TB. Flint argued that "the prevalence of the disease is less in climates either uniformly dry, or uniformly cold and dry, than in those which are moist and subject to frequent laterations of cold and warmth." Flint also considered altitude, proximity to the sea, sunlight, and temperature important. Flint, *Treatise*, 296.

73. Frank Donaldson, "The Influence of City Life and Occupations in Developing Pulmonary Consumption," *Public Health* 2 (1874–1875): 113.

74. Wiley, "Pulmonary Consumption," 87–88. See also Ludwig Bremer, "The Bearing of the Discovery of the Tubercle Bacillus on Public Hygiene," *St. Louis Medical and Surgical Journal* 47 (1884): 496. Further discussion of the understanding that consumption was a disease of urban civilization is provided in René Dubos and Jean Dubos, *The White Plague*, especially chapter 15; and Nan Marie McMurry, "'And I? I Am in a Consumption': The Tuberculosis Patient, 1780–1930" (Ph.D. diss., Duke University, 1985), chapter 9.

75. Henry Ingersoll Bowditch, review of *Medical Communications of the Massachusetts Medical Society at Its Annual Meeting, May 1862, AJMS* 45 (1863): 140; see also Bristowe, *Treatise*, 432; Flint, *Treatise*.

76. Henry Ingersoll Bowditch, "An Inquiry Concerning the Means of Preventing Consumption" (1871). Peter H. Bryce quoted Bowditch in his essay "Some Reasons Why So Many Persons Die of Consumption," which was contained in Ontario, Legislative Assembly, "Second Annual Report of the Ontario Provincial Board of Health, 1883," *Sessional Papers* 2 (1884): 354–355.

77. Donaldson, "The Influence of City Life."

78. Flint, *Treatise*, 297.

79. Shattuck, *Report*. Donaldson, "Influence of City Life," exemplified these concerns. So did tracts in standard medical texts. See also Frank Donaldson, "City Air and City Life Injurious to Consumptives," *Transactions of the American Climatological Association* 1 (1884): 70–85; C. W. Chancellor, "Impure Air and Unhealthy Occupations as Predisposing Causes of Pulmonary Consumption," *Public Health* 9 (1885): 67–96; Flint, *Treatise*, 297.

80. "Trades Producing Phthisis," *BMSJ* 5 (1831): 288–289.

81. "The Forms of Consumption Peculiar to Age and Sex," *Medical and Surgical Reporter* 39 (1878): 189. For further discussion of male and female variations in TB, see Edward B. Foote, *Plain Home Talk about the Human System, the Habits of Men and Women— the Causes and Prevention of Disease* (New York: Murray Hill, 1882).

82. "Employment of Women and Children in Agriculture," *BMSJ* 28 (1843): 491.

83. Flint, *Treatise*, 297.

84. The best statement of these sentiments is provided in a later piece: Bremer, "Bearing of the Discovery," 496.

85. Rush "Thoughts," 249.

86. E. L. Trudeau, "The History of the Tuberculosis Work at Saranac Lake, New York," *Medical News* 83 (1903): 2.

87. Julius Wilson, "'Daily Sanatorium Routine Was the Treatment,'" *American Lung Association Bulletin* (March 1982): 7–10.

88. The ways in which mid-nineteenth century campaigns against disease combined moralism with medicine are more fully explicated in Charles Rosenberg, *The Cholera Years* (Chicago: University of Chicago Press, 1962); Charles Rosenberg and Carroll Smith Rosenberg, "Piety and Social Action: Some Origins of the American Public Health Movement," in Charles Rosenberg, ed., *No Other Gods: On Science and American Social Thought* (Baltimore: Johns Hopkins University Press, 1976), 109–122; Barbara G. Rosenkrantz, *Public Health and the State*, especially chapters 1 and 3; Margaret Humphreys, *Yellow Fever and the South* (New Brunswick, N.J.: Rutgers University Press, 1992). See also Morton Keller, *Affairs of State: Public Life in Late Nineteenth Century America* (Cambridge, Mass.: Harvard University Press, 1977), chapters 12 and 13.

CHAPTER 2: COPING WITH KOCH'S CHALLENGES

1. Joseph Eichberg, "The Etiology of Tuberculosis, Being a Translation of the Original Article of Dr. Robert Koch as Presented at the Meeting of the Berlin Medical Society," *CLC* 49–50 (1883): 439; hereafter referred to as Koch, "Aetiologie," Eichberg trans.

2. Koch, "Die Aetiologie der Tuberculose."

3. On the social authority of science, see Wiebe, *Search for Order;* Charles Rosenberg, *No Other Gods: On Science and American Social Thought* (Baltimore: Johns Hopkins University Press, 1979). For a discussion of education and the middle classes, see Paul Axelrod, *Making a Middle Class* (Montreal: McGill-Queen's University Press, 1991).

4. Rosenberg, *No Other Gods*; Daniel Walker Howe, ed., *Victorian America* (Philadelphia: University of Pennsylvania Press, 1976); Carl Berger, *Science, God and Nature in Victorian Canada* (Toronto: University of Toronto Press, 1983); Suzanne Zeller, *Inventing Canada* (Toronto: University of Toronto Press, 1983); Richard Jarrell, "Science as Culture in Victorian Toronto," *Atkinson Journal of Canadian Studies* 1 (1982): 5–12.

5. Blumin, *Emergence of the Middle Class*, 8–9. Once again, this discussion of the middle classes is derivative of Blumin and of Giddens, *Class Structure*.

6. Koch, "Aetiologie," Eichberg trans., 439.

7. The centenary of Koch's identification in 1882 stimulated many such accounts. See, for example, Saul Benison, "Celebration and History: The Centenary of Robert Koch's Discovery of the Tubercle Bacillus," *BHM* 56 (1982): 157–159; T. M. Daniel, "Robert Koch, Tuberculosis and the Subsequent History of Medicine," *American Review of Respiratory Diseases* 125 (1982): 1–3; G. L. Gale, "Tuberculosis in Canada: A Century of Progress," *Canadian Medical Association Journal (CMAJ)* 126 (1982): 526–529; Russell C. Maulitz, "Robert Koch and American Medicine," *Annals of Internal Medicine* 97 (1982): 761–766. For an excellent discussion of Koch's concept of "causation," see K. Codell Carter, "The Koch-Pasteur Dispute on Establishing the Cause of Anthrax," *BHM* 62 (1988): 45–57.

8. Russell C. Maulitz, "'Physician versus Bacteriologist': The Ideology of Science in Clinical Medicine," in M. Vogel and C. Rosenberg, eds., *The Therapeutic Revolution* (Philadelphia: University of Pennsylvania Press, 1979), 91–107; Russell C. Maulitz, "Robert Koch in the United States of America," *NTM: Schriftenreihe für Geschichte der*

Naturwissenschaften, Technik, und Medizin 1 (1983): 75–84; Donald Fleming, *William H. Welch and the Rise of Modern Medicine* (Baltimore: Johns Hopkins University Press, 1954; reprinted 1987).

9. Rosen, "Bacteriologic," 483–484.

10. Edward Livingston Trudeau, *An Autobiography* (Philadelphia: Lea and Febiger, 1915), 184. Others have appreciated the cautiousness of the American response to Koch; see H.R.M. Landis, "The Reception of Koch's Discovery in the United States," *Annals of Medical History n.s.* 4 (1932): 531–537; Maulitz, "Robert Koch in the United States"; Fleming, *William Welch*, 47–76; C.E.A. Winslow, *The Life of Hermann Biggs* (Philadelphia: Lea and Febiger, 1929), 55. A classic example of the ways in which American reactions to Koch were recast in hindsight is apparent in the differences between Trudeau's account of his reception of Koch's bacillus and that provided by Russell C. Maulitz in "Robert Koch and American Medicine," *Annals of Internal Medicine* 97 (1982): 762.

11. Maulitz, "Koch in the United States"; Fleming, *William Welch*, 47–76; Winslow, *The Life of Herman Biggs*, 54–85.

12. For a discussion of the ways in which memory served the interests of professional identity, see John Harley Warner, "Remembering Paris: Memory and the Disciples of French Medicine in the Nineteenth Century," *BHM* 65 (1991): 301–325.

13. *New York Times* (May 7, 1882), 8. For further discussion of the early reception of Koch's bacillus in the United States, see Landis, "Reception," 531–537; Maulitz, "Robert Koch and American Medicine," 761–766; Richard Harrison Shryock, *The National Tuberculosis Association, 1904–1954* (1957; reprint, New York: Arno Press, 1977), 25, 48.

14. In April 1882, several newspapers reprinted a *London Times* summary of Koch's "discovery," which was the first formal attention paid his work.

15. Examples include "Koch and the Etiology of Tuberculosis," *CLC* 42 (1882): 422; "Koch's Discovery of the Bacillus of Tuberculosis," *CLC* 47 (1882): 433; excerpt from the *BMSJ* in *CLC* 47 (1882): 369; "The Etiology of Tuberculosis," *Philadelphia Medical Times*, 12 (1882): 843–851. A brief summary of Koch's paper, culled from a British source, appeared without commentary in the July issue of the *AJMS* (1882).

16. Robert Koch, "The Aetiology of Tuberculosis. An Address Delivered by Dr. Robert Koch before the Physiological Society of Berlin," trans. W. D. Oakley, *Canadian Medical and Surgical Journal* 10 (1882): 649–655, 705–718.

17. Koch, "Aetiologie," Eichberg trans.

18. "Report of the 15th Annual Meeting of the Canadian Medical Association," *Canada Medical Record* 10 (1881–1882): 277.

19. R. C. Kedzie, "President's Address: On Bacteria and Sanitary Science," *Public Health* 8 (1882): 9.

20. Peter H. Bryce, "Typhoid and Some Other Zymotic Diseases, Their Causes and Prevention, a Lecture Delivered under the Auspices of the Mechanics' Institute of Galt, October 10, 1882" in Ontario, Legislative Assembly, "First Annual Report of the Ontario Provincial Board of Health, 1882," *Sessional Papers* 13 (1883): 157.

21. For a discussion of the development of public health in Ontario, see Heather MacDougall, *Activists and Advocates: Toronto's Health Department, 1883–1983* (Toronto: Dundurn, 1990).

22. This standard American reaction to the importation of German knowledge occurred in the social sciences as well. The pattern of knowledge transfer and development in public health was, in many ways, far more akin to that which occurred in the social sciences than in the natural sciences. See Dorothy Ross, *The Origins of American Social Science* (Cambridge: Cambridge University Press, 1991); Thomas Bonner, *American Doctors and German Universities. A Chapter in International Intellectual Relations, 1870–1914*

(Lincoln: University of Nebraska Press, 1963); Elizabeth Fee, *Disease and Discovery: A History of the Johns Hopkins School of Public Health, 1916–1939* (Baltimore: Johns Hopkins University Press, 1987); Rosenkrantz, *Public Health and the State*; Leavitt, *Healthiest City*.

23. T. Mitchell Prudden, "On the Occurrence of the Bacillus Tuberculosis in Tuberculous Lesions," *Medical Record*, (New York) 23 (1883): 400. Sternberg cited similar observations in an article that appeared in the *Medical News*, (Philadelphia) 42 (1882).

24. See Fleming, *William Welch*.

25. H. F. Formad, "The Bacillus Tuberculosis and Some Anatomical Points Which Suggest the Refutation of Its Etiological Relation with Tuberculosis," *Philadelphia Medical Times* 13 (1882): 110. See also H. F. Formad, "The Bacillus Tuberculosis and the Etiology of Tuberculosis, Is Consumption Contagious?" *Philadelphia Medical Times* 14 (1883–1884): 337–338; Maulitz, "Physician versus Bacteriologist." These concerns so commonly resonated throughout Europe and North America that in 1883 Koch found himself obliged to respond to them. Robert Koch, "Kritische Besprechung der gegen die Bedeutung der Tuberkelbazillen gerichteten Publikationen," *Deutsche Medizinische Wochenschrift (DMW)* 9 (1883): 137–141.

26. See Robert Koch, "Antrittsrede in der Akademie der Wissenschaften am 1 Juli 1909," *DMW* 29 (1909), reprinted in G. Gaffky and E. Pfuhl, eds., *Gesammelte Werke von Robert Koch* (Leipzig: Georg Thieme, 1912), 1–4. In this speech, Koch explained that the science of bacteriology was rooted in botany and dealt first with classification. The practical interests of researchers had transformed the discipline, but Koch maintained his interests in its initial goals.

Several biographers comment on Koch's early fascination with natural history and collecting. See Richard Bochalli, *Robert Koch: Der Schöpfer der modernen Bakteriologie* (Stuttgart: Wissenschaftliche Veralgesellschaft MBH, 1982), 7–11; Martin Kirchner, *Robert Koch* (Berlin and Vienna: Springer Verlag, 1924), 7–9; Wolfgang Genschorek, *Robert Koch* (Leipzig: S. Hirzel, 1982), 9–13. For context, see William Bulloch, *The History of Bacteriology* (1938; reprint, New York: Dover, 1979); C.E.A. Winslow, *The Conquest of Epidemic Disease: A Chapter in the History of Ideas* (Princeton, N.J.: Princeton University Press, 1943), chapter 14; Shryock, *Development of Modern Medicine*, chapter 11.

27. Bulloch, *History*; Winslow, *Conquest*. The best histories of nineteenth-century debates over spontaneous generation are provided in John Farley, *The Spontaneous Generation Controversy from Descartes to Oparin* (Baltimore: Johns Hopkins University Press, 1977); John Farley and Gerald Geison, "Science, Politics and Spontaneous Generation in Nineteenth Century France: The Pasteur-Pouchet Debate," *BHM* 48 (1974): 161–198.

28. Robert Koch, "Die Ätiologie der Milzbrandkrankheit, begründet auf die Entwicklungsgeschichte des Bacillus Antharacis," *Beiträge zur Biologie der Pflanzen* 2 (1876): 277–311, in Gaffky and Pfuhl, *Gesammelte Werke*, 6. Koch had not directed the results of his studies of the etiology of anthrax to a medical audience. He presented them, instead, as an elucidation of the life history of the organism that would be of primary interest to those who studied botany and classification, and he published them, accordingly, in a botanical journal.

29. Robert Koch, *Untersuchungen über die Aetiologie der Wundinfektionskrankheiten* (Leipzig: Georg Thieme, 1878); translation: Sir William Watson Cheyne, *Investigations into the Etiology of Traumatic Infective Diseases* (London: New Sydenham Society, 1880). Koch's studies of anthrax convinced him that bacteria neither could nor did undergo a radical transformation. In subsequent studies of wound infections and in a harsh critique of Carl von Nägeli's *Die niederen Pilze in ihren Beziehungen zu den Infektionskrankheiten und der Gesundheitspflege* (1877), he insisted that bacteria existed in specific types that could be sorted into distinct categories that differed sharply from one another. These categories were fixed; within them, organisms varied but little from the archetype. Robert Koch,

"Referat von Carl von Nägeli, *Die niederen Pilze in ihren Beziehungen zu den Infektionskrankheiten und der Gesundheitspflege*" (1878) in Gaffky and Pfuhl, *Gesammelte Werke*, 55. See also Carl von Nägeli, "Die Individualität in der Natur, mit vozüglicher Berucksichtigung der Planzenreiches," *Monatsschrift der Wissenschaftlisches Vereins* 2 (1856): 172–212. For discussion of Nägeli's views on bacterial species see Pauline M. Mazumdar, "Karl Landsteiner and the Problem of Species, 1838–1968 (Ph.D. diss., Johns Hopkins University, 1976), 15–37.

30. See, for example, Bryce, "Typhoid and Some Other Zymotic Diseases," 155–167; Peter H. Bryce, "Zymotic Diseases, Their Nature, Methods for Their Prevention and the Results Thereof, Address Delivered before the Hamilton Literary Association," in Ontario, Legislative Assembly, "Second Annual Report," 379–393.

31. Bryce, "Zymotic Diseases," 386.

32. For a contemporary discussion of these debates, see George Sternberg, "Bacterial Organisms," *Western Lancet* 11 (1882): 198–203. The text of an address to the State Medical Society of California (1882), this was one of a series of articles in which Sternberg discussed the links between bacteriology and the spontaneous-generation debate.

33. Formad, "The Bacillus Tuberculosis and the Etiology of Tuberculosis," 338; see also Formad, "The Bacillus Tuberculosis and Some Anatomical Points," 109–119.

34. Koch merely sketched this argument in the 1882 version of his paper. Koch "Aetiologie," Eichberg trans., 493. He developed the argument more fully in the 1884 version of that work. R. Koch, "Die Aetiologie der Tuberculose," *Mittheilungen aus dem Gesundheitsamt* 2 (1884): 1–88; translation: Stanley Boyd, "The Etiology of Tuberculosis," in Wm. Watson Cheyne, ed., *Recent Essays on Bacteria in Relation to Disease* (London: New Sydenham Society, 1886), 67–204, see especially 123, 134; hereafter referred to as Koch, "Aetiologie," Boyd trans.

35. Koch, "Aetiologie," Eichberg trans., 473.

36. "Discussion on Tuberculosis at the American Medical Association, 35th Annual Meeting, May 1884—Remarks of Dr. Formad," *Medical News* (Philadelphia) 44 (1884): 584–585. A series of articles that Sternberg wrote between 1882 and 1884 demonstrated that debates over the spontaneous generation of pathogenic microorganisms were still very much alive. See, for example, Sternberg, "Bacterial Organisms."

37. W. F. Peck, "Address of the Chairman of the Section on Surgery and Anatomy Read to the Meeting of the American Medical Association in June, 1883," *Journal of the American Medical Association (JAMA)* 1 (1883): 129.

38. John J. H. Hollister, "Address of the Chairman of the Section on Practice of Medicine, Materia Medica and Physiology to the Annual Meeting of the American Medical Association, June 6, 1883," *JAMA* 1 (1883): 67.

39. Ezra M. Hunt, "Hygiene and Its Scope, Its Progress and Its Leading Aims" (President's Address to the Eleventh Annual Meeting of the American Public Health Association), *Public Health* 9 (1883): 1–16.

40. Formad, "The Bacillus Tuberculosis and the Etiology of Tuberculosis," 338.

41. Prudden, "On the Occurrence," 400. In 1884, Sternberg developed the evolutionary and religious contexts of the debate. George Sternberg, "Disease Germs," *Public Health* 10 (1884): 69–70.

42. Prudden, "On the Occurrence," 398.

43. Henry Ingersoll Bowditch, *Is Consumption Contagious?* (Boston: Ticknor and Fields, 1864). The classic account of American opposition to contagionism remains Erwin Ackerknecht, "Anticontagionism between 1821 and 1867," *BHM* 22 (1948): 562–593. More recent discussions include Humphreys, *Yellow Fever and the South*; Charles Rosenberg, *The Cholera Years* (Chicago: University of Chicago Press, 1962); Phyllis Allen Richmond,

"American Attitudes toward the Germ Theory of Disease (1860–1880)," in Gert H. Brieger, ed., *Theory and Practice in American Medicine* (New York: Neale Watson, 1976), 58–84; Phyllis Allen Richmond, "Some Variant Theories in Opposition to the Germ Theory of Disease," *JHM* 9 (1954): 290–300; Nancy Tomes, "The Private Side of Public Health: Sanitary Science, Domestic Hygiene and the Germ Theory, 1870–1900," *BHM* 64 (1990): 509–539.

44. For representative articles, see W. H. Webb, "Is Phthisis Pulmonalis Contagious, and Does It Belong to the Zymotic Group?" *AJMS* 75 (1878): 434; Edgar Holden, "Is Consumption Contagious?" *AJMS* 76 (1878): 145–159. Holden suggested that clinicians whose primary interest was pulmonary diseases frequently supported the view that consumption was contagious, while "those, however eminent as scientific men, whose tastes led them to other departments of medical science, adopt the now most generally accepted doctrine of non-contagion." Some of Philadelphia's most eminent physicians, Drs. C. T. Williams, J. M. da Costa, and J. Solis-Cohen among them, supported Webb.

45. Even those who accepted contagionism and germs did not always accept Koch. The *AJMS* contained several articles on the contagiousness of tuberculosis but nonetheless paid little attention to Koch or his studies. J. Stewart, "Quarterly Report on the Progress of Medical Science," *Canada Lancet* 14 (1881–1882): 291–292; compare *AJMS* 83, 84 (1882) and 85, 86 (1883), and "The Etiology of Tuberculosis, by Robert Koch," *AJMS* 84 (1882): 243.

46. Formad, "The Bacillus Tuberculosis and Some Anatomical Points," 111.

47. Ibid.

48. Hunt, "Hygiene," 17.

49. Ibid., 16.

50. Koch, "Aetiologie," Boyd trans. The metaphor of seed and soil appears again and again in late-nineteenth- and early-twentieth-century writings on tuberculosis. For examples, see Hollister, "Address," 67; Bremer, "Bearing of the Discovery," 495; William Osler, *The Principles and Practice of Medicine*, 8th ed. (New York: Appleton and Company, 1912), 156–157.

51. Koch, "Aetiologie," Boyd trans., 199; Koch, "Kritische Besprechung," 137–141.

52. Formad, "The Bacillus Tuberculosis and the Etiology of Tuberculosis." See also "Discussion on Tuberculosis at the American Medical Association," 574–586. Further commentary on the diathesis is provided in J. Eskridge, "Pre-physical Sign Stage of Phthisis Pulmonalis," *Philadelphia Medical Times* 12:183–185; see also the "Discussion" that followed at the Philadelphia County Medical Society Meeting of October 26, 1881, *Philadelphia Medical Times* 12:183–185.

53. The response to his 1884 paper, though generally quicker, broader, and more favorable than to his 1882 paper, was still not fast. The first complete American translation of Koch's work did not appear until 1889. See Robert Koch, "The Etiology of Tuberculosis"; translation: Rev. F. Sause, *American Veterinary Review* 13 (1889): 54–112, 202–214.

54. "Proceedings of the Ohio Medical Society, June 1884," *CLC*, n.s., 12 (1884): 741.

55. B. F. Westbrook, "On the Aetiology of Pulmonary Phthisis," *Transactions of the American Climatological Association* 1 (1884): 5.

56. Bremer, "Bearing of the Discovery," 492.

57. "Discussion at 12th Annual Meeting of the American Public Health Association," *Public Health* 10 (1884): 431.

58. Donald Fleming describes Flint as "an enthusiastic 'bacterian' at a time when men of his age standing in America tended to be either skeptical or hostile." He writes, moreover, that "one morning in 1882 Flint came bounding up the stairs in Welch's house waving a newspaper and crying to the dazed Welch, still in bed sleeping off a late night in the dead house, 'I knew it, I knew it!' Koch's great discovery of the tubercle bacillus had been announced in the papers" Fleming, *William Welch*, 71–72. It remains more difficult to test Biggs's and Welch's early enthusiasm for Koch's bacillus since neither man published any papers on tuberculosis before 1887. Fleming, however, does suggest that Welch remained cautious. Like Prudden, Welch did not immediately accept Koch's findings but went off to Berlin to discover the truth for himself. Fleming, *William Welch*, chapter 5, especially 71–73.

59. Austin Flint, "On the Pathological and Practical Relations of the Doctrine of the Bacillus Tuberculosis," *Medical News* (Philadelphia) 44 (1884): 63.

60. Ibid., 62.

61. "Discussion at 12th Annual Meeting of the American Public Health Association," 429–431.

62. Trudeau, *Autobiography*, 182–186, especially 183.

63. E. L. Trudeau, "Environment in Its Relation to the Progress of Bacterial Invasion in Tuberculosis," *Transactions of the American Climatological Association* (1887): 31–136.

64. E. L. Trudeau, "An Environment Experiment Repeated," *Medical News* 53 (1888): 467.

65. Bremer, "Bearing of the Discovery," 496.

66. Discussion on Tuberculosis at the American Medical Association," 574.

67. Fleming, *William Welch*, 71–72.

68. "Koch on the Causation of Tuberculosis," *Philadelphia Medical Times* 14 (1884): 545.

69. Robert Koch, "Zur Untersuchungen von pathogenen Organismen," *Mittheilungen aus dem Kaiserlichen Gesundheitsamt* 1 (1881): 1–48; translation: Victor Horley, "On the Investigation of Pathogenic Organisms," in Wm. Watson Cheyne, ed., *Recent Essays by Various Authors on Bacteria in Relation to Disease* (London: New Sydenham Society, 1886), 3–64, quote on 3.

70. Formad, "The Bacillus Tuberculosis and the Etiology of Tuberculosis," 377.

71. Eric E. Sattler, "The Present Status of the Tubercle Bacillus Question," *CLC*, n.s., 12 (1884): 410.

72. Flint expressed these concerns in "On the Pathological and Practical Relations," 64; they are best expressed in Charles V. Chapin, "What Changes Has the Acceptance of the Germ Theory Made in Measures for the Prevention and Treatment of Consumption?" Fiske Fund Prize Dissertation 38 (Providence, R.I.: Fiske Fund, 1888).

73. A concise summary of various attempts made after 1882 to produce immunity to tuberculosis is presented in E. L. Trudeau, "An Experimental Study of Preventive Inoculation in Tuberculosis," *Medical Record* 38 (1890): 565; also, A. Calmette, C. Guérin, A. Boquet, and L. Nègre, *La vaccination préventive contre la tuberculose par le "BCG"* (Paris: Masson,1927), 13–58; A. Calmette, *L'infection bacillaire et la tuberculose chez l'homme et chez les animaux* (Paris: Masson, 1928).

74. Flint, "On the Pathological and Practical Relations," 64.

75. Bremer, "Bearing of the Discovery," 496.

76. S. Adolphus Knopf, "The Modern Prophylaxis of Pulmonary Tuberculosis and Its Treatment in Special Institutions and at Home," (Alvaregna Prize of the College of Physicians of Philadelphia, 1898), 42; manuscript copy at the College of Physicians of Philadelphia (CPP).

77. See, for example, William Osler, "The Registration of Pulmonary Tuberculosis," *Philadelphia Polyclinic* 3 (1894): 66.

78. Trudeau, "Environment," 131.

79. For a discussion of specificity and of the transformation that took place in American therapeutics, see John Harley Warner, *The Therapeutic Perspective* (Cambridge, Mass.: Harvard University Press, 1987), chapter 3.

80. Warner, *Therapeutic Perspective*.

81. Sattler, "Present Status," 415.

82. A general discussion of these tensions is provided in Lloyd Stevenson, "Science Down the Drain: On the Hostility of Certain Sanitarians to Animal Experimentation, Bacteriology and Immunology," *BHM* 29 (1955): 1–26. The American context is developed in Rosenberg, *Cholera Years;* Charles Rosenberg and Carol Smith Rosenberg, "Piety and Social Action: Some Origins of the American Public Health Movement," in Rosenberg, *No Other Gods*; Rosenkrantz, *Public Health and the State*; Regina Markell Morantz, "Feminism, Professionalism and Germs: The Thought of Mary Putnam Jacobi and Elizabeth Blackwell," *American Quarterly* 34 (1982): 459–478.

83. Hunt, "Hygiene," 14.

84. Heather MacDougall, "Public Health and the Sanitary Idea in Toronto, 1866–1890," in Wendy Mitchinson and Janice Dickin McGinnis, eds., *Essays in the History of Canadian Medicine* (Toronto: McClelland and Stewart, 1988), 62–87; Heather MacDougall, "Epidemics and the Environment: The Early Development of Public Health in Toronto, 1832–1872," in R. A. Jarrell and A. E. Roos, eds., *Critical Issues in the History of Canadian Technology, Society and Medicine/ Problèmes cruciaux dans l'histoire de la science, de la technologie et de la médicine canadiennes* (Toronto: Scientia Canadensis Press, 1983), 135–151; Heather MacDougall, "Public Health in Toronto's Municipal Politics: The Canniff Years, 1883–1890," *BHM* 55 (1981): 186–202; Neil Sutherland, "'To Create a Strong and Healthy Race': School Children in the Public Health Movement, 1880–1914," in S.E.D. Shortt, ed., *Medicine in Canadian Society: Historical Perspectives* (Montreal: McGill-Queen's, 1981), 361–393.

85. Bremer, "Bearing of the Discovery," 492. For further discussion of the debate between Virchow and Koch, see Georgiana D. Feldberg, "'An Antitoxin of Self Respect'": North American Debates over Vaccination against Tuberculosis, 1890–1960," (Ph.D. diss., Harvard University, 1989), chapter 1. See also Rudolph Ludwig Virchow, *Collected Essays on Public Health and Epidemiology,* ed. and foreword by L. J. Rather (New Delhi: Amerind, 1985).

86. "Proceedings of the Ohio Medical Society," 741.

87. "Koch on the Causation of Tuberculosis," *Philadelphia Medical Times* 14 (1884): 545.

88. Trudeau, "Environment Experiment Repeated," 467.

89. The best historical account of the sanatorium cure is provided in Bates, *Bargaining for Life.*

90. Examples include Channing Home, Cullis Consumptives' Home, and House of the Good Samaritan, all in Boston, and Home for Incurables and House of Rest for Consumptives, both in New York.

91. Examples include the Glockner Sanatorium, in Colorado Springs, Colorado, which began treatment of tuberculosis in 1880.

92. Bremer, "Bearing of the Discovery," 492.

93. Joseph Walsh, "Treatment of Tuberculosis at the White Haven Sanatorium of the Free Hospital for Poor Consumptives," Walsh Papers, vol. 1, *CPP.*

94. Karl Von Ruck, "The Cure of Pulmonary Tuberculosis upon the Principles of Nutrition," *Weekly Medical Review* 24 (1891): 367. See also William Osler, "Tuberculo-

sis," in Alfred Loomis, ed., *A System of Practical Medicine* (New York: Lea Brothers, 1897), 837.

95. Von Ruck, "Cure," 368.

96. E. L. Trudeau, "Artificial Immunity in Experimental Tuberculosis," *New York Medical Journal and Philadelphia Medical Journal Consolidated* 78 (1903): 105.

97. G. M. Smith, "Wasted Sunbeams: Unused Housetops," *Medical Record* 33 (1888): 429. After 1890, studies of the effects of sunlight on the tubercle bacillus became a subdiscipline, and by 1906 a bibliography of almost 100 articles on the subject existed. John Weinzirl, "The Action of Sunlight on Bacteria with Special Reference to *b. Tuberculosis*," *Public Health* 32 (1906): 128–153. A brief history of the use of sunlight to treat tuberculosis is provided in R. I. Harris, "Heliotherapy in Surgical Tuberculosis," *American Journal of Public Health (AJPH)* 16 (1926): 689–690; see also Foote, *Plain Home Talk.*

98. Smith, "Wasted Sunbeams," 429; See also S. Adolphus Knopf, "Sunlight and Solar-Therapy in Its Relation to Tuberculosis," *American Medicine* 14 (1908): 321–322.

99. Histories of immunology are provided in Arthur M. Silverstein, *A History of Immunology* (San Diego: Academic Press, 1989). See also William Bulloch, "History of Doctrines of Immunity," in Bulloch, *History*, 255–284; William Derek Foster, *A History of Medical Bacteriology and Immunology* (London: Heineman, 1970); Henry J. Parish, *History of Immunization* (Edinburgh: E. & S. Livingstone, 1965); Henry J. Parish, *Victory with Vaccines* (London: E. & S. Livingstone, 1968). A more recent study is Pauline Mazumdar, *Immunology 1930–1980: Essays on the History of Immunology* (Toronto: Wall and Thompson, 1989).

100. Rosenkrantz, *Public Health and the State*; Wade Oliver, *The Man Who Lived for Tomorrow: A Biography of William Hallock Park, M.D.* (New York: Dutton, 1941); Victoria Harden, *Inventing the NIH Federal Biomedical Research Policy, 1887–1937* (Baltimore: Johns Hopkins University Press, 1986); Jonathan Liebenau, *Medical Science and Medical Industry, 1890–1929: The Formation of the American Pharmaceutical Industry* (London: Basingstoke/Macmillan, 1987); Ralph Chester Williams, *The United States Public Health Service, 1798–1950* (Washington, D.C.: PHS, 1951), chapter 4; Donald Swain, "The Rise of a Research Empire: NIH, 1930–1950," *Science* 138 (1962): 1223–1237.

101. A discussion of the status of biomedical research in American universities during the 1870s and 1880s is provided in Kenneth M. Ludmerer, *Learning to Heal* (New York: Basic Books, 1985), chapter 2; also, Philip J. Pauly, "The Appearance of Academic Biology in Late Nineteenth Century America," *Journal of the History of Biology* 17 (1984): 369–397.

102. Liebenau, *Medical Science*; John T. Mahoney, *The Merchants of Life. An Account of the American Pharmaceutical Industry* (New York: Harper & Row, 1959).

103. For further explanation, see United States Department of Agriculture (USDA), *Annual Report* (1881–1882), 290–295; D. E. Salmon and T. Smith, "On a New Method of Producing Immunity from Contagious Diseases," *Proceedings of the Biological Society of Washington* 3 (1886): 29–33; D. E. Salmon and T. Smith, "Experiments on the Production of Immunity by the Hypodermic Injection of Sterilized Cultures," *Transactions of the International Medical Congress* (9th session, 1887), 403–407.

104. Trudeau, "Experimental Study," 568.

105. Robert Koch, "An Address on Bacteriologic Research Delivered before the International Medical Congress Held in Berlin, August 1890," *British Medical Journal (BMJ)* (1890): 383; see also Robert Koch, "Ueber bakteriologische Forschung," *Verhandlungen der X internationalen medizinische Kongress*, vol. 1 (Berlin, 1890), 35–47.

106. Robert Koch, "Weitere Mittheilungen über ein Heilmittel gegen Tuberkulose," *DMW* 46 (1890): 1029–1032; Robert Koch, "Weitere Mittheilungen über das Tuber-

kulin," *DMW* 17 (1891): 1189–1192; R. Koch, "Fortzetzug der Mittheilungen über ein Heilmittel gegen Tuberkulose," *DMW* 17 (1891): 101.

107. Koch referred to his lymph as a *heilmittel*, which was translated into English as either remedy or cure.

108. Robert Koch, "A Further Communication on a Remedy for Tuberculosis, Translated from the Original Article Published in the *Deutsche Medizinische Wochenschrif,*" *BMJ* (November 22, 1890): 1193–1195.

109. *New York Times* (November 16, 1890). A detailed and more complete discussion of popular reactions to tuberculin is provided in David Liebowitz, "Scientific Failure in an Age of Optimism: Public Reaction to Robert Koch's Tuberculin Cure," *New York State Journal of Medicine* 93 (January 1993): 41–48.

110. The *Index Medicus* for 1891 lists over fifty articles on Koch's tuberculin and cites reports of trials conducted in small and large towns throughout the United States.

111. H. D. Geddings, "Official Experiments with Tuberculin," in U.S. Department of the Treasury, *Annual Report of the Supervising Surgeon General* (1891), 63.

112. University of Pennsylvania, Veterinary Department, "Koch's Tuberculin: Report of the Tuberculosis Commission," *American Veterinary Review* 15 (1891): 431–436.

113. For further discussion of the debate between Koch and Pasteur, see H. H. Mollaret, "Contribution à la connaissance des relations entre Koch et Pasteur," *NTM: Schriftenreihe für Geschichte der Naturwissenschaften, Technik, und Medizin* 20 (1983): 57–66.

114. Koch, "An Address on Bacteriologic Research," 380.

115. Ibid., 382.

116. Bulloch, *History*; Silverstein, *History of Immunology*; Parish, *History of Immunization*.

117. Two competing explanations for the action of tuberculin emerged. One suggested that it created an environment hostile to the growth of tubercle bacilli by destroying or causing necrosis of tissues; the alternative school proposed that tuberculin nourished the tissues, thereby rendering them impervious to bacilli. For a discussion, see S. K. Jackson, "Tuberculin, Its Value as a Scientific Discovery Apart from Its Therapeutic Importance; Together with a Consideration of the Most Rational Mode of Employing the Principle Involved in It," *JAMA* 16 (1891): 806–809.

118. Rudolph Virchow, "Remarks on the Effect of Koch's Remedy on the Internal Organs of Tuberculous Patients," *BMJ* (1891): 129.

119. John Syer Bristowe, "An Address on the Koch Method of Treatment for Tuberculosis," *BMJ* (1891): 895.

120. Ibid., 894.

121. Ibid.

122. Sir Joseph Lister, "Professor Koch's Remedy for Tuberculosis," *BMJ* (1890): 1373.

123. Ibid.

124. "The Koch Treatment," *Canada Medical Record* 19 (1891): 95–96.

125. "Inoculative Treatment of Tuberculosis," *Canada Lancet* 23 (1890): 221.

126. G. T. Ross, "Berlin Letter," *Canada Medical Record* 19 (1891): 82–84, 101–104.

127. "The Koch Treatment," 110.

128. Paul Gibier, "Dr. Koch's Discovery," *North American Review* 151 (1890): 726–731.

129. For fuller discussion, see Liebowitz, "Scientific Failure."

130. Geddings, "Official Experiments," 80.

131. University of Pennsylvania, "Koch's Tuberculin," 436.

132. Joseph W. Stickler, "Some Achievements of Koch's 'Lymph,'" *New York Medical Journal* 53 (1891): 98–104.

133. Joseph W. Stickler, "What Is the Truth about Tuberculin?" *New York Medical Journal* 56 (1892): 465; see also Knopf, "Modern Prophylaxis."

134. R. O. Beard, "The Nature Treatment of Tuberculosis," *Public Health* 25 (1899): 249.

135. Parish, *Victory with Vaccines*, 31. See also Archer Cochrane, *A Guide to the Use of Tuberculin* (New York: William Wood, 1915), 9–10; F. M. Pottenger, "A Study of Tuberculin and Allied Products with Reference to Their Action and the Proper Method of Their Administration," *Therapeutic Gazette* 27 (1903): 12–19.

136. Karl Von Ruck, "The Truth about Tuberculin," *Virginia Medical Monthly* 18 (1891–1892): 466–467.

137. Pottenger, "Study of Tuberculin," 12–19.

138. F. M. Pottenger, *Tuberculin in Diagnosis and Treatment* (St. Louis: C. Moseby, 1913), especially chapter 6.

139. Karl Von Ruck, "A Practical Method of Prophlyactic Immunization against Tuberculosis with Special Reference to Its Application in Children" (Report from the Von Ruck Research Laboratory for Tuberculosis 1, June 1, 1912, Asheville, North Carolina), NA RG 90-0425-32, Box 64.

140. W. L. Dunn, "The Dangers of the Present Tuberculin Era," *Transactions of the American Climatological Association* 25 (1909): 272–283.

141. Numerous such requests are included in the general correspondence files of the PHS. NA RG 90-0425-32, Box 64.

142. A. M. Stimson to K. Von Ruck, October 1911, NA RG 90-0425-32, Box 64.

143. Karl Von Ruck, "A Practical Method of Prophylactic Immunization against Tuberculosis, a Preliminary Announcement," *JAMA* 58 (1912): 1504; Karl Von Ruck, "A Practical Method of Prophylactic Immunization against Tuberculosis with Special Reference to Its Application in Children," *Medical Record* 82 (1912): 369.

144. U.S. Congress, Senate, *Treatment of Tuberculosis: Letter from the Secretary of the Treasury Transmitting in Response to a Senate Resolution of May 26, 1913 a Report by the USPHS of the Investigation of the Methods and Practices Employed by Doctors Karl and Silvio Von Ruck in Treating Tuberculosis and Rendering Persons Immune from Tuberculosis.* 63rd Cong., 3rd sess., 1914, S. Doc. 641, 6–10. NA RG 90-0425-32, Box 64.

145. U.S. Congress, *Treatment of Tuberculosis*, 26.

146. The debate over the Von Ruck treatment continued until 1916, as letters in support of tuberculin and against it were exchanged. See, for example, "Remarks of the Honorable Luke Lea, of Tennessee, in the Senate of the United States, Friday, September 8, 1916," NA RG 90-0425-32, Box 64.

147. Karl Von Ruck and Silvio Von Ruck, *Studies in Immunization against Tuberculosis* (New York: Paul Hoeber, 1916).

148. S. Adolphus Knopf, "The Tuberculosis Problem in the United States," *North American Review of Reviews* 174 (1902): 380.

149. Karl Von Ruck, "Should Tuberculin Be Administered in Private Practice?" *Medical News* 60 (1892): 340.

150. Knopf, "Modern Prophylaxis," 125; see also James T. Whittaker, "General Impressions from Six Years Use of the O.T.," *JAMA* 29 (1897): 951–954; Joshua Lindley Barton, "The Scientific Treatment of Tuberculosis," *Medical Record* 52 (1897): 376–379; E. L. Trudeau, "The Therapeutic Use of Tuberculin Combined with Sanitarium Treatment of Tuberculosis," *AJMS* 132 (1906): 175–186.

151. National Association for the Study and Prevention of Tuberculosis (NASPT), *Tuberculosis Directory* (New York, 1911), 237.

152. White Haven Sanatorium, Committee on Problems, "Minutes of the Third Meeting, July 7, 1909," Walsh Papers, vol. 2.

153. Von Ruck, "Should Tuberculin Be Administered in Private Practice?" 344.

154. Knopf, "Modern Prophylaxis," 127.

155. Ibid., 132.

156. E. L. Trudeau, "Observations in Adirondack Cottage Hospital on the Use of Koch's Tuberculin in the Treatment of Pulmonary Tuberculosis," *Transactions of the New York Academy of Medicine* 8 (1892): 165. See also E. L. Trudeau, "Results of the Employment of Tuberculin and Its Modifications at the Adirondack Cottage Sanitarium," *Medical News* 61 (1892): 299.

157. Trudeau, "Results of the Employment," 300.

158. Ibid.

159. E. L. Trudeau and E. R. Baldwin, "A Chemical and Experimental Research on 'Antiphthisin' (Klebs)," *Medical Record* 25 (1895): 871–874; E. L. Trudeau and E. R. Baldwin, "The Need of an Improved Technic in the Manufacture of Koch's T.R. Tuberculin," *Medical News* 71 (1897): 257–258.

160. E. L. Trudeau and E. R. Baldwin, "Experimental Studies on the Preparation and Effects of Antitoxins for Tuberculosis," *AJMS* 116 (1898): 692–707, quote on 693; "Experimental Studies on the Preparation and Effects of Antitoxins for Tuberculosis, Part II," *AJMS* 117 (1899): 56–77.

161. Vincent Y. Bowditch to E. R. Baldwin, December 18, 1905; H. D. Pease to E. R. Baldwin, November 8, 1907, and July 28, 1908; Herbert Mason King to E. R. Baldwin, July 11, 1905, December 13, 1905, and December 22, 1906; Charles D. Parfitt to E. R. Baldwin, March 25, 1903, and March 31, 1903; all in Baldwin Papers, National Library of Medicine, Washington, D.C.

162. Bowditch to Baldwin, December 18, 1905, Baldwin papers.

163. King to Baldwin, December 13, 1905, Baldwin Papers; Parfitt to Baldwin, March 25, 1903, Baldwin Papers.

164. E. L. Trudeau, "The Tuberculin Test in Incipient and Suspected Pulmonary Tuberculosis," *Medical News* 70 (1897): 687.

165. R. Koch to E. R. Baldwin, April 1902, Baldwin Papers.

166. H. K. Mulford to E. R. Baldwin, January 14, 1908, Baldwin Papers.

167. Mulford to Baldwin, January 21, 1908, Baldwin Papers.

168. Mulford to Baldwin, January 14, 1908, Baldwin Papers.

169. See, for example, F. E. Stewart, director of the Scientific Department at H. K. Mulford, to Baldwin, February 28, 1908, and Mulford to Baldwin, December 17, 1910, Baldwin Papers.

170. Stewart to Baldwin, November 16, 1910, Baldwin Papers.

171. E. L. Corman to E. R. Baldwin, June 28, 1908, Baldwin Papers.

172. For example, Secretary of the AMA Council on Pharmacy to E. R. Baldwin, January 30, 1912, Baldwin Papers. The letter said: "The Council has under consideration Tuberculin Rosenbach, manufactured by Kalle and Co. and the Council is debating whether or not the product should be accepted for New and Unofficial Remedies. Have you any experience with it?"

173. John F. Anderson, director, Hygienic Laboratory, PHS, to E. R. Baldwin, September 27, 1910, December 30, 1911, and January 4, 1912, Baldwin Papers.

174. D. G. Campbell to E. R. Baldwin, February 12, 1908, Baldwin Papers.

175. Correspondence between W. A. Griffin, superintendent, Sharon Sanatorium, and E. R. Baldwin, September 1905–August 1923; E. R. Baldwin to Horton Casparis, October 14, 1922, Baldwin Papers.

176. Salmon and Smith, "On a New Method," 33. By 1895, Smith had recognized the importance of antitoxic studies to the control of human disease. As pathologist to the Massachusetts State Board of Health, he investigated the therapeutic and preven-

tive uses of diphtheria antitoxin. William Hallock Park of the New York City Department of Health similarly endorsed antitoxic immunity and diphtheria antitoxin. Smith published numerous papers on diphtheria antitoxin; representative early papers include Theobald Smith, "Antitoxic and Microbicide Powers of the Blood Serum after Immunization with Special Reference to Diphtheria," *Albany Medical Annals* 16 (1895): 175–189; Theobald Smith, "The Production of Diphtheria Antitoxin," *Journal of the Association of Engineering Societies* 16 (1896): 83–92; Theobald Smith, "The Conditions Which Influence the Appearance of Toxin in Cultures of the Diphtheria Bacillus," *Transactions of the Association of American Physicians* 11 (1896): 37–61; T. Smith, "The Toxin of Diphtheria and Its Antitoxin," *BMSJ* 139 (1898): 157–160; 192–194.

177. Liebenau, *Medical Science*; Oliver, *Man Who Lived for Tomorrow*.

178. E. L. Trudeau and E. R. Baldwin, "A Résumé of Experimental Studies on the Preparation and Effects of Antitoxic Serum in Tuberculosis," *Transactions of the Association of American Physicians* 13 (1898): 111.

179. Ibid., 121; see also Trudeau and Baldwin, "Experimental Studies," and "Experimental Studies II."

180. Von Ruck, "Should Tuberculin Be Administered in Private Practice?" 344.

181. Paul J. Quirk, "Food and Drug Administration," in James Q. Wilson, ed., *The Politics of Regulation* (New York: Basic Books, 1980), 194.

182. Liebenau, *Medical Science*, especially chapter 6.

183. U.S. Congress, 57th Cong., 1st sess., chap. 1378: "An Act to regulate the sale of viruses, serums, toxins and analogous products in the District of Columbia, to regulate interstate traffic in said articles, and for other purposes," 728–729.

184. See *U.S. v. E. C. Knight*, 151 U.S. 1 (1895); *Champion v. Ames*, 188 U.S. 321 (1903). See also Robert McCloskey, *The American Supreme Court* (Chicago: University of Chicago Press, 1960), chapters 5 and 6; for an analysis of the more general intellectual context, see Duncan Kennedy, "Toward an Historical Understanding of Legal Consciousness: The Case of Classical Legal Thought in America, 1850–1940," *Research in Law and Sociology* 3 (1980): 3–24.

185. Koch, "An Address on Bacteriologic Research," 383.

186. Koch, "Further Communication," 1194.

187. Cochrane, *A Guide*, 9–10; Pottenger, "Study of Tuberculin," 12–19.

188. Jackson, "Tuberculin, Its Value," 809; Trudeau, "Observations," 165.

189. Frank Fremont Smith, "The Value of Koch's Remedy Employed as an Alterative—Reactive Fever Prevented," *Transactions of the American Climatological Association* 8 (1891): 222.

190. Ibid.

191. Karl Von Ruck, "The Treatment of Tuberculosis Apart from Climate," *Times and Register* (Philadelphia) (1893): 5; see also Von Ruck, "Cure," and Jackson, "Tuberculin, Its Value," 806–809.

192. Von Ruck, "Cure," 369.

193. Trudeau, "Artificial Immunity," 105; Trudeau, "Therapeutic Use," 175–186; E. L. Trudeau, "Tuberculin Immunization in the Treatment of Pulmonary Tuberculosis," *AJMS* 133 (1907): 813–829, especially 827–829.

194. W. L. Dunn, "The Dangers of the Present Tuberculin Era," *Transactions of the American Climatological Association* 25 (1909): 273.

195. Koch, "Further Communication," 1195.

196. Von Ruck, "Should Tuberculin Be Administered in Private Practice?" 342; see also K. Von Ruck, "A Contribution to the Clinical Uses of Professor Koch's Remedy for Tuberculosis," *Medical Record* 39 (1891): 592.

197. Trudeau, "Observations," 166–167.

198. Trudeau, "Therapeutic Use," 186.
199. Allen K. Krause, *Rest and Other Things* (Baltimore: Williams & Wilkins, 1923), 11.
200. Ibid., 17–18.
201. Ibid., 17.
202. Koch, "Aetiologie," Eichberg trans., 439.

CHAPTER 3: SPIT AND POLISH

1. "With a State Sanatorium Secured, What Next?" (symposium), *Transactions of the National Tuberculosis Association (Trans. NTA)* 4 (1908): 29.
2. E. L. Trudeau, "The Tuberculin Test in Incipient and Suspected Pulmonary Tuberculosis," *Medical News* 70 (1897): 687–689.
3. See, for example, Luther Emmett Holt, "A Report on One Thousand Tuberculin Tests in Young Children," *Proceedings of the Sixth International Congress on Tuberculosis* 2 (1908): 551–559; Henry Heiman, "Clinical Observations on the Von Pirquet Reaction in Children," *Proceedings of the Sixth International Congress on Tuberculosis* 2 (1908): 569–577; H. D. Chapin and T. H. Coffin, "Recent Tests in the Diagnosis of Tuberculosis in Children at the New York Post-Graduate Medical School and Hospital," *Proceedings of the Sixth International Congress on Tuberculosis* 2 (1908): 578–580; Louis Fischer, "An Aid to the Diagnosis of Tuberculosis in Infancy and Childhood by means of the Cutaneous Inoculation of Diluted Tuberculin of Pure Tuberculin (Pirquet Method)," *Proceedings of the Sixth International Congress on Tuberculosis* 2 (1908): 581–587. Von Pirquet himself had determined that 70 percent of otherwise healthy children reacted positively to tuberculin. C. Von Pirquet, "Erfahrungen über die kutane Tuberkulinreaktion an 2000 obduzierten Kindern," *Proceedings of the Sixth International Congress on Tuberculosis* 2 (1908): 458–476; C. Von Pirquet, "The Frequency of Tuberculosis in Children," *Proceedings of the Sixth International Congress on Tuberculosis* 2 (1908): 559–567. See also J. A. Myers, "Exterminating Tuberculosis," *Journal of the National Education Association* 12 (1923): 50.
4. Clarence A. Lucas, *TB and Diseases Caused by Immoral and Intemperate Habits* (Indianapolis: Bookwalter-Ball, 1920), 49.
5. Allen K. Krause, *Rest and Other Things* (Baltimore: Williams & Wilkins, 1923), 87.
6. Lucas, *TB and Diseases*, 49.
7. Nancy Tomes, "The Private Side of Public Health: Sanitary Science, Domestic Hygiene and the Germ Theory, 1870–1900," *BHM* 64 (1990): 509–539.
8. Judith Walzer Leavitt, *The Healthiest City: Milwaukee and the Politics of Health Reform* (Princeton, N.J.: Princeton University Press, 1982); Barbara G. Rosenkrantz, *Public Health and the State;* Margaret Humphreys, *Yellow Fever and the South* (New Brunswick N.J.: Rutgers University Press, 1992).
9. Rothman, *Living in the Shadow*, 188.
10. Ibid., 187.
11. Krause, *Rest and Other Things*, 100.
12. For discussions of the states' police powers and public health, see Steven M. Fleisher, "The Law of Basic Public Health Activities: Police Power and Constitutional Limitations," in Ruth Roemer and George McKray, eds., *Legal Aspects of Health Policy* (Westport, Conn.: Greenwood Press, 1980), 5–32; Milton I. Roemer, "Government's Role in American Medicine: A Brief Historical Survey," in Chester R. Burns, ed., *Legacies in Law and Medicine* (New York: Science History Publications, 1977), 183–205; Moris Kagan, "Federal Public Health: A Reflection of the Changing Constitution," in Burns, *Legacies*, 206–229. A contemporary discussion of the ways in which the police powers

applied to control of tuberculosis is found in James A. Tobey, *A Manual of Tuberculosis Legislation* (New York: NTA, 1928).

For discussions of opposition to quarantine and registration, see Erwin H. Ackerknecht, "Anticontagionism between 1821 and 1867," *BHM*, 22 (1948): 562–593; Warner, *Government, Medicine and Society*; John Blake, "The Inoculation Controversy in Boston," *New England Quarterly* 25 (1952): 489–506; Martin Kaufman, "The American Anti-vaccinationists and Their Arguments." *BHM* 41 (1967): 463–478; Leavitt, *Healthiest City*; Rosenkrantz, *Public Health and the State*.

13. William Osler, "The Registration of Pulmonary Tuberculosis," *Philadelphia Polyclinic* 3 (1894): 66. See also Hermann M. Biggs, "The Administrative Control of Tuberculosis," *First Annual Report of the Henry Phipps Institute* (1905), 170–171. For an extended discussion of the debate over reporting, see Daniel Fox, "Social Policy and City Politics: Tuberculosis Reporting in New York City, 1889–1900." *BHM* 49 (1975): 169–195.

14. Quoted in Biggs, "Administrative Control," 171.

15. Tuberculosis did not become reportable in Albany until 1907; Buffalo declared tuberculosis reportable in 1902, Rochester in 1900, and Syracuse in 1908. Similarly, in Massachusetts Boston made tuberculosis reportable in 1900, Fall River in 1906, and Lowell in 1903. The State of Massachustetts did not make tuberculosis reportable until 1907. See NASPT, *Tuberculosis Directory* (1911), especially 231–243; Rosenkrantz, *Public Health and the State*; New York City, Department of Health, *Annual Report* (1925), 44.

16. George Jasper Wherrett, *The Miracle of the Empty Beds: A History of Tuberculosis in Canada* (Toronto: University of Toronto Press, 1977), 201.

17. Quoted in Tobey, *Manual of Tuberculosis Legislation*, 8, 12.

18. New York City, Department of Health, *Annual Report* (1925), 44.

19. New York City, Department of Health, *Contagious Consumption: Rules to Be Observed for the Prevention and Spread of Consumption*, (1889).

20. See Luther Emmett Holt, *Food and Growth: A Discussion of the Nutrition of Children* (New York: Macmillan, 1922), 22; see also H. E. Kleinschmidt, "Publicity Campaign of National Scope," *AJPH* 18 (1928): 1369–1374.

21. Charles V. Chapin, "State Control of Tuberculosis," Fiske Fund Prize Dissertation 44 (Providence, R.I.: Fiske Fund, 1900), 25; see also Lawrence Flick, "Report of the Committee on Tuberculosis," *Public Health* 30 (1905): 106–112; Marshall I. Price, "Supplemental Report of the Committee on Tuberculosis," *Public Health* 30 (1905): 113–121; NASPT, *Tuberculosis Directory* (1911) 218–256.

22. E. L. Trudeau, "Address of the President to the First Annual Meeting of the National Association for the Study and Prevention of Tuberculosis," *Transactions of the National Association for the Study and Prevention of Tuberculosis (Trans. NASPT)* 1 (1906): 15.

23. Ibid.

24. Karl Von Ruck, "The Prophylaxis of Tuberculosis," *Therapeutic Gazette* 14 (1890): 221–222.

25. Leavitt, *Healthiest City;* see also Naomi Rogers, *Dirt and Disease: Polio before FDR* (New Brunswick, N.J.: Rutgers University Press, 1992).

26. "An Act defining the powers and duties of local health officers and boards of health in the matter of the protection of the people of the State of New York from the disease known as tuberculosis" sect. 326 (May 19, 1908), cited in NASPT, *Tuberculosis Directory* (1911).

27. Quote from a 1906 South Bend, Indiana, ordinance cited in NASPT, *Tuberculosis Directory* (1911), 226.

28. New York City, *Sanitary Code* (1898), quoted in ibid., 242.

29. Rogers, *Dirt and Disease*; also, Leavitt, *Healthiest City*. Physicians frequently de-

bated the merits of legislation that attempted to control spitting and thereby limit infection. For examples, see Lawrence Flick, "Report of the Committee on Tuberculosis," *Public Health* 30 (1905): 106–121; Lawrence Flick, "Present Status of the Tuberculosis Campaign and the Essentials for Thorough and Prompt Success," reprint from *New York Medical Journal* 85 (1910), in Flick Pamphlets, CPP; Wm. Charles White, "The Official Responsibility of the State in the Tuberculosis Problem," *Trans. NTA* 11 (1915): 273.

30. "An Act defining. . . ." San Francisco, Minneapolis, and other municipalities similarly presented spitting as a nuisance. See People of the City and County of San Francisco, Bill 1112, Ordinance 975, "Providing methods for the prevention of the spread of tuberculosis," Sect. 7 (December 6, 1909); City Council of Minneapolis, "An Ordinance relating to the preservation of health and the prevention and suppression of disease in the city of Minneapolis," Sect. 7 (August 26, 1905)—all cited in NASPT, *Tuberculosis Directory* (1911).

31. General Assembly of Virginia, "An Act prohibiting expectorating or spitting in public places . . . " (March 17, 1906), cited in NASPT, *Tuberculosis Directory* (1911).

32. NASPT, *Tuberculosis Directory* (1911), 232.

33. Krause, *Rest and Other Things*, 86.

34. Lawrason Brown, *Rules for Recovery from Pulmonary Tuberculosis* (Philadelphia: Lea and Fabiger, 1917), 8.

35. New York City, Department of Health *Contagious Consumption* (1889); compare "Circular Issued by the New York City Department of Health," in *A Handbook on the Prevention of Tuberculosis* (New York: Charity Organization Society, 1903) and Joseph Walsh "Circular of Information Regarding Pulmonary TB or Consumption for the NASPT" (1904) *Walsh Papers* Vol 3: 59.

36. NASPT, *Tuberculosis Directory* (1911), 226.

37. Ibid., 274–275.

38. Ibid., 218, 227, 235.

39. Calculated from data provided in ibid., 217–256.

40. Wiebe, *Search for Order*, 149. See also Michael B. Katz, *In the Shadow of the Poor House: A Social History of Welfare in America* (New York: Basic Books, 1986). Classic discussions of the ways in which the desire to create self-reliance shaped American attempts to relieve poverty are provided in Robert H. Bremner, *From the Depths: The Discovery of Poverty in the United States* (New York: New York University Press, 1956); Paul Boyer, *Urban Masses and Moral Order in America* (Cambridge, Mass.: Harvard University Press, 1978); Hace Tishler, *Self Reliance and Social Security, 1870–1917* (New York: Kennikat Press, 1971); and James T. Patterson, *America's Struggle against Poverty* (Cambridge, Mass.: Harvard University Press, 1981).

41. S. Adolphus Knopf, "The Tuberculosis Problem in the United States," *North American Review of Reviews* 1 (1902): 170–171.

42. Krause, *Rest and Other Things*, 87.

43. Ibid., 101.

44. Ibid. Here, Krause sounded much like Hunter, who in his 1904 work *Poverty* spoke of the need to "increase incentive by more nearly equalizing opportunity." Robert Hunter, *Poverty* (New York, 1904), quoted in Richard Hofstadter, *The Progressive Movement, 1900–1915* (Englewood Cliffs, N.J.: Prentice-Hall, 1963), 58.

45. B. J. Lloyd, "Centralized Control of Tuberculosis through the United States Public Health Service," *Trans. NTA* 15 (1919): 337–339; see also Eugene R. Kelley, "Centralized Control of Tuberculosis by State Commissions or Divisions of Tuberculosis," *Trans. NTA* 15 (1919): 340–342; Gordon Dickinson, "Centralized Control of Tuberculosis by Divisions of Tuberculosis in County or City Boards of Health," *Trans.*

NTA 15 (1919): 343–344; "Discussion of Papers by Dr. Lloyd, Dr. Kelley, and Dr. Dickinson," *Trans. NTA* 15 (1919): 344–363.

46. See Bates, *Bargaining for Life;* Rothman, *Living in the Shadow.* Classic discussions of asylums and other correctional institutions are provided in David J. Rothman, *The Discovery of the Asylum* (Boston: Little, Brown, 1971), especially xiii–xiv; David J. Rothman, *Conscience and Convenience: The Asylum and Its Alternatives in Progressive America* (Boston: Little, Brown, 1980); Nancy Tomes, *A Generous Confidence: Thomas Story Kirkbride and the Art of Asylum-Keeping* (Cambridge and New York: Cambridge University Press, 1984). See also Bremner, *From the Depths,* 18.

47. William H. Ross, "Teaching and Control of the Tuberculosis Patient," *Texas State Journal of Medicine* 21 (1925–1926): 472.

48. Quoted in Julius Wilson, "'Daily Sanatorium Routine Was the Treatment,'" *American Lung Association Bulletin* (March 1982), 8.

49. Allen K. Krause, "Antituberculosis Measures," in Krause, *Rest and Other Things,* 77; Wilson, "Daily Sanatorium Routine," 8.

50. Wilson, "Daily Sanatorium Routine," 8; see also 7–10.

51. Joseph Walsh, "Treatment of Tuberculosis at the White Haven Sanatorium of the Free Hospital for Poor Consumptives," Walsh Papers, vol. 1.

52. A fuller account of Flick's efforts is provided in Feldberg, "'An Antitoxin.'" His work also forms the subject of Bates, *Bargaining for Life,* which provides a rich analysis of Flick's achievements.

53. Quoted in Walsh, "Treatment," [2].

54. "Minutes of the Annual Meeting of the Medical Administrative Council of White Haven, October 26, 1910," Walsh Papers, vol. 1, item 4; see also "Rules of the Free Hospital for Poor Consumptives and the White Haven Sanatorium Association," Walsh Papers, vol. 1, item 5.

55. "Rules of the Free Hospital for Poor Consumptives."

56. See J. Dickin McGinnis, "The White Plague in Calgary: Sanatorium Care in Southern Alberta," *Alberta History* 28 (1980): 1–15; H. E. MacDermott, *A Short History of the Royal Edward Institution* (Montreal: Royal Edward Chest Hospital, 1965); Marjorie Freeman Campbell, *Holbrook of the San* (Toronto: Ryerson Press, 1953); Godfrey Gale, *The Changing Years: The Toronto Hospital and the Fight against Tuberculosis* (Toronto: West Park Hospital, 1979). Apparent differences in the intentions and activities of American and Canadian sanatoria may be more historiographic than real. Studies of the London Sanatorium suggest that the classic works, cited above, unduly emphasized the medical and therapeutic functions of Canadian sanatoria; compare J. J. Connor, "Prescribed Reading: Patients' Libraries in North American Tuberculosis Institutions," *Libraries and Culture* 27 (1992): 252–278; and J.T.H. Connor, *A Heritage of Healing: The London Health Association and Its Hospitals* (London, Ontario: University Hospitals, 1990).

57. See, for example, "Rules of the Free Hospital for Poor Consumptives" and "Card of Instructions for Patients," Walsh Papers, vol. 1, 652.

58. "Minutes of the Annual Meeting of the White Haven Staff, May 23, 1907," Walsh Papers, vol. 1, item 4.

59. Lawrence Flick, "General Letter Regarding the Admission of Patients to White Haven, March 27, 1908," Walsh Papers, vol. 1, 328.

60. "Memo from the Free Hospital for Poor Consumptives, March 28, 1905," Walsh Papers, vol. 1, 117. See also Flick, "General Letter"; "Minutes of the Meeting of the Medical Administrative Council, October 26, 1910," Walsh Papers, vol. 1, 333.

61. "Training School Graduation," *Philadelphia North American* (February 11, 1906), in Walsh Papers, vol. 1.

62. "Dr. Flick on the Value of Cured Consumptives as Nurses," *Philadelphia North*

American (February 11, 1906), "First Class of Tuberculosis Nurses Ever Graduated," *Philadelphia North American* (February 11, 1906), in Vol. 1.

63. Flick, "General Letter"; "Minutes of the Meeting of the Medical Administrative Council."

64. See "Rules of the Free Hospital for Poor Consumptives" and "Card of Instructions for Patients."

65. For examples of legislation, see NASPT, *Tuberculosis Directory* (1911). Debate about the advisability of employing consumptives or allowing them to marry took place often and at many levels, as individual physicians, medical and public health organizations, governmental agencies, and voluntary agencies pondered the legislative control of TB. For examples, see Paul Paquin, "Should the Marriage of Consumptives Be Discouraged?" *Public Health* 20 (1894): 144–165; S. Adolphus Knopf, "Some Newer Problems and Some Newer Phases of the Anti-tuberculosis Problem in the U.S.," *Medical Record* (February 1, 1913); CPP, "Minutes of the Meetings of the Section on Public Health and Industrial Medicine," 1924–1937, CPP; J. H. Landis, "The Control of Tuberculosis," reprint from *CLC* 43 (1913) in Flick Pamphlets, CPP. The debate about whether consumptives should marry also became part of the broader eugenic appeal for child welfare; see George M. Korber, "The Child and the Home," *Trans. NTA* 11 (1915): 41–47, especially 46–47.

66. See, for example, "Letter from Dr. Lewis H. Taylor to Dr. Joseph Walsh re Miss MacFarlane," Walsh Papers, vol. 1, 111; "Case of Miss Ewing, a Nurse at White Haven Asked to Resign Because of an Indiscretion, June 10, 1908," Walsh Papers, vol. 1, 390; Wm. G. Townsend to Dr. Walsh, June 10, 1908, Walsh Papers, vol. 1, 390; "Concerned Patient to Dr. Walsh, July 8, 1908," Walsh Papers, vol. 1, 415.

67. Earlier versions of this argument were presented in Feldberg, " 'An Antitoxin,' " 105–109; Georgina Feldberg, "Bacteriology and the Dilemmas of Caring for Consumptives" (paper presented to the Canadian Society for the History of Medicine, Annual Meeting, Victoria, B.C., May 25, 1990); Georgina Feldberg, "Now You See 'Em, Now You Don't: The Gender Dynamics of Biomedical Research" (paper presented to the History of Science Society, Annual Meeting, Madison, Wis., November 1991). Again, further discussion of tuberculosis nursing can be found in Bates, *Bargaining for Life*.

68. "Circulars of Information, Special Course in the Nursing of Tuberculosis" Walsh Papers, vol. 2.

69. "Flyer, October 3, 1904," Walsh Papers, vol. 2.

70. "Exam for First Year Class, May 11, 1910," Walsh Papers, vol. 2.

71. Joseph Walsh, "Circular of Information Regarding Pulmonary TB or Consumption for Distribution in Philadelphia," 1906, Walsh Papers, vol. 3, 59.

72. See "Training School for Nurses," undated, Walsh Papers, vol. 1, item 6; "Dr. Flick on the Value of Cured Consumptives as Nurses." Comments from the staff of White Haven on nurses who failed to follow rules are referred to in note 66 above.

73. Letter to Joseph Walsh, July 8, 1908, Walsh Papers, vol. 1, 415.

74. "Rules of the Free Hospital for Poor Consumptives."

75. "Investigation into the Behavior of Miss Heibel, Nurse at White Haven," 1909, Walsh Papers, vol. 1, 588.

76. Wm. G. Townsend to Joseph Walsh, June 10, 1908, Walsh Papers, vol. 1, 390.

77. "Dr. Flick on the Value of Cured Consumptives as Nurses."

78. "Training School for Nurses." A "Circular of Information" for the Special Course in the Nursing of Tuberculosis, offered by the Philadelphia Hospital, similarly advertised that this course "is intended to afford an opportunity for self support and useful career to women who have had tuberculosis." Walsh Papers, vol. 2.

79. This numerical assessment is based on analysis of the list of sanatoria in the United States and Canada provided in NASPT, *Tuberculosis Directory* (1911), 11–68, 298–301.

80. "Sanatoria (1901)," in Flick Pamphlets, CPP. See also Herbert M. King and Henry B. Neagle, "Sanatorium Provision with Industrial Opportunities for Indigent Consumptives," *Trans. NASPT* 1 (1906): 325–332; Herbert C. Clapp, "What Cases Are Suitable for Admission to a State Sanatorium for Tuberculosis, Especially in New England," *Trans. NASPT* 1 (1906): 339–348; Vincent Y. Bowditch and Henry B. Dunham, "Six Years' Experience at the Massachusetts State Sanatorium for Tuberculosis at Rutland Mass," *Trans. NASPT* 1 (1906): 349–358; Alfred Meyer, "History and Work of the Bedrock Sanitarium for Consumptives," *Trans. NASPT* 1 (1906): 438–450.

81. Knopf, "Some Newer Problems."

82. See NASPT, *Tuberculosis Directory* (1911), 11–68. Members of both the Senate and the House of Representatives repeatedly introduced bills pertaining to the care of "indigent" consumptives, usually at the behest of their constituents, who felt the need for intervention. The federal government responded by establishing special sanatoria for veterans (1899) and for indigent consumptives. The Office of Indian Affairs also established fifteen sanatoria for the care of Native Americans with tuberculosis.

83. Christopher Easton in "With a State Sanatorium Secured," 36; H. Wirt Steele in "With a State Sanatorium Secured," 42.

84. A. E. Kepford in "With a State Sanatorium Secured," 33.

85. Easton in "With a State Sanatorium Secured," 36.

86. William H. Baldwin, "Progress of the Sanatorium Movement in America," *Trans. NASPT* 1 (1905): 72.

87. Knopf, "The Modern Prophylaxis," 20; see also Baldwin, "Progress," 72.

88. Baldwin, "Progress," 72.

89. E. L. Trudeau, "History of the Tuberculosis Work," 2.

90. E. R. Baldwin to H. A. Burns, superintendent of the Minnesota State Sanatorium, February 4, 1930, Baldwin Papers.

91. Louis M. Warfield in "With a State Sanatorium Secured," 30.

92. This summary is based, once again, on analysis of the list of sanatoria provided in NASPT, *Tuberculosis Directory* (1911), 11–68.

93. Classic discussions are Sheila Rothman, *Woman's Proper Place: A History of Changing Ideals and Practices, 1870–the Present* (New York: Basic Books, 1978); Julia Wrigley, "Do Young Children Need Intellectual Stimulation? Experts' Advice to Parents, 1900–1985," *History of Education Quarterly* 29 (1989): 41–75; Barbara Ehrenreich and Deirdre English, *For Her Own Good: 150 Years of Experts' Advice to Women* (Garden City, N.Y.: Anchor, Doubleday, 1978). For more recent reinterpretations, see Molly Ladd-Taylor, "Federal Help for Mothers: The Rise and Fall of the Sheppard Towner Act," in Dorothy Helly and Susan Reverby, eds., *Gendered Domains: Rethinking Public and Private in Women's History* (Ithaca, N.Y.: Cornell University Press, 1992), 217–227. See also Molly Ladd-Taylor, *Motherwork: Women, Child Welfare and the State, 1890–1930* (Urbana and Chicago: University of Illinois Press, 1994); Richard Meckel, *"Save the Babies": American Public Health Reform and the Prevention of Infant Mortality, 1890–1950* (Baltimore: Johns Hopkins University Press, 1990); Rima D. Apple, *Mothers and Medicine: A Social History of Infant Feeding, 1890–1950* (Madison: University of Wisconsin Press, 1987).

94. Krause, *Rest and Other Things*; Brown, *Rules for Recovery.*

95. William Charles White to Joseph Walsh, August 4, 1908, Walsh Papers, vol. 1, 424.

96. New York City, Department of Health, "Guarding the Health of Seven Mil-

lion People," *Annual Report* (1929), 17. For a discussion of the dispensary's history, see Charles Rosenberg, "Social Class and Medical Care in 19th Century America: The Rise and Fall of the Dispensary," *JHM* 29 (1974): 32–54.

97. Warfield in "With a State Sanatorium Secured," 30.

98. A summary of these efforts is found in NASPT, *Tuberculosis Directory* (1911). The New York City Department of Health provided a brief history of its tuberculosis control efforts in its report for 1929. New York City, Department of Health, "Guarding the Health of Seven Million People," 57.

99. New York City, Department of Health, *Annual Report* (1918), 57

100. New York City, Department of Health, *Annual Report* (1916), 54; see also New York City, Department of Health, "Guarding the Health of Seven Million People," 84.

101. Lloyd, "Centralized Control," 337.

102. New York City, Department of Health, *Annual Report* (1929), 82; see also Ellen La Motte, *The Tuberculosis Nurse* (1915; reprint, New York: Garland, 1985).

103. White, "Official Responsibility," 270.

104. Hermann Biggs, "A War Tuberculosis Program for the Nation," *Am. Rev. TB* 1 (1917–1918): 257–266.

105. Don B. Armstrong, "Medical Aspects of the Framingham Community Demonstration," *Am. Rev. TB* 2 (1918–1919): 203. Armstrong observed that "of special interest were the findings according to nationalities." These ranged as follows: Italian 51 percent, Irish 30 percent, Jewish 30 percent, American 18 percent, others 27 percent.

106. Ibid.

107. Albert G. Love and Charles B. Davenport, *Defects Found in Drafted Men* (Washington, D.C.: GPO, 1919), 29–30.

108. Karl Pearson, *Tuberculosis, Heredity and Environment* (London: Dulau, 1912).

109. Summaries of these data, along with criticisms, are presented in James A. Tobey, "Why Is There Less Tuberculosis?" *American Mercury* 4 (January 1925): 76; E. Opie and F. M. MacPhedran, "The Contagion of Tuberculosis," *Am. Rev. TB* 14 (1926): 347; E. Opie and F. M. MacPhedran, "Spread of Tuberculosis within Families," *JAMA* 87 (1926): 1549–1551.

110. Charles Rosenberg, "Charles Benedict Davenport and the Irony of American Eugenics," in Rosenberg, *No Other Gods*, 89–97; Daniel Kevles, *In the Name of Eugenics* (Berkeley: University of California Press, 1985), chapter 3.

111. Debates over restricting the immigration of tuberculous people are documented in NA RG 90-0425-32TB, Box 64. See also Kevles, *In the Name of Eugenics*, 56.

112. Tobey, "Why Is There Less Tuberculosis?" 76.

113. Ibid., 77.

114. Krause, *Rest and Other Things*, 86.

115. Allen K. Krause, *Environment and Resistance in Tuberculosis* (Baltimore: Williams & Wilkins, 1923), 8.

116. Ibid., 9, 12.

117. Krause, *Rest and Other Things*, 101.

118. Ibid.

119. White, "Official Responsibility," 269.

120. In 1914, a bill was introduced in the House of Representatives (H.R. 8352) "to standardize the treatment of tuberculosis," and a bill was introduced in the Senate (S. 4370) "to provide hospitals for the tubercular poor." See also Bills H.R. 11864 (1916)—"to provide State Support for Indigent Consumptives"—and S. 3202 (1916)—"to Standardize the Treatment of Tuberculosis in the United States, to Provide Federal Aid in Caring of Indigent Tuberculous Persons, and for Other Purposes."

121. C. V. Craster, M.D., "Discussion of John A. Lapp, Social Insurance as a Means of Relieving Poverty," *Trans. NTA* 15 (1919): 424.

122. White, "Official Responsibility," 269.

123. The tension between state responsibility and individual freedom became particularly marked in Progressive discourse. The strongest testimony to that tension is the repeal of smallpox vaccination laws in the Progressive states of Wisconsin and Minnesota. See also Sidney Fine, *Laissez Faire and the General Welfare State* (Ann Arbor: University of Michigan Press, 1976), chapter 11; Eric Goldman, *Rendezvous with Destiny* (New York: Knopf, 1952); Morton Keller, *Affairs of the State* (Cambridge, Mass.: Harvard University Press, 1977), especially Conclusion; Robert Wiebe, "The Social Functions of Public Education," *American Quarterly* 21 (1969): 147–164.

124. The quotations, representative of the views of a spectrum of reformers, come from Hunter, *Poverty*, quoted in Hofstadter, *The Progressive Movement*, 58. Discussions of the ways in which the desire to create self reliance shaped American attempts to relieve poverty are provided in Bremner, *From the Depths*; Paul Boyer, *Urban Masses and Moral Order in America* (Cambridge, Mass.: Harvard University Press, 1978); Katz, *In the Shadow*; Hace Tishler, *Self Reliance and Social Security, 1870–1917* (New York: Kennikat Press, 1971); and James T. Patterson, *America's Struggle against Poverty* (Cambridge, Mass.: Harvard University Press, 1981).

125. Lloyd, "Centralized Control," 337–338. Also see references listed in note 45 above.

126. Kelley, "Centralized Control of Tuberculosis," 341; John A. Lapp, "Social Insurance as a Means of Relieving Poverty," *Trans. NTA* 15 (1919): 416–423. See also Craster, "Discussion of John A. Lapp," 424.

127. Craster, "Discussion of John A. Lapp," 425.

128. Ibid., 424.

129. Lloyd, "Centralized Control," 336.

130. For discussions of the attention children needed, see ibid. and Holt, *Food and Growth*, 8–15; see also George M. Kober, "The Child and the Home," *Trans. NTA* 11 (1915): 41; Charles C. Browning, "Discussion of Paper by Dr. Kober," *Trans. NTA* 11 (1915): 45–46.

131. "Circular Issued by the New York City Department of Health."

132. David Lyman, "The Control of the Careless Consumptive," *Am. Rev. TB* 2 (1918–1919): 42.

133. Holt, *Food and Growth*, 34.

134. Ibid., 33–34; see also Herbert M. King, "An Experiment in Diet at the Annex of the Loomis Sanatorium," *Proceedings of the Sixth International Congress on Tuberculosis* 3 (1908): 719–724; Maurice I. Smith, "Tuberculosis and Vitamine Requirements in the Nutrition of the White Rat," *Trans. NTA* 19 (1924): 274.

135. R. I. Harris, "Heliotherapy in Surgical Tuberculosis," *AJPH* 16 (1926), and Woods Hutchinson, "Light Refreshments," *Saturday Evening Post* 197 (May 2, 1925), provide typical examples. The quote comes from Hutchinson, 16–17.

136. Gerald B. Webb, "Address of the President," *Trans. NTA* 16 (1921): 26. During the 1920s and 1930s, nutritional studies funded by the NTA included M. M. Steinbach (Columbia University), "Diabetes and Tuberculosis"; M. C. Winternitz (Yale University), "Tissue Reaction in Tuberculosis and Enzymes in Resistance"; E. B. Fred (University of Wisconsin), "Cod-Liver Oil in Skin Tuberculosis"; S. J. Klein (Columbia University), "Vitamin C Absorption and Resistance to Tuberculosis." This list is culled from the summary of grants awarded by the NTA and the list of projects provided in Dorothy White Nicholson, *Twenty Years of Medical Research* (New York: NTA, 1943), 61–94. An extensive bibliography of studies of nutrition can also be found in Esmond Long,

"Constitution and Related Factors in Resistance to Tuberculosis," *Archives of Pathology* 32 (1941): 286–298.

137. For a discussion of the Sheppard-Towner Act, see Ladd-Taylor, "Federal Help for Mothers"; Ladd-Taylor, *Motherwork.* See also Appel, *Mothers and Medicine*; Meckel, "*Save the Babies.*"

138. Holt published the Lane Lectures in his *Food and Growth.* See Holt, *Food and Growth*, 5.

139. M. Grace Osborne, "The Crusade in the School and the Community," *Trans. NTA* 16 (1920): 474. The NTA outlined the objectives of the Modern Health Crusade in a series of pamphlets. NTA, *The Modern Health Crusade* (New York, 1920, 1921, 1923). Shryock provides a brief history of the crusade in his history of the NTA. Richard Harrison Shryock, *The Development of Modern Medicine: An Interpretation of the Social and Scientific Factors Involved* (1939; reprint, Madison: University of Wisconsin Press, 1979), 170–173.

140. Osborne, "Crusade in the School," 474.

141. NTA, "Health Rules for Modern Crusaders," in Shryock, *Development of Modern Medicine*, 170.

142. S. Adolphus Knopf, "Essentials of the Prevention of Tuberculosis in Infancy and Childhood," *JAMA* 88 (1927): 1059.

143. Ibid., 1058.

144. H. S. Cumming to E. A. Meyerding, executive secretary of the Minnesota Public Health Association, December 4, 1928, NA RG 90-0425-32, Box 64.

145. S. Adolphus Knopf, "Tuberculosis among Young Women," *JAMA* 90 (1928): 533.

146. For discussions of images of female consumptives, see Nan Marie McMurry, "'And I? I Am in a Consumption': The Tuberculosis Patient, 1780–1930." (Ph.D. diss., Duke University, 1985).

147. Knopf, "Tuberculois among Young Women," 533.

148. Eleanor Roosevelt, *This Is My Story* (New York: Doubleday, 1937), 209–211.

149. Blanche Wiesen Cook, *Eleanor Roosevelt*, vol. 1: *1884–1933* (New York: Penguin, 1992), 235.

150. Knopf, "Tuberculosis among Young Women," 534.

151. Holt, *Food and Growth*, 216–229.

152. A general discussion of medical advice columns is offered in Julia Wrigley, "Do Young Children Need Intellectual Stimulation? Experts' Advice to Parents, 1900–1985," *History of Education Quarterly* 29 (1989): 41–75.

153. See, for example, "Light Cure," *Literary Digest* 75 (December 22, 1923): 1; "Babies and Sunshine," *Literary Digest* 79 (December 1, 1923): 27; A. F. Hess, "Relation of Hygiene, More Particularly Light to the Health of the Child," *Home Economics* 15 (July 1923): 311–314; E. E. Slosson, "Sun Cure," *Scientific Monthly* 16 (1923): 555–557; "Sunshine as a Medicine," *Literary Digest* 80 (March 22, 1924): 69–70; Hutchinson, "Light Refreshments," 16–17; S. Josephine Baker, "Sun Baths for the Youngest Generation," *Ladies' Home Journal* (June 1928), 198; Paul deKruif, "Old Doctor Sun," *Ladies' Home Journal* (October 1931), 6.

154. Logan Clendening, "Breakfastless Children and Tuberculous Youths," *Ladies' Home Journal* (November 1929), 23.

155. Ibid.

156. Thoughtful and important reinterpretations of women's activism and welfare are provided in Theda Skocpol, *Protecting Soldiers and Mothers: The Political Origins of Social Policy in the United States* (Cambridge: Belknap, 1992); Ladd-Taylor, "Federal Help for Mothers"; Ladd-Taylor, *Motherwork.*

157. Florence Deakins Becker, "TB: General Correspondence and Writing," Becker Papers, Box 7, Library of Congress, Washington, D.C.

158. Krause, *Rest and Other Things*, 86.

159. Baldwin, "Progress," 72.

160. Trudeau, "Address of the President," 15.

161. "Henry Phipps Institute, Feb. 24, 1910" (newspaper article, source unknown), Walsh Papers, vol. 2.

162. Trudeau, "Address of the President," 15.

163. Chapin, "State Control of Tuberculosis," 24.

164. A discussion of Biggs's efforts is provided in Knopf, "Essentials of the Prevention"; Holt, *Food and Growth*; Kleinschmidt, "Publicity Campaign."

CHAPTER 4: MEDICINE, SCIENCE, AND THE NATIONAL INTEREST

1. E. L. Trudeau, "Relative Immunity in Tuberculosis and the Use of Tuberculin," *British Journal of Tuberculosis* 10 (1916): 29–30.

2. "Tells of a Vaccine for Tuberculosis: Professor Calmette Reports His Discovery to the Academy of Paris," *New York Times* (June 26, 1924), 25.

3. "Experts Discuss Calmette Vaccine," *New York Times* (June 27, 1924), 18.

4. Albert Calmette and C. Guérin, "Sur l'immunisation contre la tuberculose," *Proceedings of the Sixth International Congress on Tuberculosis* 1 (1908): 181–187.

5. Dr. E. A. Watson, chief pathologist at the Department of Agriculture, Ottawa, and Dr. A. C. Rankin, professor of bacteriology, director of the Provincial Laboratory, and dean of the Faculty of Medicine at the University of Alberta, first conducted these trials. By 1925, BCG was "already made in considerable quantity in Canada." See National Research Council of Canada (NRCC), Associate Committee on Tuberculosis Research (ACTR), *Minutes of the Second Meeting* (1925), 38–45. See also Wherrett, *Miracle of the Empty Beds*, 59–60.

6. "Experts Discuss Calmette Vaccine," 18.

7. "Tells of a Vaccine," 25.

8. "Preventive Not Curative," *New York Times* (June 27, 1924), 18.

9. [Allen K. Krause], "Calmette's Protective Inoculation against Tuberculosis," *Am. Rev. TB* 10 (1924–1925): 224–225.

10. Emil von Behring, P. Römer, and W. G. Ruppel, "Tuberkulose," *Beiträge zur experimentellen Therapie* 5 (1902): 1–84.

11. The best discussion of this concept was later provided by Theobald Smith, *Parasitism and Disease* (Princeton, N.J.: Princeton University Press, 1934), especially 29–30.

12. E. R. Baldwin, "Immunity in Tuberculosis," *Proceedings of the Sixth International Congress on Tuberculosis* 1 (1908): 176.

13. For further explanation, see USDA, *Annual Report* (1881–1982), 290–295; Salmon and Smith, "On a New Method," 29–33; Salmon and Smith, "Experiments on the Production of Immunity," 403–407.

14. Theobald Smith, "Two Varieties of the Tubercle Bacillus from Mammals," *Transactions of the Association of American Physicians* 11 (1896): 75–97.

15. T. Smith, "The Vaccination of Cattle against Tuberculosis," *Journal of Medical Research* 8 (1908): 451–458; also T. Smith, "Certain Aspects of Natural and Acquired Resistance to Tuberculosis and Their Bearing on Preventive Measures," *JAMA* 68 (1917): 669–674, 764–769.

16. Smith, "Certain Aspects," 766.

17. Smith, "Vaccination of Cattle," 481.

18. E. R. Baldwin, "Immunity in Tuberculosis," *Proceedings of the Sixth International Congress on Tuberculosis* 1 (1908): 176.

19. G. B. Webb and Wm. W. Williams, "Immunity in Tuberculosis: Its Production in Monkeys and Children," *JAMA* 57 (1911): 1431–1434.

20. U.S. Congress, Senate, *Dr. Friedmann's New Treatment for Tuberculosis: Message from the President of the United States Transmitting in Response to Senate Resolution of January 2, 1913, a Memorandum of the Secretary of State Submitting a Report by the Consul General at Berlin Relative to the Friedmann Cure for Tuberculosis*, 62d Cong., 3rd sess., 1913, S. Doc. 1018.

21. William Charles White, *Natural and Artificial Cure of Tuberculosis*, Technical Series (New York: NTA, 1925), 10.

22. William Charles White, "Chemical Treatment of Tuberculosis and Vaccines in Immunization against Tuberculosis," *AJPH* 16 (1926): 532.

23. Comments of A. Calmette, "Conference on the Relations of Tuberculosis of Animals and of Man," *Proceeding of the Sixth International Congress on Tuberculosis* 4 (1908): 749. Calmette and Guérin artificially infected the teats of female goats, then allowed their newborn kids to suckle. The kids rapidly developed intestinal tuberculosis, from which many recovered, but later in life some developed pulmonary disease. A. Calmette and C. Guérin, "Origine intestinale de la tuberculose pulmonaire et mechanisme de l'infection tuberculose," *Annales de l'Institut Pasteur (Anns. Inst. Past.)* 19 (1905): 601–618, and 20 (1906): 353–378. See also A. Calmette, A. Boquet, and L. Nègre, "Essai de vaccination contre l'infection tuberculeuse par voi buccale chez les petits animaux de laboratoire." *Anns. Inst. Past.* 38 (1924): 399–400.

24. Calmette in "Conference on the Relations," 749–750. Calmette's argument did not convince Koch, who responded, "As regards the views expressed by Calmette, I have expected long since that somebody would put forward the argument that the bacilli change their character on the way from the mesentery to the lungs. But this, gentlemen, is a mere hypothesis, supported by nothing. On the contrary, everything we know at present on this subject speaks against this hypothesis; for it is a proved fact that the bovine tubercle bacillus keeps its character for a very long time." Comments of R. Koch, "Conference on the Relations," 752.

25. See Dorothy White Nicholson, *20 Years of Medical Research* (New York: NTA, 1943); Virginia Cameron and Esmond R. Long, *Tuberculosis Medical Research: National Tuberculosis Association, 1904–1955* (New York: NTA, 1959).

26. A. Calmette, C. Guérin, A. Boquet, and L. Nègre, "Sur la vaccination préventive des enfants nouveau nés contre la tuberculose par le BCG, *Anns. Inst. Past.* 41 (1927): 204. All translations from the French in this chapter are the author's.

27. Albert Calmette, C. Guérin, A. Boquet, and L. Nègre, *La vaccination préventive contre la tuberculose par le BCG* (Paris: Masson et Cie, 1927), 6.

28. A. Calmette, C. Guérin and B. Weill-Hallé, "Immunisation contre l'infection tuberculeuse," *Anns. Inst. Past.* 38 (1924), 392. On this point, Calmette also drew from the work of A. Marafan, who suggested that a mild, natural infection might produce immunity to TB. A. Marafan, "De l'immunité conféré par la guérison d'une tuberculose pour la phthise pulmonaire." *Archives Générales de Médicine* 17 (1886): 423.

29. Calmette et al., *La vaccination préventive*, 5; Calmette provides a summary of these various efforts on 13–58. See also Henry J. Parish, *History of Immunization* (Edinburgh: E. & S. Livingstone, 1965), chapter 8.

30. Over a period of thirteen years, Calmette and Guérin passed Noccard's bovine bacillus through 230 generations on a 5 percent ox-bile and glycerine medium in order to culture an organism that retained the essential physiological characteristics of tubercle bacilli but had none of their virulence.

31. A. Calmette and C. Guérin, "Nouvelles recherches expérimentelles sur la vaccination des bovides contre la tuberculose," *Anns. Inst. Past.* 34 (1920): 37; A. Calmette, A. Boquet, and L. Nègre, "Contribution à l'étude du bacille tuberculeux bilié," *Anns. Inst. Past.* 35 (1921): 261. See also Calmette et al., "Immunisation contre l'infection," 390.

32. NRCC, ACTR, *Minutes of the First Meeting* (1924), 12.

33. S. A. Petroff, "A New Analysis of the Value and Safety of Protective Immunization with BCG," *Am. Rev. TB* 20 (1929): 275–296.

34. Quoted in ibid., 289

35. A. Calmette, *Tubercle Bacillus Infection and Tuberculosis in Man and Animals* (Baltimore: Williams & Wilkins, 1924), 294, quoted in Petroff, "New Analysis," 289. See also Albert Calmette, "Do There Exist in Nature or Can There Be Artificially Produced Saprophytic Varieties of Koch's Tubercle Bacillus Which Possess the Property of Becoming Virulent Tubercle Bacilli?", excerpted in Canadian Tuberculosis Association (CTA), *Annual Report* 24 (1924): 23–24.

36. Petroff, "New Analysis," 289.

37. Ibid., 295.

38. Ibid., 277.

39. Watson cultured three separate strains of BCG, obtained directly from Calmette and Guérin, into 145 substrains descending to the 121st generation. Forty percent of the 500 guinea pigs he injected later developed "slight or localized lesions, or apparently arrested or healed lesions." Watson could not attribute the infections to spontaneous tuberculosis or contamination and therefore concluded that 6 of the 145 cultures had become virulent. E. A. Watson, "Studies on Bacillus Calmette-Guérin and Vaccination against Tuberculosis," *Canadian Journal of Research* 9 (1933): 133–135; see also E. A. Watson, "Research on Bacillus Calmette-Guérin and Experimental Vaccination against Bovine Tuberculosis," *Journal of the American Veterinary Medical Association* 73 (1928): 799–816.

40. Watson, "Studies on Bacillus," 135.

41. Esmond Long, who later assumed the directorship of the Phipps Institute, was probably the best known of the Americans who undertook such analyses. See Esmond Long, "Cultural Differences among Acid-Fast Bacteria," *Transactions of the Chicago Pathological Society* 11 (1922): 266–283; Esmond Long, "Chemical Evidence on the Phylogenetic Classification of the Tubercle Bacillus: The Plant or Animal Question," *Am. Rev. TB* 8 (1923): 195–213.

42. Petroff, "New Analysis," 278.

43. George Vincent, president of the Rockefeller Foundation, to Florence Deakins Becker, July 28, 1921, in "TB: General Correspondence and Writings," Becker Papers, Box 7.

44. A. Calmette, "Enquête sur l'epidémiologie de la tuberculose dans les colonies Françaises," *Anns. l'Inst. Past.* 26 (1912): 497–514. See also Calmette et al., *La vaccination préventive* , 173–175.

45. Calmette et al., *La vaccination préventive*, 172–177.

46. Ibid., 61–127.

47. Calmette, Boquet, and Nègre, "Essai de vaccination," 399–400.

48. Ibid.

49. Calmette et al., *La vaccination prevéntive*, 186–187.

50. B. Weill-Hallé and R. Turpin, "Sur la vaccination antituberculeuse de l'enfant par le BCG," *Anns. Inst. Past.* 49 (1927): 256.

51. Calmette et al., *La vaccination préventive*, 176.

52. Ibid., 187.

53. A. Calmette, C. Guérin, B. Weill-Hallé, and R. Turpin, "Essais d'immunisation contre l'infection tuberculeuse," *Bulletin de l'Académie de Médicine de Paris* 91 (1924): 787–796.

54. Weill-Hallé and Turpin, "Sur la vaccination antituberculeuse," 253–270.

55. Of 303 vaccinated children born to tubercular mothers, 269 were under two years of age. Of these 2—or 0.7 percent—died of tubercular diseases; the general mortality for this group was 6.3 percent. Among children born to tubercular fathers, mortality among those vaccinated was 1.14 percent; in the general population, it was 5.69 percent. Mortality for children in the general population born to two tubercular parents was 12.9 percent; mortality for the vaccinated children in this category was 0 percent. Calmette et al., *La vaccination préventive* , 191–195.

56. Biraud found that general mortality among the children under two years of age raised in tubercular families was 7.6/100, and among those with tubercular mothers it was 6.6/100. In the vaccinated population mortality was 1.55/100 and 2.46/100, respectively. Calmette et al., *La vaccination préventive*, 195.

57. Ibid., 196.

58. Ibid., 197–199; also, Calmette et al., "Sur la vaccination préventive," 219.

59. Calmette et al., *La vaccination préventive* , 222.

60. Ibid., 207–213. Many of these trials are also abstracted and reviewed in the *Bulletin Institut Pasteur* 27 (1929): 300–309.

61. "Vaccination against Tuberculosis." (editorial), *JAMA* 84 (1925), 1575.

62. White, "Chemical Treatment of Tuberculosis," 535.

63. [William Charles White], "Vaccination of the New-Born against Tuberculosis with Bacillus Calmette-Guérin," *JAMA* 89 (1927): 115. See also Wm. Charles White, "Questions Relative to Immunization against Tuberculosis," 1928, 2, NA RG 90–0425–32, Box 64.

64. M. J. King and William H. Park, "Effect of Calmette's BCG Vaccine on Experimental Animals," *AJPH* 19 (1929): 179–192.

65. Though Canadian researchers had moved quickly to test and employ BCG, they had not done so without any reservations; as they proceeded they too called for careful scrutiny and verification of Calmette's claims that BCG was harmless to all species of animals. NRCC, ACTR, *Minutes of the Second Meeting* (1925), 35. See also F. B. Smith, "Tuberculosis and Bureaucracy: Bacille Calmette Guérin: Its Troubled Path to Acceptance in Britain and Australia." *Medical Journal of Australia* 159 (1993): 408–411.

66. [Allen Krause], "Calmette's Protective Inoculation against Tuberculosis," *Am. Rev. TB* 10 (1924–1925), 225.

67. NRCC, ACTR, *Minutes of the Second Meeting* (1925), 35.

68. [Krause], "Calmette's Protective Inoculation," 225.

69. [White], "Vaccination of the New-Born," 116.

70. White, "Questions Relative to Immunization," 2.

71. Wm. Charles White, "Investigations of TB Research in Europe," May 16, 1927, NA RG 90-0425–32 TB, Box 64.

72. For general discussions of American views on the links between science and progress, see Wiebe, *Search for Order,* especially chapter 6; Rosenberg, *No Other Gods,* especially 2–4; Nathan Reingold, ed., *Science in America since 1820* (New York: Science History Publications, 1976).

73. [Krause], "Calmette's Protective Inoculation," 224. For discussion of the development of a national research agenda, see Victoria Harden, *Inventing the NIH: Federal Biomedical Research Policy, 1887–1937* (Baltimore: Johns Hopkins University Press, 1986).

74. For example, in his presidential address to the first annual meeting of the NTA, Trudeau made a plea for laboratory research that went unheeded. Edward L. Trudeau,

"Address of the President to the First Annual Meeting of the National Association for the Study and Prevention of Tuberculosis," *Trans. NASPT* 1 (1896): 15. In 1916 Baldwin once again called for research. "The duty of the United States," he wrote, "is to . . . put forth more research." Baldwin made this appeal more for the sake of publicity than for the good of the antituberculosis crusade. He was not dissatisfied with the accomplishments of that crusade, and he admitted that great strides had been made. He called for research to sustain the campaign rather than to give it new direction. "If we wish to maintain the present interest of the public in the subject," he argued, "we must broaden scientific standards and secure their sympathy and support." E. R. Baldwin, "Address of the President," *Trans. NASPT* 12 (1916): 19–23.

75. Columbia University, School of Hygiene, Division of Public Health Education, "Interview with Esmond R. Long, July 26, 1963." Long Papers, 57, National Library of Medicine, Washington, D.C. Hereafter referred to as Long Interview.

76. In the years after 1921, the NTA continued to emphasize studies of resistance. Forty-four percent, or 213, of the 486 studies that it funded during the period 1921–1950 dealt with topics in immunity and resistance; in contrast, 9 percent—or 43 of 486—were devoted to the study of chemotherapy and other measures that would destroy the microbial sources of infection. This summary is based on an analysis of the projects funded by the NTA as listed in the appendix to Nicholson, *20 Years of Medical Research*, 61–95. Studies of sunlight, which Koch had demonstrated would kill tubercle bacilli and which other researchers subsequently found would heal tuberculous lesions and stimulate metabolism, defined one important theme of this research. These studies included Wilton R. Earle, "Degeneration in vitro of Leucocytes and Connective Tissue under the Influence of Light," *Procceedings of the Society for Experimental Biology and Medicine* 24 (1927): 611–614; Wilton R. Earle, "Studies of the Effect of Light on Blood and Tissue Cells. I. The Action of Light on White Blood Cells in Vitro," *Journal of Experimental Medicine* 48 (1928): 457; Wilton R. Earle, "Studies of the Effect of Light on Blood and Tissue Cells. II. The Action of Light on Erythrocytes in Vitro," *Journal of Experimental Medicine* 48 (1928): 667; Wilton R. Earle, "Studies of the Effect of Light on Blood and Tissue Cells. III. The Action of Light on Fibroblasts in Vitro," *Journal of Experimental Medicine* 48 (1928): 683; Kenneth C. Smithburn and George I. Lavin, "The Effects of Ultraviolet Radiation on Tubercle Bacilli," *Am. Rev. TB* 39 (1939): 782. See also Cameron and Long, *Tuberculosis Medical Research*.

77. Wherrett, *Miracle of the Empty Beds*, chapter 8; George Jasper Wherrett, *Tuberculosis in Canada*, Royal Commission on Health Services (Ottawa: Queen's Printer, 1965).

78. NRCC, *Report of the President* (1924–1925), 24.

79. Honorary Advisory Council for Scientific and Industrial Research (Canada), *Report of the Administrative Chairman* (1920–1921), 21.

80. Robert C. Vipond, "Constitutional Politics and the Legacy of the Provincial Rights Movement in Canada," *Canadian Journal of Political Science* 18 (1985): 267–291; Robert C. Vipond, *Liberty and Community: Canadian Federalism and the Failure of Constitutional Vision* (Albany: State University of New York Press, 1991); Peter H. Russell, Rainer Knopf, and F. L. Morton, *Federalism and the Charter* (Ottawa: Carleton University Press, 1989), part 1.

81. For further discussion of these issues, see Georgina Feldberg, "The Origins of Organized Canadian Medical Research: The National Research Council's Associate Committee on Tuberculosis Research, 1924–1938," *Scientia Canadensis* 15 (1991): 53–69.

82. In 1938, the ACTR became the Associate Committee on Medical Research of the NRCC. In 1960, that committee was reconstituted as the Medical Research Council of the National Research Council, and in 1967 it became the Medical Research

Council. See NRCC, ACTR, *Report of the Seventh Meeting* (1936), especially 15; see also Armand Frappier, *Fifty Years of Study and Use of BCG in Canada, 1924–1974* (Montreal: Institut Armand-Frappier, 1979), 3–4.

83. Long Interview, 51–57. See also Cameron and Long, *Tuberculosis Medical Research*, 4.

84. This is not to suggest that the federal government had no interest in TB. The various federal agencies responsible for Indian affairs, veterans, and trade and commerce all participated in the control of TB, and through its States Services Division, the PHS assisted states and voluntary agencies in their efforts to determine the extent of the tuberculosis problem. See Ralph Chester Williams, *The United States Public Health Service 1798–1950* (Washington D.C.: Commissioned Officers Association of the United States Public Health Service, 1951), 280–282, 344.

85. The most comprehensive published discussions of the federal tuberculosis-control efforts initiated by the PHS—or the lack thereof—are provided in, ibid., especially chapter 4, and Bess Furman, *A Profile of the United States Public Health Service* (Bethesda, Md.: NIH, 1973). See also Long Interview, 20.

86. U.S. Department of the Treasury, Marine Hospital Service, *Annual Report of the Surgeon General* (1922); Nicholson, *20 Years of Medical Research*; Cameron and Long, *Tuberculosis Medical Research*.

87. See, for example, "The New Treatment for Tuberculosis," *JAMA* 81 (1923): 310; "Specific Treatment of Tuberculosis," *JAMA* 81 (1923): 864.

88. For articles in the popular press, see, for example, Watson Davis, "Inoculation for Tuberculosis," *Current History* 24 (May 1926): 257–258; Watson Davis, "The New Vaccine against Tuberculosis," *Current History* 25 (November 1926): 231–232; "Science and Invention—Vaccination for Tuberculosis," *Literary Digest* 84 (March 14, 1925): 81–82; "A Vaccine against Tuberculosis," *Current Opinion* 77 (October 1924): 498. For an example of a letter, see Florence Campbell Forester to Allen K. Krause, May 20, 1930, Becker Papers, Box 7.

89. Samuel B. English to PHS and Wm. McCoy to S. B. English, November 19 and 24, 1928, NA RG 90-0470, Box 6.

90. "Investigations of Sanocrysin, 1926–1939, NA RG 52A–208, Box 13.

91. For a discussion of changing relations between the government and industry on matters of testing and scientific standards, see Charles O. Jackson, *Food and Drug Legislation in the New Deal* (Princeton, N.J.: Princeton University Press, 1970); Victoria Harden, *Inventing the NIH.*

92. For further discussion of McCoy and the development of a national research agenda, see Harden, *Inventing the NIH.*

93. G. W. McCoy to E. M. Houghton, February 11, 1925, NA RG 52A–208, Box 13.

94. Ibid.

95. Houghton to McCoy, April 15, 1925, NA RG 52A–208, Box 13.

96. O. W. Smith to G. W. McCoy, April 17, 1925, NA RG 52A–208, Box 13.

97. Stimson to McCoy, July 6, 1925, NA RG 52A–208, Box 13.

98. William Charles White to the director of NIH, August 30, 1939, NA RG 52A–208, Box 13. See also J. Burns Amberson, B. T. McMahon, and M. Pinner, "A Clinical Trial of Sanocrysin in Pulmonary TB," *Am. Rev. TB* 24 (1931): 401–435; Benjamin Brock, "The Sanocrysin Treatment of Pulmonary TB in the White and Negro Races," *Am. Rev. TB* 24 (1931): 436–445.

99. Correspondence between O. W. Smith and G. W. McCoy, June through August 1925, NA RG 52A–208, Box 13.

100. NRCC, ACTR, *Minutes of the Second Meeting* (1925). 61–64. See also Robert D.

Defries, *The First Forty Years, 1914–1955: Connaught Medical Research Laboratories, University of Toronto* (Toronto: University of Toronto Press, 1968).

101. G. W. McCoy to H. S. Cumming, September 1, 1931, NA RG 90-0470-132, Box 70. In 1935, R. E. Dyer, acting director of the Division of Scientific Research of the NIH, complained to the assistant surgeon general that "we have no actual experience with this product [BCG]." He too attributed this state of affairs, at least in part, to the influence of drug companies. BCG, Dyer explained, "has not been licensed under the biologics law, nor has application for such a licence been made." Memo from R. E. Dyer, acting director, Division of Scientific Research, to S. L. Christian, assistant surgeon general, September 26, 1935, NA RG 52A–208, Box 13. Merck, Sharpe and Dohme, and its predecessors, similarly steered clear of BCG, as did H. K. Mulford and its successors.

102. Smith also notes the symbolic importance of Lübeck and argues that "hearsay calumnies about reactivated virulence and French arrogance and deceit prejudiced anglophone opinion until at least 1980." Smith, "Tuberculosis and Bureaucracy," 410.

103. M. J. King and William H. Park, "Effect of Calmette's BCG Vaccine on Experimental Animals," *A JPH* 19 (1929): 179–192.

104. Watson had little interest in the questions of species transformation that so perturbed Americans; he worried that only 5 percent of the animals that he had injected with BCG developed progressive tuberculosis. In subsequent studies Watson found that his cultures had lost their ability to produce TB; none of his experimental animals developed disease, and all attempts to restore BCG to virulence failed. Hence, Watson ultimately conceded that his own laboratory error may have been a cause of the earlier results and that in any case his reservations about the safety of BCG applied only to cultures distributed between 1924 and 1928. Satisfied that BCG had been permanently, hereditarily fixed, Watson publicly stated that it was "incapable of causing progressive, reinoculable tuberculosis in laboratory test animals." Watson, "Studies on Bacillus," 128, 136.

105. Petroff, "New Analysis," 276.

106. " 'Preventive Vaccination' Discussion from the International Union against Tuberculosis, Oslo, August 13–15," *Lancet* 219 (September 6, 1930): 529–530.

107. "Discussion of Preventive Vaccination against Tuberculosis at the Seventh Conference of the International Union against Tuberculosis, held at Oslo, August 13–15, 1930; Report by Eugene Opie," 8, Opie Papers, file: "BCG," American Philosophical Society, Philadelphia.

108. Ibid., 9.

109. Ibid., 3.

110. Eugene Opie, "Report of the Director of the Laboratory of the Henry Phipps Institute, 1930," Opie Papers, file: "Tuberculosis—Phipps Institute, 1930."

111. Eugene Opie to Albert Calmette, December 22, 1930, Opie Papers, file: "BCG."

112. "Eugene Opie's Response to the Lübeck Tragedy," *Ledger of the Philadelphia College Medical Society*, October 21, 1931, Opie Papers, file: "BCG Vaccine."

113. McCoy to Cumming, September 1, 1931.

114. Edward T. Devine, "Travel Notes to the Board of Managers of the Bellevue-Yorkville Health Demonstration Concerning Opinions of BCG in Europe," in *BCG Vaccination against Tuberculosis* (New York: New York Tuberculosis and Health Association, 1930), 8–9; manuscript copy in Opie Papers, file: "BCG Vaccine."

115. Ibid., 11.

116. Paul de Kruif, "BCG: Toward the White Plague's End," *Ladies' Home Journal* (March 1931), 71.

117. Ibid.

118. For example, Paul de Kruif, *Microbe Hunters* (New York: Harcourt Brace, 1926).

119. de Kruif, "BCG," 8.

120. Ibid.

121. E. T. Devine to Dr. Witter Barnard, July 20, 1930, in Devine, "Travel Notes," 13; manuscript copy in Opie Papers, file: "BCG Vaccine."

122. Petroff, "New Analysis," 295.

123. S. A. Knopf, "Birth Control in Disease," *Nation* (January 27, 1932), 109–110.

124. S. Adolphus Knopf, "Essentials in Prevention of Tuberculosis in Infancy and Childhood," *JAMA* 88 (1927): 1058–1060.

125. S. Adolphus Knopf, "Preventive Inoculation in Children with BCG," in S. Adolphus Knopf, *Report to the United States Government on Tuberculosis with Some Therapeutic and Prophylactic Suggestions* (New York: NTA, 1933), 43.

CHAPTER 5: FOR COWS, BOYS, AND INDIANS

1. Petroff, "New Analysis," 276.

2. These were not the only trials. Investigators in both countries additionally tested BCG in populations of nurses and medical students, in asylums for the mentally disturbed, and in prisons. The trials on cattle, children, and Native Americans, however, provided the basis for policy decisions and hence emerge as the most significant.

3. [White], "Vaccination of the New-Born," 115–116.

4. Fewer than half of those whom Park vaccinated orally became tuberculin positive, but the laboratory animals that he injected interally reacted quickly and consistently to tuberculin. M. J. King and W. H. Park, "Effect of Calmette's BCG Vaccine on Experimental Animals," *AJPH* 29 (1929): 179–192; C. Kereszturi and W. H. Park, "Oral Vaccination with BCG on Human Beings in NYC," *Am. Rev. TB* 20 (1929): 297; C. Kereszturi, W. Park, M. Levine, P. Vogel, and M. Sackett, "Clinical Study of BCG Vaccination," *New York State Journal of Medicine* 33 (1933): 376.

5. Eugene Opie, "Discussion of Dr. Joseph D. Aronson, the Present Status of Immunization against Tuberculosis with B.C.G.," [1930], Opie Papers, file: "Tuberculosis—Protective Inoculation BCG."

6. Petroff, "New Analysis," 285.

7. "His Preventive Not Enough" *New York Times* (June 28, 1924), 12.

8. S. A. Petroff and A. Branch, "Bacillus Calmette Guérin (BCG): Animal Experimentation and Prophylactic Immunization of Children," *AJPH* 18 (1928): 863.

9. Petroff, "New Analysis," 290.

10. In France alone, 21,200 children had been vaccinated; additional vaccinees in Belgium, Romania, Greece, Algeria, and Indochina raised the number to 43,283. For discussion of these trials, see the special edition of *Anns. Inst. Past.* (March 1927) and [White], "Vaccination of the New-Born," 115–116.

11. William Charles White, "Investigations of TB Research in Europe, 16 May, 1927," NA RG 90-0425-32, Box 64.

12. [White], "Vaccination of the New-Born," 115. The editorial noted that "these figures are based on reports as far back as 1913, and for Stuttgart as far back as 1889."

13. Ibid.

14. Petroff, "New Analysis," 292.

15. "Discussion of Preventive Vaccination," 9–10.

16. [White], "Vaccination of the New-Born," 115. Opie similarly found that if one looked closely at the French studies, mortality from all causes was lower in the test population than among the controls. He too leapt to the conclusion that the two populations must consequently be different.

17. In 1893, after the city of Lawrence, Massachusetts, had introduced a filtered and purified water supply as part of their campaign against typhoid, Hiram Mills, an engineer and a member of the State Board of Health, observed "that a marked decrease in the general death-rate of the city and not merely in the death-rate from typhoid fever, was taking place." In Hamburg, Germany, Dr. J. J. Reinke made similar observations, so that by 1910 public health officials widely recognized that when water was purified to combat typhoid, a general reduction in mortality followed. W. T. Sedgwick and J. Scott MacNutt, "On the Mills-Reinke Phenomenon and Hazen's Theorem Concerning the Decrease in Mortality from Diseases Other than Typhoid Fever Following the Purification of Public Water-Supplies," *Journal of Infectious Diseases* 7 (1910): 489–564.

18. [White], "Vaccination of the New-Born," 115.

19. Petroff, "New Analysis," 293.

20. Ibid., 295.

21. Opie, for one, recognized the possibilities of alternatives. Director of the laboratory at the Henry Phipps Institute, Opie began in the late 1920s to experiment with a killed vaccine. See Opie Papers, files: "Tuberculosis—Protective Inoculation" and "Protective Inoculation—Resistance."

22. NRCC, ACTR, *Report of the First Meeting* (1924), 62. Its priorities were "A) the ultimate fate of living bacilli inoculated into animals for prophylactic purposes, B) the fate of tubercle bacilli introduced into an already infected animal, C) whether living tubercle bacilli attenuated by artificial means (or bacilli of weak virulence) and employed for vaccinating purposes are able, by passage through animals or other means, to recover their former or original virulence," and BCG.

23. Further discussion of the origins of the ACTR can be found in Feldberg, "'An Antitoxin'"; Feldberg, "The Origins of Organized Canadian Medical Research."

24. NRCC, ACTR, *Report of the First Meeting* (1924), 62.

25. NRCC, ACTR, "Memorandum re BCG Vaccine by Dr. Rankin," *Report of the Second Meeting* (1925), 46.

26. E. A. Watson, "Report on BCG and Tuberculin in the Campaign against Bovine TB," in NRCC, ACTR, *Report of the Second Meeting* (1925), 188–190.

27. NRCC, ACTR, *Report of the Second Meeting* (1925), 205–211; see also J. A. Baudouin, "Vaccination against Tuberculosis with the BCG Vaccine," *Canadian Journal of Public Health* 27 (1936): 20.

28. A fuller account of these events is provided in Frappier, *Fifty Years of Study and Use of BCG;* an elegant summary of the use of BCG in Canada is also provided in Wherrett, *Miracle of the Empty Beds*, chapter 4.

29. *Report of the Technical Conference on the Study of Vaccination against Tuberculosis with BCG*, Publication 111/17 (Geneva: League of Nations Health Organization, 1928), 50.

30. J. A. Baudouin, "Vaccination against Tuberculosis with the BCG Vaccine," *Canadian Journal of Public Health* 27 (1936), 24.

31. Ibid.

32. Ibid., 26.

33. Ibid.

34. J. A. Baudouin, "La vaccination antituberculeuse au B.C.G., résumé du rapport . . . ," *L'Union Médicale du Canada* 70 (1941): 750–751; 71 (1942): 375–378; 73 (1943): 826–830.

35. J. W. Hopkins, "BCG Vaccination in Montreal," *Am. Rev. TB* 43 (1941): 597.

36. See J. A. Baudouin, "Etude du BCG faite au Canada," in *Premier Congrès International du BCG* (Paris: Institut Pasteur, 1948), 213; A. Frappier and R. Guy, "The Use

of BCG," *CMAJ* 61 (1949): 18; A. Frappier, L. Frappier-Davignon, M. Cantin, and J. St.-Pierre, "Influence de la vaccination par le BCG sur la mortalité par méninige tuberculeuse des enfants de 0 à 10 ans dans la Province de Québec," *CMAJ* 86 (1962): 934–941.

37. CTA, *Annual Report* (1950), 23.

38. CTA, *Annual Report* (1924), 18; CTA, *Annual Report* (1925), 137.

39. A fine biography of Ferguson is provided by C. Stuart Houston, *R. G. Ferguson* (Toronto: Hannah/Dundurn, 1991).

40. CTA, *Annual Report* (1926), 15–17; NRCC, ACTR, *Report of the Second Meeting* (1925), 50, 175. A more complete discussion of Canadian efforts to confront the problems of tubercular disease in the native populations is provided in Wherrett, *Miracle of the Empty Beds*, chapter 7.

41. CTA, *Annual Report* (1926), 17.

42. The argument that tuberculosis was different diseases with many manifestations was used to explain the high mortality from tuberculosis in both black and Native American populations. In the case of Native Americans, environmental explanations usually predominated, but the question of a "separate disease" remained important. See Herbert A. Burns, "Tuberculosis in the Indian," *Am. Rev. TB* 26 (1932): 498–506; David A. Stewart, "The Red Man and the White Plague," in CTA, *Annual Report* (1936), 18–22. Some of the arguments that pertain to tuberculosis among blacks are summarized in Marion Torchia, "Tuberculosis among American Negroes: Medical Research on a Racial Disease, 1830–1950," *Journal of the History of Medicine and Allied Sciences* 32 (1977): 252–279; Marion Torchia, "The Tuberculosis Movement and the Race Question," *BHM* 49 (1975): 152–168.

43. R. G. Ferguson, "Tuberculosis Study among the Indians of Saskatchewan," in CTA, *Annual Report* (1928), 28.

44. CTA, *Annual Report* (1926), 17.

45. Wherrett, *Miracle of the Empty Beds*, 60–61. Among Canada's native peoples, infant mortality, an important general indicator of health status, had soared to over 1000/100,000 population.

46. R. G. Ferguson and A. B. Simes, "BCG Vaccination of Indian Infants in Saskatchewan," *Tubercle* 30 (1949): 7.

47. R. G. Ferguson, "Tuberculosis Research at the Fort Qu'Appelle Indian Health Unit," in CTA, *Annual Report* (1934), 20–21. The Indian Health Unit was established in 1930 with funds supplied jointly by the NRCC, the Department of Indian Affairs, and the Saskatchewan Anti-Tuberculosis League to "determine the value of practical preventive health measures in reducing the morbidity and mortality of tuberculosis among the Indians."

48. R. G. Ferguson, "Tuberculosis Research at the Fort Qu'Appelle Sanatorium," in CTA, *Annual Report* (1933), 25.

49. "Report of the Sub-committee on BCG," in CTA, *Annual Report* (1931), 26.

50. R. G. Ferguson, "Tuberculosis Research at the Qu'Appelle Indian Health Unit," in CTA, *Annual Report* (1935), 27–28.

51. Ferguson articulated this position in a variety of ways. Ferguson, "Tuberculosis Study among the Indians of Saskatchewan"; R. G. Ferguson, "BCG Vaccination in Hospitals and Sanatoria of Saskatchewan," *Am. Rev. TB* 54 (1946): 325–329.

52. Ferguson and Simes, "BCG Vaccination of Indian Infants," 6.

53. Noted in Ferguson, "BCG Vaccination in Hospitals and Sanatoria," 326.

54. Ibid., 337.

55. Ferguson and Simes, "BCG Vaccination of Indian Infants," 8.

56. Ibid, 10.

57. The federal tuberculosis-control budget devoted far less to vaccination programs between 1948 and 1953 than to sanatoria, diagnosis, and case finding. At most, 6 percent was spent. Still, the number of vaccinees increased dramatically, from 43,000 in 1947 to 74,000 in 1949. See "Number of BCG Vaccinations in Canada," in CTA, *Annual Report* (1949), 23; CTA, *Annual Report* (1953), 126–127.

58. Petroff, "New Analysis," 295.

59. J. A. Baudouin, "Vaccination contre la tuberculose par le BCG à Montréal," in *Vaccination préventive de la tuberculose de l'homme et des animaux par le BCG*, 6th ed. (Paris: Masson et Cie, 1932), 103–113. Also, Baudouin, "Vaccination against Tuberculosis," 20–26. For a more complete discussion of the significance of these trials, see Frappier, *Fifty Years of Study and Use of BCG,* especially 5–10.

60. Kereszturi and Park, "Oral Vaccination," 302.

61. Ibid., 305, and Kereszturi et al., "Clinical Study of BCG Vaccination," 378.

62. "Discussion of Preventive Vaccination," 10.

63. Kereszturi and Park, "Oral Vaccination," 305.

64. Ibid., 302.

65. Ibid., 305. In fact, the controls showed a slight advantage over the vaccinees. Nontuberculous mortality was 6.4 percent among the controls and 6.6 percent among the vaccinees or, when age-adjusted, 6.7 percent for controls to 9.1 percent for vaccinees. Ibid., 304.

66. Kereszturi et al., "Clinical Study of BCG Vaccination," 380.

67. Ibid.

68. Ibid., 379.

69. K. Birkhaug, "Discussion of C. Kereszturi and W. Park, et al., 'Clinical Study of BCG Vaccination,'" *New York State Journal of Medicine* 33 (1933): 381.

70. A brief discussion of tuberculosis among Native Americans is provided in McMurry, "'And I?'" 218–233.

71. Morton Keller, *Affairs of State* (Cambridge, Mass.: Harvard University Press, 1977), 457–461.

72. In 1912, Congress appropriated funds for a survey of the prevalence of TB and other diseases among Native Americans. This report highlighted the problem. Ralph Chester Williams, *The United States Public Health Service 1798–1950* (Washington, D.C.: Commissioned Officers Association of the United States Public Health Service, 1951), 422, 427. Contemporary and modern studies of tuberculosis among Native Americans are numerous. A good example is Ales Hrdlicka, *Tuberculosis among Certain Indian Tribes of the U.S.* (Washington, D.C.: GPO, 1909).

73. U.S. Congress, Senate, *Report of the National Tuberculosis Association to U.S. Senate on Tuberculosis among North American Indians,* 67th Cong., 4th sess., 1923. The NTA commission on tuberculosis among the Indians immediately cited "economic conditions" as the major cause of high mortality.

74. Reported in J. G. Townsend, Joseph D. Aronson, Robert Saylor, and Irma Parr, "Tuberculosis Control among the North American Indians," *Am. Rev. TB* 45 (1942): 43.

75. William Hallock Park to Eugene Opie, September 26, 1935; Eugene Opie, Oscar Scholls, and James Miller, "Report of Subcommittee on the Proposal for B.C.G. Vaccination Experiment," 1935, Opie Papers, file: "Tuberculosis, Public Health Committee."

76. Eugene Opie to Albert Calmette, December 22, 1930, Opie Papers, file: "BCG Vaccine"; Calmette to Opie, November 22, 1930, Opie Papers, file: "BCG Vaccine."

77. Eugene Opie, "Report on Study of Protective Inoculation against Tuberculosis in Jamaica," n.d. [post-1940], Opie Papers, file: "Opie, E. L."

78. Long Interview; a representative sample of Long's papers include: E. R. Long and F. Seibert, "Tuberculin and the Tuberculin Reaction," *Trans. NTA* 16 (1925): 388; E. R. Long and F. Seibert, "Tuberculin: Chemical Composition of the Active Principle and the Nature of the Tuberculin Reaction," *JAMA* 85 (1925): 650; E. R. Long and F. Seibert, "Chemical Composition of the Active Principle and Nature of the Tuberculin Reaction, I–VI," *Am. Rev. TB* 13 (1936): 393. Long's own work on the nutrition and metabolism of the tubercle bacillus includes E. R. Long, "Chemical Problems in the Bacteriology of the Tubercle Bacillus," *Am. Rev. TB* 5 (1921): 705; E. R. Long, "The Nutrition of Acid-Fast Bacteria," *Am. Rev. TB* 5 (1921): 857; E. R. Long, "A Chemical View of the Pathogenesis of Tuberculosis," *Am. Rev. TB* 22 (1930): 467.

79. Long Interview, 50.

80. E. R. Long and H. W. Hetherington, "A Tuberculosis Survey in the Papago Indian Area of Southern Arizona," *Am. Rev. TB* 33 (1936): 407. See also E. R. Long, "A Brief Comparison of Tuberculosis in the White, Indian and Negro Races," *Am. Rev. TB* 35 (1937): 1–5.

81. E. R. Long, "Tuberculosis Control in Indians and Negroes—A Report to Surgeon General L. R. Thompson," May 3, 1937, NA RG 443, Box 110.

82. J. D. Aronson, "Protective Vaccination against Tuberculosis with Special Reference to BCG Vaccination," *Am. Rev. TB* 58 (1948): 261.

83. Ibid.

84. Townsend, Aronson, et al., "Tuberculosis Control," 51.

85. Ibid.

86. J. D. Aronson and Carroll E. Palmer, "Experience with BCG Vaccine in the Control of Tuberculosis among North American Indians," *Public Health Reports* 61 (1946): 819–820. Aronson wrote more favorable and less inhibited reports of his trial to Opie. See letters from J. D. Aronson to Eugene Opie, 1942–1946, Opie Papers, file: "Aronson." See also the progress reports presented to the director of NIH, January 22, 1938, December 24, 1938, June 30, 1939, December 31, 1939, April 30, 1940, NA RG 443, Box 110.

87. Aronson and Palmer, "Experience with BCG Vaccine," 811.

88. Anthony M. Lowell, *Tuberculosis* (Cambridge, Mass.: Harvard University Press, (1969), 68–69. Mortality in nonwhite males dropped from 194/100,000 in 1930 to 139/100,000 in 1940. In nonwhite females, it dropped from 189/100,000 in 1930 to 117/100,000 in 1940. This decline may be misleading however. Data on infection rates are hard to come by, but the new case rate during this period rose from 78/100,000 to 91/100,000 (ibid., 46). While the new-case rate is in many ways a reflection of patterns of reporting, it should also be closely tied to the infection rate.

89. Editorial, "BCG Vaccination against Tuberculosis," *Public Health Reports* (June 7, 1946): 801–802. These concerns are raised most forcefully in correspondence among Aronson, Long, and Opie. Letters from J. D. Aronson to E. R. Long, Long Papers; letters from J. D. Aronson to Eugene Opie, Opie Papers, file: "Aronson."

90. J. D. Aronson and C. F. Aronson, "Appraisal of the Protective Value of BCG Vaccination," *JAMA* 149 (1952): 334.

91. J. D. Aronson and Helen C. Taylor, "The Trend of Tuberculous Infection among Some Indian Tribes and the Influence of BCG Vaccination on the Tuberculin Test," *Am. Rev. TB* 72 (1955): 35.

92. Townsend, Aronson, et al., "Tuberculosis Control," 43–44.

93. Ibid., 46.

94. Aronson and Taylor, "Trend of Tuberculosis," 53.

95. Baudouin, admittedly, did not provide extensive data on the background of his subjects, but case histories and socioeconomic data were available, and Baudouin did

endeavor to match his subjects and controls closely. See Baudouin references in note 34 above.

96. M. Levine and M. Sackett, "Results of BCG Immunization in New York City," *Am. Rev. TB* 53 (1946): 530.

97. Ibid., 523–525.

CHAPTER 6: "NOT A SUBSTITUTE FOR APPROVED HYGIENIC MEASURES"

1. Milton I. Roemer, "Tuberculosis and Its Control in Rural Areas," *Public Health Reports* 64 (October 7, 1949): 1269.

2. Ibid.

3. Personal communication, Dr. George Comstock, August 1985; Bess Furman, *A Profile of the United States Public Health Service* (Bethesda, Md.: NIH, 1973), 410–411.

4. The new-case rate per 100,000—based on reporting from forty-eight states and the District of Columbia—rose from 79.3 in 1941 to 87.5 in 1942 and to 95 in 1944. The death rate per 100,000 for the same area declined from 44.5 in 1941 to 43.1 in 1942 and to 41.2 in 1944. This represented an average rate of decline of 2.5 percent per annum as compared to an average rate of decline of 5 percent per annum in the five years between 1936 and 1940. See Lowell, *Tuberculosis*, 46, Table 3.2.

5. Williams, *United States Public Health Service*, 640: "the disease most frequently discovered at the time of inspection was pulmonary tuberculosis."

6. Esmond R. Long and Seymour Jablon, *Tuberculosis in the Army of the United States in World War II* (Washington, D.C.: GPO, 1955), 1.

7. On July 3, 1939, Congressman Warren Magnuson forwarded to the surgeon general a petition that he had received in support of Bill S. 2547. Signed by numerous constituents from Seattle, the petition called for prompt action on the question of "a separate tuberculosis commission for the control of tuberculosis." See Thomas Parran to Warren G. Magnuson, July 8, 1939, NA RG 90-0425, Box 51. Over the next five years, the surgeon general continued to receive correspondence of this kind. See also Residents of San Antonio, Jr. Chamber of Commerce to Thomas Parran, March 4, 1941, NA RG 90-0425, Box 51.

8. Stephen B. Gibbons, acting Secretary of the Treasury, to Pat Harrison, chairman of the Senate Committee on Finance, re: S. 2547, June 30, 1939, NA RG 90-0425, Box 51.

9. Parran to Magnuson, July 8, 1939.

10. Ibid.

11. Ibid. Parran's view was not atypical. Long similarly linked tuberculosis control to "public relief" and, on these grounds, believed that "as a matter of principle" TB control "is largely a *state* responsibility. But travelling transient problem is certainly Federal." See Holmer Folks to E. R. Long, January 31, 1938, with Long response attached, Long Papers, Box 5.

12. Letters from Thomas Parran, re: H.R. 3968, March 12 and 18, 1941, NA RG 90-0425, Box 51.

13. Ibid.

14. Bills H.R. 3463 and H.R. 3492 (1941) both addressed the issue of a separate tuberculosis-control section. Parran's memos and correspondence on this subject are included in NA RG 90-0425, Box 51.

15. Memo from Herman Hilleboe to Thomas Parran, "Tuberculosis Control Program of the Public Health Service," December 15, 1942, NA RG 90-0425, Box 51.

16. Thomas Parran, "Health Is Everybody's Business," 1944, preliminary unpub-

lished draft of Parran, "New Horizons in Public Health," June 15, 1945, 18, in "Parran Speeches," Pritchard Papers, Box 4, National Library of Medicine, Washington, D.C. See also Thomas Parran, "Report of the Surgeon General," in U.S. Federal Security Agency, *Annual Report of the USPHS* (*Ann. Rpt. USPHS*) (1944), v–vi.

17. U.S. Congress, "An Act to Consolidate and Revise the Laws Relating to the Public Health Service . . . " (hereafter referred to as the PHS Act), 78th Cong., 2d sess., July 1, 1944, *U.S. Statutes at Large* 58 (1944), Public Law 410, sec. 314(b), ch. 373, 693–694; see also Parran, "Report of the Surgeon General," ix.

18. Allan Brandt, *No Magic Bullet: A Social History of Venereal Disease in the United States* (Oxford: Oxford University Press, 1986), chapter 4.

19. Parran, "Report of the Surgeon General," 8–9.

20. U.S. Federal Security Agency, "Report of the Tuberculosis Control Division," *Ann. Rpt. USPHS* (1945), 107.

21. Parran, "New Horizons in Public Health," June 15, 1945, Pritchard Papers, Box 4. In an earlier version of this speech, "Health Is Everybody's Business," Parran put the point more bluntly: "Full employment, with a continuing high level of national income, is an inseparable factor in progress toward better national health. So also are programs of healthful housing and improved nutrition." See also Parran, "Report to the Surgeon General," 18.

22. The chairman of the ACTR, H. M. Tory, was president of the NRCC, and most of the committee members were research scientists. See NRCC, ACTR, *Report of the First Meeting* (1924), 1–2.

23. Born in Minnesota in 1903, Palmer took his undergraduate degrees in chemistry and biology at the local Hamline University. He completed a Ph.D. in anatomy with subfields in pediatrics and biostatistics in 1929, then moved to Johns Hopkins. He later became a consultant to the Child Hygiene Office of the PHS, where he contributed extensively to the Hagerstown studies of the growth and development of children. He later moved to the Tuberculosis Control Division. See George Comstock, "Ripples in a Pond: How the Work of One Scientist Can Influence Public Health around the World," Delta Omega Lecture, April 6, 1982. I thank Dr. Comstock for generously providing his time and a typescript of that lecture.

24. U.S. Federal Security Agency," Report of the Tuberculosis Control Division" (1945), 107.

25. Ibid.

26. Nicholson, *20 Years of Medical Research*, 63.

27. A formal statement of the goals of the division is presented in PHS Act, chs. 371–373, 682–706. A summary of this legislation is also provided in Williams, *United States Public Service*, and Bess Furman, *A Profile of the United States Public Health Service*.

28. Williams, *United States Public Health Service*, 542.

29. "Report of a Conference on BCG Vaccination," September 7, 1946, 1–2, NA RG 90-62A-177, Box 7.

30. Ibid., 3.

31. "Report of a Conference on BCG Vaccination—Conclusions and Recommendations," 1946, NA RG 90-62A-177, Box 7.

32. Ibid.

33. J. Arthur Myers, "Exterminating Tuberculosis," *National Education Association Journal*, 12 (1923): 50.

34. Ibid.

35. J. Arthur Myers and Francis E. Harrington, "The Effect of Initial Tuberculous Infection on Subsequent Tuberculous Lesions," *JAMA* 103 (1934): 1535.

36. G. W. McCoy to H. S. Cumming, September 1, 1931. NA RG 90-0470-132, Box 70.

37. "Tuberculosis Control: Report of Assistant Commissioner Robert Plunket," in New York State, Department of Health, *Annual Report* (1946), 19.

38. New York State, Department of Health, *Annual Report* (1946), 74.

39. New York State, Department of Health, *Annual Report* (1947), 72.

40. Ibid.

41. U.S. Federal Security Agency, "Report of the Tuberculosis Control Division" (1947), 416–417.

42. "Tuberculosis Mortality Relationships—Age, Race and Sex, 1947," *Public Health Reports* 64 (October 7, 1949): 1261–1269; Milton I. Roemer, "Tuberculosis and Its Control in Rural Areas," *Public Health Reports* 64 (1949): 1269–1278.

43. Tuberculosis remained a much more serious disease among blacks. See M. H. Burke, H. C. Schenck and J. A. Thrash, "Tuberculosis Studies in Muscogee County, Georgia. II. X-Ray Findings in a Community-wide Survey and Its Coverage as Determined by a Population Census," *Public Health Reports* 64 (March 4, 1949): 263–290, especially 269–272. For discussion of social determinants, see Roemer, "Tuberculosis," 1272; George W. Comstock, "Tuberculosis Studies in Muscogee County, Georgia," *Public Health Reports* 64 (March 4, 1949): 260.

44. Roemer, "Tuberculosis," 1269.

45. Ibid., 1271.

46. Ibid.

47. Pastor J. Rodriguez and J. L. Janer, "Tuberculosis in the Island of Puerto Rico," *Am. Rev. TB* 67 (1953): 132.

48. Roemer, "Tuberculosis," 1270. For later data, see also Lowell, *Tuberculosis*, 79.

49. Comstock, "Tuberculosis Studies in Muscogee," 260.

50. This debate is best presented in an interchange between E. R. Long and L. L. Lumsden, medical director of the New Orleans office of the PHS, that took place in August 1938. See Lumsden to Long, August 27, 1938, and Long to Lumsden, August 29, 1938, Long Papers, Box. 15.

51. Carroll Palmer and Thomas B. McKneely, "Preliminary Report of the Hagerstown Tuberculosis Conference," 1938, especially 1–3, 17–18, Long Papers, Box 15. See also "Minutes of the Hagerstown Tuberculosis Conference, September 26–October 1, 1938," Long Papers, Box 15; "The Hagerstown Tuberculosis Conference of 1938: A Retrospective Opinion" (editorial), *American Review of Respiratory Diseases* 99 (1969): 119–120.

52. Lumsden to Long, August 27, 1938, 2, Long Papers, Box 15.

53. Hilleboe to Myers, July 29, 1944, NA RG 90-0425, Box 51.

54. Because they presumed that sensitivity to tuberculin afforded some protection, Canadians recommended BCG vaccination for tuberculin-negative nurses. See R. G. Ferguson, "BCG Vaccination in Hospitals and Sanatoria of Saskatchewan," *Am. Rev. TB* 54 (1946): 325–339; G. F. Kincade, "BCG Vaccination Program for Student Nurses in British Columbia," *Canadian Nurse* 49 (1953):110–113. The same policy was advocated in some parts of the United States. In 1940, Rosenthal began to vaccinate student nurses at the Cook County Hospital (Illinois). Sol Roy Rosenthal, "Recent Advances in BCG Vaccine," presented to 1955 BCG Conference, October 17, 1955, NA RG 90-62A-177, Box 7. In 1949, BCG was recommended for nurses entering training in Boston, Lewiston (Maine), and Washington D.C. U.S. Federal Security Agency, *Ann. Rep. USPHS* (1949), 121. It had also become "routine practice in New York to BCG vaccinate tuberculin negative student nurses, medical students and hospital personnel." New York State, Department of Health, *Annual Report* (1949), 13.

55. Lawrence W. Shaw, "Field Studies on Immunization against Tuberculosis. I: Tuberculin Allergy Following BCG Vaccination of School Children in Muscogee County, Georgia," *Public Health Reports* 66 (1951): 1416.

56. Ibid., 1420.

57. An induration of 5 mm or more was considered a positive response. The majority of the subjects had reactions of "erythema only" or of less than 5 mm. Ibid., 1420.

58. Ibid., 1421–1422.

59. Johannes Holm, "General Introduction to Field Operations," *Second Annual Report of the International Tuberculosis Campaign* (Copenhagen, 1950), 123; Shaw, "Field Studies," 1422.

60. Shaw, "Field Studies," 1424.

61. Ibid., 1422.

62. Carroll E. Palmer, Lawrence W. Shaw, and George W. Comstock, "Community Trials of BCG Vaccination," *Am. Rev. TB* 77 (1958): 877–907, especially 878–879.

63. Carroll E. Palmer and Lawrence W. Shaw, "Present Status of BCG Studies," *Am. Rev. TB* 68 (1953): 465.

64. Ibid. The data are unclear. Palmer and Shaw report that mortality was 1/700 for the controls and 4/4,500 for the vaccinees. Adjusted per 1000 population, these rates would be 1.42 for the controls and 0.89 for the vaccinees. The authors do not indicate whether the percentage difference might be significant. Moreover, twice as many vaccinees as controls participated in the study, but the rates seem not to have been adjusted for population.

65. Palmer and Shaw, "Present Status," 466.

66. Ibid., 465.

67. Wade Hampton Frost, "Age Selection of Mortality from Tuberculosis in Successive Decades" (1939), in Kenneth F. Maxcy, ed., *Papers of Wade Hampton Frost, M.D.: A Contribution to Epidemiological Method* (New York: Commonwealth Fund, 1941), 600. See also Wade Hampton Frost, "How Much Control of Tuberculosis?" (1937), in Maxcy, *Papers of Wade Hampton Frost*, 602–612.

68. Frost, "Age Selection," 594.

69. "Editorial: BCG Vaccination against Tuberculosis," *Public Health Reports* 61 (June 7, 1946): 802.

70. Palmer and Shaw, "Present Status," 466.

71. Frost, "How Much Control," 607.

72. Comstock, "Tuberculosis Studies in Muscogee" 260.

73. Ibid., 262.

74. U.S. Congress, House, Committee on Interstate and Foreign Commerce, *Health Inquiry*, 81st Cong., 2d sess., 1953, 552.

75. Ibid., 557.

76. Ibid., 576.

77. Ibid., 578–579.

78. U.S. Federal Security Agency, *Ann. Rept. USPHS* (1949), 117.

79. U.S. Federal Security Agency, *Ann. Rept. USPHS* (1952), 56.

80. Ibid.

81. U.S. Congress, *Health Inquiry*, 584.

82. Ibid.

83. New York State, Department of Health, "Report of the Director of the Division of Laboratories and Research," *Annual Report of the Division of Laboratories and Research* (1953), 3–4.

84. Memo from David Gold, senior assistant surgeon general, Tuberculosis Control Division, to George R. Groppe, U.S. Maritime Commission, July 24, 1944, and Thomas Parran to W. T. Harrison, medical director, PHS District 5, California, November 28, 1944, NA RG 90-0425, Box 51.

85. In the years immediately following its release, physicians disagreed about the ways in which streptomycin worked. Though it was generally recognized to be bactericidal, some researchers—Dubos among them—also believed that streptomycin had bacteriostatic action. See R. Dubos, *Bacterial and Mycotic Infections of Man*, 2d ed. (Philadelphia: Lippincott, 1952), 344.

86. Shirley H. Ferebee to J. Burns Amberson, October 20, 1948, Long Papers, Box 15; also, personal communication, August 30, 1985.

87. NIH, Steering Committee of Tuberculosis Study Section, "Statement of Policy on Cooperative Clinical Streptomycin Evaluation in Therapy of Pulmonary Tuberculosis," n.d. Long Papers, [presumed 1948], Box 15.

88. C. E. Sunderlin, "Technical Memorandum on the Chemotherapy of Tuberculosis," March 1, 1949, 5, Long Papers, Box 7.

89. A concise explanation of the effects of streptomycin and PAS is provided in Dubos, *Bacterial and Mycotic Infections*, 344–345, 771–772.

90. Walsh McDermott to E. R. Long, March 7, 1947, Long Papers, Box 6.

91. McDermott to Long (1947), 2.

92. "PHS Tuberculosis Program Report: Mrs. Ferebee's Comments: Meeting of Committee on Co-operation [of the NTA] with Federal Agencies," September 13, 1955, NA RG 90-62A-177, Box 7. A full account of the preventative and therapeutic actions of isoniazid is provided in the United States Pharmaceutical Industry, *Drug Information for the Health Care Practitioner*, 7th ed. (1987), 1034–1036; see also *The Physicians Desk Reference*, 42nd ed. (Montvale, N.J.: Medical Economics Data Service, (1987), 869–870.

93. U.S. Federal Security Agency, *Ann. Rept. USPHS* (1954), 147–148.

94. U.S. Federal Security Agency, *Ann. Rept. USPHS* (1955), 123; also, Memo to members of the 14th Conference on the Chemotherapy of Tuberculosis from the Committee on the Chemotherapy of Tuberculosis, Veterans Administration Central Office, "Account of the Conference, February 23, 1955," especially 2–3, 6–8, NA RG 90-62A-177, Box 7.

95. E. R. Long to James Perkins, June 2, 1966, Long Papers, Box 5.

96. See, for example, James J. Waring, "Impact of Modern Therapy on Tuberculosis," *JAMA* 161 (1956): 1368–1371. Also, Herman Hilleboe and Robert E. Plunkett, Division of Tuberculosis Control, State of New York Department of Health, to county, city, and district health officers, "Current Concepts on the Drug Treatment of Nonhospitalized Tuberculosis Patients," March 9, 1955, especially 5, NA RG 90-62A-177, Box 7.

97. Waring, "Impact of Modern Therapy," 1370.

98. J. D. Aronson and C. F. Aronson, "Appraisal of Protective Value of BCG Vaccination," *JAMA* 149 (1952): 334; Samuel Stein and J. D. Aronson, "The Occurrence of Pulmonary Lesions in BCG Vaccinated and Unvaccinated Persons," *Am. Rev. TB* 68 (1953): 699–709; J. D. Aronson and Helen C. Taylor, "The Trend of Tuberculosis Infection among Some Indian Tribes and the Influence of BCG Vaccination on the Tuberculin Test," *Am. Rev. TB.* 72 (1955): 35-52.

99. See R. J. Anderson to Leonard Scheele, surgeon general, re: "BCG Conference, New York City (1955)," October 17, 1955, August 15, 1955, January 13, 1956, NA RG 90-62A-177, Box 7.

100. Ibid.

101. Because the PHS did not sponsor Rosenthal's trials, they have not been included in this discussion. See Sol Roy Rosenthal, *BCG Vaccine against Tuberculosis* (Boston and Toronto: Little, Brown, 1957); Rosenthal, "Recent Advances."

102. Anderson to Scheele, August 15, 1955, NA RG 90-62A-177, Box 7. Two years later, when the PHS organized yet another meeting on BCG, participants addressed

the question of Rosenthal's impartiality specifically. Reporting to his superiors on a conversation he had had about "possible participants in a future meeting on BCG vaccination," Bloomquist, medical director of the Tuberculosis Program, wrote: "Dr. Sol Rosenthal's name was mentioned at the end of the conversation. I gained the impression that Dr. Cogeshall felt that he need not be invited because of his vested interest in BCG." E. T. Bloomquist to Chief, Bureau of State Services, and Chief, Tuberculosis Program, January 4, 1957, NA RG 90-62A-177, Box 7.

103. More compelling were data that Palmer began to collect after 1956. By screening large numbers of Navy recruits, school children, college students, and adults, Palmer found a "low rate of tuberculin reactors among almost all the young people tested." These findings were not presented until the 1960s, however, and the extent of the decline in reactivity is hard to gauge. See Lydia B. Edwards and Carroll E. Palmer, "Tuberculous Infection," in American Public Health Association, *Tuberculosis* (1969), 125-179, especially 176.

104. J. A. Myers, "Pathogenesis of Tuberculosis," *JAMA* 161 (1956): 1386. See also J. A. Myers, "A Summary of the Views Opposing BCG," *Advances in Tuberculosis Research* 8 (1957): 272–303.

105. Palmer and Shaw, "Present Status," 465–466.

106. The best summary of the Puerto Rico trial is provided in Palmer, Shaw, and Comstock, "Community Trials," 877–907, especially 886–896, 904.

107. Palmer and Shaw, "Present Status," 462.

108. J. D. Aronson, "The Status of BCG Vaccination in the United States and Canada," *Advances in Tuberculosis Research* 8 (1957): 150–151.

109. Opie to Aronson, handwritten response below Aronson to Opie, June 19, 1958, Opie Papers, file: "Aronson." Similar sentiments were voiced on many occasions. Long, in a much later letter, best summarized the position. "Since so much is made of the loss of the tuberculin test as an indicator of infection," he wrote to Rosenthal, "in the opinion of many persons, this has not been proved to the detriment claimed by some to be the case, and that other, nontuberculous infections, acquired spontaneously, and widely prevalent, have a similar effect." Esmond Long to Sol Roy Rosenthal, June 6, 1967, Long Papers, Box 5.

110. Myers and Harrington, "Effect of Initial Tuberculous," 1535.

111. Carroll E. Palmer, "Tuberculin Sensitivity and Contact with Tuberculosis: Further Evidence of Non-specific Sensitivity," *Am. Rev. TB* 68 (1953): 678.

112. Ibid.

113. Aronson, "The Status of BCG," 131–153.

114. Palmer, Shaw, and Comstock, "Community Trials," 877–907, especially 880–883.

115. Ibid., 884.

116. For a discussion of the Swedish trial, see "Tuberculosis in Sweden and the Fight against It in Recent Years," *Public Health Reports* 61 (June 7, 1946): 828. Palmer's concerns about this method are presented in Palmer and Shaw, "Present Status"; also, personal communication, Shirley Ferebee Woolpert, August 30, 1985.

117. Quoted in Palmer and Shaw, "Present Status," 462.

118. Palmer, Shaw, and Comstock, "Community Trials," 878.

119. See M. Greenwood, "Professor Calmette's Statistical Study of BCG Vaccine," *BMJ* (1928), 793; "Editorial," *BMJ* (1933), 571. Brief historical accounts of the use of BCG in Great Britain are provided in Linda Bryder, *Below the Magic Mountain* (Oxford: Oxford University Press, 1988), 138–142, 243–245, 264–265; F. B. Smith, *The Retreat of Tuberculosis* (London: Croom Helm, 1988), 194–203.

120. "BCG and Vole Bacillus Vaccines in the Prevention of Tuberculosis in Adoles-

cents—First (Progress) Report to the Medical Research Council by Their Tuberculosis Vaccines Clinical Trials Committee," *BMJ* (1956), 413–427.

121. Ad Hoc Advisory Committee on BCG to the Surgeon General, June 14, 1957, NA RG 90-62A-177, Box 7.

122. Ibid.

123. "Present Policy of the American Trudeau Society on BCG Vaccination," *Am. Rev. TB* 57 (1948): 544.

124. Ibid., 545.

125. "Ibid., 544.

126. Edward T. Bloomquist, medical director, Tuberculosis Program, "Trip Report," September 13–16, 1956, NA RG 90-62A-177, Box 7.

127. "Statement of Ad Hoc Advisory Committee on BCG," June 1957, NA RG 90-62A-177, Box 7.

128. Ibid. Also, "Statement of the Ad Hoc Advisory Group on BCG Vaccination, 1957," *Am. Rev. TB* 76 (1957): 728. This statement was later quoted in "PHS Recommendations on the Use of BCG in the U.S.," *Mortality and Morbidity Weekly Report* (October 15, 1966): 350.

129. "BCG and Vole Bacillus Vaccines in the Prevention of Tuberculosis in Adolescents—Second (Progress) Report to the Medical Research Council by Their Tuberculosis Vaccines Clinical Trials Committee," *BMJ* 2 (1959): 379–396; "BCG and Vole Bacillus Vaccines in the Prevention of Tuberculosis in Adolescence and Early Adult Life—Third (Progress) Report to the Medical Research Council by Their Tuberculosis Vaccines Clinical Trials Committee," *BMJ* 1 (1963): 973–978.

130. John Davies, "BCG Vaccination—Its Place in Canada," *Canadian Journal of Public Health* 56 (1965): 252.

131. USDHEW, *Arden House,* 5–6.

132. Ibid, especially 1–5.

133. "Appropriations and Budgets, 1945-1960," NA RG 90 64A-645, Box 387.

134. Personal communication, Shirley Ferebee Woolpert, August 30, 1985.

135. Hilleboe and Plunkett, "Current Concepts," 6.

136. U.S. Federal Security Agency, *Ann. Rep. USPHS* (1959), 123.

137. "Public Health Service Recommendations on the Use of BCG Vaccination in the United States," *Morbidity and Mortality Weekly Report* (October 15, 1966): 350.

138. Cited in Jerry Brimberry, acting director, Tuberculosis Control Section, Kentucky Department of Health to John C. Taylor, commissioner, Department of Corrections, February 8, 1971, NA RG 90-73E-0058, Box 107. On the costs of screening programs and other services, see also "Statement on Changes in State Policies on Mass Casefinding for Tuberculosis," October 24, 1958, especially 7–8, NA RG 90-64A-645, Box 387; USDHEW, *Tuberculosis in the United States, Status of the Disease in the Early Sixties,* PHS Publication 1036 (Washington, D.C.: GPO, 1963), especially 23–24.

139. NIH, "Statement of Policy"; see also discussions of streptomycin in Long Papers.

140. McDermott to Long, March 7, 1947, 2–3, Long Papers.

141. Ibid., 2.

142. Hilleboe and Plunkett, "Current Concepts," 3.

143. Robert Anderson, "New Drugs for Tuberculosis: Information for Professional Staff," March 18, 1952, RG 90-68A-2748, Box 1. See also USDHEW, "Report of the Meeting of the Tuberculosis Control Officers and Sanatorium Directors, May 1955," NA RG 90-62A-177, Box 7.

144. Hilleboe and Plunkett, "Current Concepts," 3.

145. Waring, "Impact of Modern Therapy," 1369.

146. James W. Raleigh, "Chemotherapy Rings the TB Bell," *American Lung Association Bulletin* (March 1982): 17: "Until the 1960s drug therapy for tuberculosis had been considered an adjunct to the basic bed-rest treatment at hospitals and sanatoriums. As patients improved dramatically and consistently on chemotherapy, the amount of decreed rest in a patient's day decreased."

147. Ibid. Physicians prescribed drug therapy with rest more than twice as often as either drug therapy or rest alone. See Paul A. Pamplona, senior surgeon, Tuberculosis Program, PHS, "The Problems and Challenges of Tuberculosis Control" (paper presented at the annual meeting of the Massachusetts Tuberculosis and Health Society, Boston, May 11, 1956), 9. NA RG 90-62A-177, Box 7.

148. Pan American Health Organization, Advisory Committee on Medical Research, "Re-evaluation of Research Needs in Tuberculosis," *Proceedings of the Second Meeting of the Pan American Health Organization,* June 17–21, 1963 (Washington, D.C.), 10.

149. USDHEW, *Arden House*, 5.

150. Hilleboe and Plunkett, "Current Concepts," 4.

151. Ibid.

152. Ibid.

153. Ibid.

154. "Present Policy," 544.

CONCLUSION

1. Timothy Beardsley, "Paradise Lost? Microbes Mount a Comeback as Drug Resistance Spreads," *Scientific American* 26 (November 1992): 18–20; Ken Chowder, "TB: The Disease That Rose from Its Grave," *Smithsonian* 23 (November 1992): 180–196. See also a series of articles in the *New York Times* (October 11–15, 1993).

2. "TB Easily transmitted, Adds a Peril to Medicine," *New York Times* (October 12, 1992), 1, B2.

3. "Confinement for TB: Weighing Rights vs. Health," *New York Times* (November 21, 1993), A1, 45.

4. Jerry L. Brimberry, acting director, Tuberculosis Control Section, Kentucky Department of Health, "INH Prison Study," February 8, 1971, NA RG 90-73E-0058, Box 107.

5. Hilleboe and Plunkett, "Current Concepts," 5.

6. Andrew Theodore to Shirley Ferebee, April 19, 1967, NA RG 90-73E-0058, Box 107.

7. "New Drug Resistant TB Strain Appears: Officials Fear American-Style Outbreak," *Winnipeg Free Press* (August 15, 1992), A3; "Deadly, Untreatable TB Strain Plaguing US Puts Canadian Health Officials on Red Alert," *Montreal Gazette* (October 4, 1992), A1, A6; "Ottawa to Vaccinate Prisoners against TB," *Montreal Gazette* (November 2, 1992). The *CMAJ* also reprinted an earlier article on the use of BCG. Armand Frappier and Roland Guy, "Use of BCG," *CMAJ* 146 (1992): 529-535; originally *CMAJ* 61 (1949): 18–24.

8. *New York Times* (October 15, 1992), B4.

9. "Scientists Crack Code of Organism Causing TB," *Toronto Globe and Mail* (September 10, 1993), A10.

10. In Canada, in 1945, the tuberculous death rate stood at 48/100,000; in the United States it was 38/100,000. By 1951, the two rates had met, and, in 1960, the Canadian death rate had dropped to 4.6/100,000 while the American rate remained at 6.0/100,000. Lowell, *Tuberculosis*, 96–97; Lowell does not provide the base for the 1960 rate, but one presumes that it is 100,000.

11. Canadian and American sources differ on this point. See John W. Davies, "BCG Vaccination—Its Place in Canada," *Canadian Journal of Public Health* 56 (1965): passim. Compare Lowell, *Tuberculosis*, 95, and U.S. Federal Security Agency, *Ann. Rep. USPHS* (1952), 56.

12. In 1955, the death rate among Native Americans was reported at 46/100,000 and among Alaskans at 100/100,000. U.S. Federal Security Agency, *Ann. Rep. USPHS* (1957), 118; Lowell, *Tuberculosis*; USDHEW, *Tuberculosis in the United States: Status of the Disease in the Early Sixties*, PHS Publication 1036 (Washington, D.C.: GPO, 1964). Compare George Jasper Wherrett, *The Miracle of the Empty Beds* (Toronto: University of Toronto Press, 1977), 252.

13. Davies, "BCG Vaccination," 252.

14. Ibid.

15. James Patterson, *America's Struggle against Poverty* (Cambridge, Mass.: Harvard University Press, 1981), chapter 12. See also Sidney Fine, *Laissez Faire and the General Welfare State: A Study of Conflict in American Thought* (Ann Arbor: University of Michigan Press, 1976), chapter 10; Roy Lubove, *The Struggle for Social Security* (Cambridge, Mass., Harvard University Press, 1968), especially the introduction by Oscar Handlin; Stephen Skowroneck, *Building a New American State: The Expansion of National Administrative Capacities, 1877–1936* (Cambridge and New York: Cambridge University Press, 1982); Samuel H. Beer, "In Search of a New Public Philosophy," in Anthony King, ed., *The New American Political System* (Washington, D.C.: American Enterprise Institute, 1978). Beer argues that New Deal programs, like earlier programs of reform, attempted to effect change not by charity but by the redistribution of power. They were designed to enable individuals to improve their own lot. See also Morton Keller, *Affairs of State* (Cambridge, Mass.: Harvard University Press, 1977), 600, where it is argued that the New Deal failed to resolve many of the earlier tensions that had marked American social reform.

16. Linda Bryder, "Papworth Village Settlement—A Unique Experiment in the Treatment and Care of Tuberculosis?" *Medical History* 28 (1984): 372-390; also informative but less concise is E. M. Breiger, *The Papworth Families: A 25 Year Survey* (London: Heinemann, 1944).

17. Dalhgren's proposal and reactions to it are summarized in PHS correspondence, September to December 1954. See especially Robert Anderson to Congressman Edgar Hiestand, California, December 3, 1954, NA RG 90-62A-177, Box 7.

18. Paul A. Pamplona, "Letter from William Dahlgren," September 9, 1954, NA RG 90-62A-177, Box 7.

19. Edward T. Bloomquist to William Frank Oechsli, public health analyst, Los Angeles County Tuberculosis and Health Association, December 23, 1954, NA RG 90-62A-177, Box 7.

20. U.S. Federal Security Agency, *Ann. Rept. USPHS* (1951), 150.

21. Leonard Scheele, "Report of the Surgeon General," in U.S. Federal Security Agency, *Ann. Rept. PHS* (1949), 7.

22. See, for example, Hilleboe and Plunkett, "Current Concepts," passim, but especially 4. Also, Robert Anderson, "Tuberculois Morbidity and Mortality—The Situation Today" (draft of a paper presented to the Annual Meeting of the NTA, May 1955), 3–4. NA RG 90-62A-177, Box 7.

23. "Minutes of the NTA-PHS Joint Staff Meeting, June 18, 1957," 2, NA RG 90-62A-177, Box 7.

24. For a discussion of inequities in the provision of medical services, see David E. Rogers and Eli Ginzberg, eds., *Medical Care and the Health of the Poor* (Boulder, Colo.: Westview Press, 1993).

25. "Infections by Health Worker Spur Tuberculosis Warning," *Toronto Globe and Mail* (August 12, 1994), A5.

Index

bacteriologic revolution, 4, 37, 44, 48, 81, 218n15

ACTR, *see* Associate Committee on Tuberculosis Research

Adirondack Cottage Sanitarium, *see* Saranac Lake, Trudeau Sanitarium

administrative control, *see* state

African Americans, *see* blacks

agrarianism, 6, 7, 25, 27, 30, 91

AIDS, 1, 6, 7, 214

allopaths, 15

American Climatological Association, 46

American exceptionalism, *see* nationalism

American Medical Association (AMA), 39, 43, 48, 74

American Public Health Association (APHA), 30, 39, 43, 46, 51

American Trudeau Society (ATS), 3, 196

Anderson, Robert, 184, 192–193, 205, 212

antibiotics, 194–196, 202–207, 212; costs of, 203; and drug-resistant tubercle bacilli, 196, 208; toxicity of, 194, 195, 202

antiphthisin, Klebs, 72

antitoxins, *see* vaccines: antitoxic

Arden House (Harriman, N.Y.), 202

Aronson, J. D., 169–174, 181, 198, 192, 199

Associate Committee on Tuberculosis Research (ACTR), 126, 140–141, 158–159, 163–165, 180, 213, 249n82

Atkinson, Thomas, 26, 27

bacteria, *see* bacteriology; germs; tubercle bacillus

bacteriologic revolution, 4, 37, 44, 48, 81, 218n15

bacteriology, 37; and botany, 41–44, 226nn26, 28; and debates over species transformation, 41–42, 59, 60, 130, 133–134, 226n29; 246n24; and debates over spontaneous generation, 41, 44; and medical practice, 37–40, 44, 47–51, 82, 84–85; and public health practice, 83–90

Baker, S. Josephine, 118, 119

Baldwin, E. R., 72–75, 102, 128, 169

Bates, Barbara, 9, 90, 92

Baudouin, J. A., 159–162, 166, 174

BCG (bacillus Calmette-Guérin), 2, 5, 10, 209; American response to, 8, 9, chap. 4–6 *passim;* attenuation of, 130–131, 246n30; Canadian reaction to, 3, 126, 132, 136, 158–165, 202, 248n65; defined, 3, 125–126; efficacy of, 3, 154–158, 160–162, 164–165, 171, 174, 188–189, 200; efficacy, relative, 153, 158, 166–167, 171–175, 185, 201; international reaction to, 3, 126, 136, 146–150, 168; recommendations for use of, 3, 162, 164, 181–184, 200–202, 210, 212; and reduction of mortality, general, 154–158, 171, 252n4, 255n65; and reduction of mortality, tuberculous, 135–136, 164, 167, 190, 200; and resistance, 150–152, 203–208; safety of, 133–134, 145–152; trials, animals,

Wilson, Julius, 90–91

Winyah Sanatorium (Asheville, N.C.), 52, 53; and tuberculin, 64–71

Wohler, Friedrich, 41

women, 6, 7, 12, 31–32, 68, 82, 94–97, 106, 113–120, 170; and food, 113, 114–118; and household work, 32–33, 88; and sexuality, 113–114

working class, 7, 82, 88, 108, 113

World Health Organization, 3

X-rays, 105, 172, 186, 187, 198–199

yellow fever, 19, 20, 22, 23, 24, 44

ABOUT THE AUTHOR

Georgina Feldberg is the director of the York University Centre for Health Studies in North York, Ontario. She received her B.A. with honors in biology and her Ph.D. in the history of science at Harvard University. She also pursued graduate coursework in public health and in reproductive physiology and biochemistry at the Harvard Schools of Medicine and Public Health. She has written on science, medicine, and gender and on the restructuring of health-care systems. Professor Feldberg lives in Toronto and teaches in the Division of Social Science at York University, where she also holds the position of coordinator of the Programme in Health and Society.